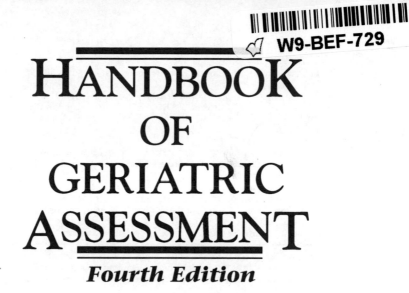

# HANDBOOK OF GERIATRIC ASSESSMENT

## *Fourth Edition*

**Edited by**

**Joseph J. Gallo, MD, MPH**
Associate Professor
Department of Family Practice and Community Medicine
Department of Psychiatry
University of Pennsylvania School of Medicine
Philadelphia, Pennsylvania

**Hillary R. Bogner, MD, MSCE**
Assistant Professor
Department of Family Practice and Community Medicine
University of Pennsylvania School of Medicine
Philadelphia, Pennsylvania

**Terry Fulmer, PhD, RN, FAAN**
The Erline Perkins McGriff Professor &
Head, Division of Nursing
New York University
New York, New York

**Gregory J. Paveza, MSW, PhD**
Interim Associate Vice President for Academic Affairs
University of South Florida – Lakeland
Lakeland, Florida

**JONES AND BARTLETT PUBLISHERS**
*Sudbury, Massachusetts*
BOSTON    TORONTO    LONDON    SINGAPORE

*World Headquarters*

| | | |
|---|---|---|
| Jones and Bartlett Publishers | Jones and Bartlett Publishers | Jones and Bartlett Publishers |
| 40 Tall Pine Drive | Canada | International |
| Sudbury, MA 01776 | 6339 Ormindale Way | Barb House, Barb Mews |
| 978-443-5000 | Mississauga, ON L5V 1J2 | London W6 7PA |
| info@jbpub.com | CANADA | UK |
| www.jbpub.com | | |

Jones and Bartlett's books and products are available through most bookstores and online booksellers. To contact Jones and Bartlett Publishers directly, call 800-832-0034, fax 978-443-8000, or visit our website at www.jbpub.com.

Substantial discounts on bulk quantities of Jones and Bartlett's publications are available to corporations, professional associations, and other qualified organizations. For details and specific discount information, contact the special sales department at Jones and Bartlett via the above contact information or send an email to specialsales@jbpub.com.

The authors, editor, and publisher have made every effort to provide accurate information. However, they are not responsible for errors, omissions, or for any outcomes related to the use of the contents of this book and take no responsibility for the use of the products and procedures described. Treatments and side effects described in this book may not be applicable to all people; likewise, some people may require a dose or experience a side effect that is not described herein. Drugs and medical devices are discussed that may have limited availability controlled by the Food and Drug Administration (FDA) for use only in a research study or clinical trial. Research, clinical practice, and government regulations often change the accepted standard in this field. When consideration is being given to use of any drug in the clinical setting, the health care provider or reader is responsible for determining FDA status of the drug, reading the package insert, and reviewing prescribing information for the most up-to-date recommendations on dose, precautions, and contraindications, and determining the appropriate usage for the product. This is especially important in the case of drugs that are new or seldom used.

Copyright © 2006 by Jones and Bartlett Publishers, Inc.

ISBN-13: 978-0-7637-9452-1
ISBN-10: 0-7637-9452-x

**Library of Congress Cataloging-in-Publication Data**
Handbook of geriatric assessment / edited by Joseph J. Gallo ... [et al.].— 4th ed.
    p. ; cm.
  Includes bibliographical references and index.
  ISBN 0-7637-3056-4 (case bound)
  1. Older people—Diseases—Diagnosis—Handbooks, manuals, etc. 2. Older people—Psychological testing—Handbooks, manuals, etc. 3. Older people—Care—United States—Handbooks, manuals, etc.
  [DNLM: 1. Geriatric Assessment. WT 30 H2374 2006] I. Gallo, Joseph J.
  RC953.G34 2006
  618.97'075—dc22
6048                                                                              005008303

**Production Credits**
Acquisitions Editor: Kevin Sullivan
Associate Editor: Amy Sibley
Production Director: Amy Rose
Production Assistant: Kate Hennessy
Marketing Manager: Emily Ekle
Manufacturing Buyer: Amy Bacus
Composition: Graphic World
Cover Design: Anne Spencer
Printing and Binding: Malloy, Inc.
Cover Printing: Malloy, Inc.

Printed in the United States of America
10 09 08 07 06     10 9 8 7 6 5 4 3 2

# Contents

# *Contributors*

**Hillary R. Bogner, MD, MSCE**
Assistant Professor
Department of Family Practice and Community Medicine
University of Pennsylvania School of Medicine
Philadelphia, Pennsylvania

**Marguarette M. Bolton, BA**
Program Coordinator
Elder Mistreatment Training Project
Division of Nursing
New York University
New York, New York

**David Carr, MD**
Associate Professor of Medicine and Neurology
Department of Medicine and Neurology
Washington University
St. Louis, Missouri

**Monica K. Crane, MD**
Fellow
Geriatrics Division, Department of Internal Medicine
University of Pennsylvania School of Medicine
Philadelphia, Pennsylvania

**David J. Doukas, MD**
Professor and
William Ray Moore Endowed Chair of Family Medicine and Medical
Humanism
Department of Family and Geriatric Medicine,
Institute of Bioethics, Health Policy, and Law
University of Louisville
Louisville, Kentucky

**Carmel Bitondo Dyer, MD, FACP, AGSF**
Associate Professor of Medicine
Baylor College of Medicine
Director, Geriatrics Program
Harris County Hospital District
Co-director of the Texas Elder Abuse and Mistreatment Institute
Houston, Texas

**Yolanda B. Esparza, MSW**
Program Manager
On Lok Senior Health
Fremont, California

**Adolfo Firpo, MD, MPA, FCAP**
Director
Elder Mistreatment Training Project
Division of Nursing
New York University
New York, New York

**Terry Fulmer, PhD, RN, FAAN**
The Erline Perkins McGriff Professor &
Head, Division of Nursing
New York University
New York, New York

**Joseph J. Gallo, MD, MPH**
Associate Professor
Department of Family Practice and Community Medicine
Department of Psychiatry
University of Pennsylvania School of Medicine
Philadelphia, Pennsylvania

**Carrie Guttman, BSNc**
Baccalaureate Nursing Student
School of Nursing
Fairfield University
Fairfield, Connecticut

**Lucia C. Kim, MD, MPH**
Assistant Professor of Medicine
Baylor College of Medicine
Houston, Texas

**Marilyn Lopez, MA, APRN, BC, GNP**
Geriatric Nurse Practioner
New York University Medical Center
New York, New York

**Barbara Morano, LCSW-C, MSW, CMC**
Geriatric Consultant
Morano Consultants
New York, New York

**Carmen Morano, PhD, LCSW-C**
Associate Professor, Chair Aging Specialization
School of Social Work
University of Maryland
Baltimore, Maryland

**Charles P. Mouton, MD, MS**
Professor and Chair
Department of Community Health and Family Practice
Howard University College of Medicine
Washington, DC

**Laurence B. McCullough, PhD**
Professor of Medicine and Medical Ethics,
Center for Medical Ethics and Health Policy
Baylor College of Medicine
Houston, Texas

**David Nicklin, MD**
Assistant Professor
Department of Family Practice and Community Medicine
University of Pennsylvania School of Medicine
Philadelphia, Pennsylvania

**David Oslin, MD**
Associate Professor
Department of Psychiatry
Division of Geriatric Psychiatry
University of Pennsylvania
Philadelphia, Pennsylvania

**Gregory J. Paveza, MSW, PhD**
Interim Associate Vice President for Academic Affairs
University of South Florida – Lakeland
Lakeland, Florida

**Ian Portelli, PhD(c), MSc, CRA, BSc, SRN**
Large Scale Emergency Readiness (LaSER) Project Director
Steinhardt School of Education
New York University & CCPR
New York, New York

**George W. Rebok, PhD**
Professor
Department of Mental Health
Bloomberg School of Public Health
The Johns Hopkins University
Baltimore, Maryland

**James P. Richardson, MD, MPH, AGSF**
Chief, Geriatric Medicine
Union Memorial Hospital
Baltimore, Maryland

**Miriam B. Rodin, MD, PhD**
Assistant Professor of Geriatrics
Department of Medicine
University of Chicago
Chicago, Illinois

**Arthur Sanders, MD, MHA**
Professor
Department of Emergency Medicine
University of Arizona
Tuscon, Arizona

**Joyce Shea, DNSc, APRN, BC**
Assistant Professor
School of Nursing
Fairfield University
Fairfield, Connecticut

**Eugenia L. Siegler, MD**
Associate Professor of Clinical Medicine
Division of Geriatrics and Gerontology
Weill Medical College of Cornell University
New York, New York

**Chad VanDerHeyden, MD, MS**
Senior Resident
Department of Emergency Medicine
University of Arizona
Tuscon, Arizona

**Carla VandeWeerd, PhD**
Research Assistant Professor
Department of Community and Family Health
College of Public Health
University of South Florida
Tampa, Florida

**Meredith Wallace, PhD, APRN**
Assistant Professor & Adult Nurse Practitioner Specialty Program
Coordinator
School of Nursing
Fairfield University
Fairfield, Connecticut

**Marsha N. Wittink, MD, MBE**
Assistant Professor
Department of Family Practice and Community Medicine
University of Pennsylvania School of Medicine
Philadelphia, Pennsylvania

**Faika Zanjani, PhD**
Post-doctoral Fellow
Department of Psychiatry
Division of Geriatric Psychiatry
University of Pennsylvania
Philadelphia, Pennsylvania

# *Preface*

The original concept for a book about multidimensional assessment in primary care geriatrics arose from the experience of William Reichel, MD working with the assessment program of the Baltimore County Department of Health of Baltimore County, Maryland, from 1970 until 1988, and from the experience of establishing a geriatric assessment program at Franklin Square Hospital Center in Baltimore, Maryland, in 1985–1986 (Joseph J. Gallo and William Reichel). Since the first edition, geriatric assessment has taken hold as evidenced by a growing literature suggesting that assessing multiple domains is essential in caring for older adults, with renewed interest in the prevention of functional decline.

This fourth edition of the *Handbook of Geriatric Assessment,* with new and revised chapters, again emphasizes material that has practical application in primary care settings in order to encourage a multidimensional approach in the care of older persons. As was the intent of the earlier editions, the fourth edition fosters a multidimensional approach by discussing the assessment of domains that have a significant bearing on the life of older persons. Although this book was never meant to be a comprehensive guide to all assessment instruments, we want to provide readers with instruments, questionnaires, and concepts that can be employed in designing clinical assessment procedures. We have been gratified that many professionals have found previous editions of the *Handbook of Geriatric Assessment* useful in their clinical work. At the same time, the healthcare system continues to undergo change, driven, in part, by the pressures of caring for a growing population of older adults. Guidelines, evidence-based medicine, clinical pathways, managed care, and disease management have become commonplace terms. Whether these ideas will have a lasting effect on health care in the future is anybody's guess. The power and promise of the Internet for managing information is likely to play an integral role in how these changes play out. As the roles of nurses and other professional caregivers in the healthcare system continue to undergo transformation, the notion of multidimensional assessment takes on additional salience. By drawing discussions of the domains of geriatric assessment into one place, we hope that clinicians will continue to find practical and useful ideas to take into their daily work with older people.

Joseph J. Gallo  
Hillary R. Bogner  
Terry Fulmer  
Gregory J. Paveza

# *Acknowledgment*

The editors gratefully acknowledge the competent and diligent assistance provided by Grace Kim-Lee in carrying out the many tasks that went into the production of this book.

Joseph J. Gallo
Hillary R. Bogner
Terry Fulmer
Gregory J. Paveza

# Section I
# The Context of Assessment

# 1

# *The Context of Geriatric Care*

Joseph J. Gallo and Hillary R. Bogner

As the 21st century begins, the projected growth of the world's aged population is unprecedented. From 1970 to 1997, the proportion of persons aged 65 years and older in the United States has grown from 10% to 13%, and by 2050, 20% of all adults are expected to be 65 years old and older.[1] The proportion of persons aged 85 years and older is also growing rapidly.[2] Some estimate that more older persons are alive on the earth now than have reached old age in all of history.[3] The rate of growth in the proportion of older persons from minority groups is much faster than the rate of growth in the older white population of the United States. This increasing ethnic diversity of the aged will have important implications for how health care is organized and delivered.[4] Aging is a worldwide phenomenon. Each month, of the 1.2 million people around the world who reach later life, 1 million live in developing countries.[5] The age, ethnic, and cultural diversity of the older population suffuses into all the domains of geriatric assessment.

## THE CONTEXT OF GERIATRIC CARE

Because geriatric assessment places a premium on uncovering deficits, we should call to mind a wider worldview. The role of older people in other societies has often been more clearly defined than in

3

modern American culture. In preindustrial society, older persons frequently had considerable wealth and power, which they passed on to the younger members of the group at the appropriate time. Often some special functions were performed by the older members, who knew about family histories and sacred rituals and how to mediate with ancestors. In addition, older persons may have provided some services to the community, such as serving as judges or as experts in child rearing. Even in a technologic society, older people are a valuable resource. In contrast to the stereotypes, older people contribute much as informal helpers and unpaid volunteer workers. When all forms of productive activity are combined, the amount of work done by older men and women is substantial.[6,7] Without exposure to productive older people, younger people (including the middle-aged) lose their sense of history. The aging process becomes something to be feared, even a taboo topic, because the values of society place great emphasis on youth. It is tempting to view growing older as something to be ashamed of, as if old age means nothing but static existence or worse only decline and deterioration.

In contrast, older adults have significant developmental work to do. Persons who are successfully aging have made remarkable adaptations and show considerable resiliency. Erikson[8] summarized this developmental work as the dichotomy of ego integrity versus ego despair: despair, when one looks back on life with regret, not having accomplished what was wanted; and integrity, when one looks back on life and is able to accept it as a unique life in history, one that had to be.

Erikson's first "age of man" relates to the infant's development of "basic trust versus basic mistrust" in the world. The life cycle comes full circle in the relation of ego integrity and basic trust because "healthy children will not fear life if their elders have integrity enough not to fear death."[8] The older person also integrates, in "age-appropriate" ways, the psychosocial themes from previous stages, reflecting back over the entire life cycle. For example, "intimacy and isolation" in young adulthood refers to the development of the ability to be intimate with another versus a failure to develop such relationships. The older adult also faces this issue because the person must deal with the restructuring of relationships.[9]

Growing old marks a time of significant growth for many persons. Among the considerable developmental and adaptive tasks of older adults are dealing with the loss through death or relocation of family and friends, adjusting to changes in living arrangements, retiring, managing with less income, changing social roles, increasing leisure time, and changing sexual and physical functioning, and finally, accepting the inevitability of death. The gracefully aging older person who is able to integrate all of these aspects has a great deal to teach younger persons about life.

Successful aging occurs along multiple dimensions, including maintenance of active involvement with life and achieving a sense of psychological well-being.[10] One model of "successful aging" consists of "selective optimization with compensation."[11] Selection refers to prioritizing one's activities to the most important or pleasurable and adjusting of expectations. Optimization refers to maximization of the chosen behaviors through practice and by accommodating conditions to the ability of the older person; compensation refers to use of strategies that compensate for aging-related losses. Baltes[11] noted strategies of the pianist Rubenstein as an illustration of selective optimization with compensation. Rubenstein selects a smaller number of pieces to play, rehearses more often, and slows down before allegro movements to give the listener the impression of speed. Perhaps the strategies of successful aging can be taught.[12]

In the future, the role of older adults in society may undergo further development and evolution. Toffler[13] has called the technologic revolution that includes the proliferation of computers as the third wave. In contrast to expectations engendered by Orwell's *1984*, this revolution could lead to increased freedom and leisure time. During the first wave (preindustrial society), each household formed an economic unit. The home or the field was the focus of work, and families worked together. Home life and work were intimately related. The second wave was marked by the industrial revolution. Work now took place in the factory. Behavior became dictated by schedules and the division of labor. Consequently, there is less need for older people as repositories of history and culture. The third wave is marked by the advent of the "electronic cottage," with smaller work units and persons working at home. Work again will become less centralized, as it was in the agricultural society of the first wave. Because employees will have the ability to work at home, centralized places of work may become a thing of the past. The implication for the family is that children will once again be near their working parents, a situation that has not been common since the agricultural age. Family roles may then undergo transformation.

Persons may have more than one career over the course of a lifetime. The experience that the older persons have would be invaluable in helping younger workers apply theory to practical problems. Technologic change will also demand that education continue throughout life. It may not be unusual for persons to move in and out of formal educational situations at different ages. Older persons may again be seen as "mentors" to the young.[14]

Expectations about medical care will likely be different as well. For example, older adults in the future may have other ideas about the role of the family in caring for the impaired adult. In a mobile society, informal social networks may be strained. Expectations about retirement may be different so that a lower standard of living or poor health will not be tolerated. Better educated older persons, especially regarding health matters, might question their physicians more than today's older population does and perhaps would want to participate to a greater degree in decisions, seeing themselves as more responsible for the quality of their own health. The Internet has become a source and clearinghouse for health-related information for professionals and patients. In addition, the Internet is providing a forum for discussion and support of caregivers and homebound older adults. At the same time, the health care system is redefining itself. Governments all over the world are grappling with the issue of resource allocation in planning health care services for populations that include greater proportions of older people. It is against this changing backdrop that today's older adults require care.

## MULTIDIMENSIONAL ASSESSMENT

Caring for older patients can be a challenging task for clinicians. The clinician is frequently called on to assist older patients and their families in decisions that can have a direct effect on quality of life. Small changes in the ability of an older person to perform daily activities or in the ability of a caregiver to provide support can have an impact on major life decisions. Older persons are vulnerable to reversible problems that contribute to disability, but even small improvement in functional status can have significant positive effects. Therefore, caring for the older person requires that the clinician assess functional, social, and other aspects of the patient's condition in addition to the usual focus on medical issues.

The domains of multidimensional assessment, such as mental health, physical health, functioning, and social situation, set the field of geriatrics apart from other fields of medicine. The purpose of this book is to assist health care professionals who work with older patients to include these domains in assessment. The author and contributors are mindful of the primary care practitioner whose time with the patient is limited and hope that assessment instruments that are useful in everyday practice may become part of routine care and ultimately save time. Not all older persons who could benefit from multidisciplinary assessment will have access to a team, but practicing physicians and other health care professionals can use community expertise and standardized instruments.[15] Instruments found in this book, such as the Folstein Mini-Mental State Examination[16] and the Instrumental Activities of Daily Living Screen,[17] can be incorporated into the office evaluation of older persons.[18,19]

A number of strategies can be employed to bring the facets of geriatric assessment into geriatric care despite the time and reimbursement barriers that confront the primary care physician and others who care for older adults.[20] At the same time, health care professionals working individually can arrive at the same recommendations as a multidisciplinary team, targeting specific problems for intervention.[21,22] Geriatric assessment has reached a stage of development where incorporation into the practices of physicians and other health professionals is practical. The use of computerized assessment capability may facilitate the integration of the components of geriatric assessment into care settings. Approaches described in this book can improve the outpatient recognition and management of functional and medical problems.[19,21–30] The remaining sections of this introductory chapter set the stage for understanding the domains of assessment and the other chapters that follow.

## Ethnicity and Assessment

The increasing need to care for older persons from diverse cultures and ethnic groups means that clinicians must consider how assessment and development of a treatment plan are modified to avoid misunderstanding or ineffective care. Users of assessment instruments should be aware of the issues involved when drawing conclusions from test scores for questionnaires derived for persons of a different cultural background from which the instruments were developed and tested. In addition, it is important to try to elicit the beliefs, attitudes, and goals about illness that older adults may have that may differ from what is expected.

## Mental Status Assessment

Although much can be gleaned from observation of the speech and mannerisms of the patient, formal evaluation with school-like tests of cognitive status can yield valuable information that is accessible to all who use the chart. In the office, the use of standardized questions to assess mental function may be particularly important for older patients who are experiencing difficulty in performing certain daily tasks, such as using the telephone or handling money. Mental status testing at the time of admission to the hospital or nursing home serves to establish a baseline and heightens awareness to the onset of delirium. The effect on mental state of depression, substance abuse, adverse effects of prescribed and over-the-counter medications, and other medical conditions should also be considered. The role of depression on functional impairment, especially among older persons with chronic medical conditions, has become increasingly recognized. Our new edition now highlights specific aspects of mental health among older adults, namely, cognition, depression, and substance use.

## Functional Assessment Including Driving

Functional assessment includes the ability to perform various tasks of daily life, such as dressing and housework, as well as the more cognitively complex and physically demanding tasks, such as grocery shopping. Because the ability to function is closely tied to the quality of life, assessing functioning is a central element of geriatric assessment. Function can be both a signal of illness and a focus for preventive efforts. Aside from specific medical diagnoses, functional status is independently associated with the care the patient needs, the risk for institutionalization, and mortality. The ability to drive an automobile safely is an important but often neglected aspect of functional assessment of older ambulatory patients. The evaluation of the older driver presents one of the most difficult clinical situations faced by the practicing primary care physician for which guidance can be found in a chapter devoted to assessment of the older driver.

## Social Assessment

Older persons often present with problems of daily living and require a comprehensive outlook—one that includes the family of the patient within the physician's purview. In some cases, the health of the caregiver may be of great importance to the patient's well-being. Most long-term care is provided by caregivers who often need physical and emotional support in order to maintain the older person at home. Frequently, the caregiver is a woman, especially daughters and daughters-in-law. In contrast to the common myth that families "dump" their older members in institutions, clinical experience shows that families tend to go "above and beyond the call of duty" in providing care for their older relatives. Evaluation of the older person cannot be complete without some assessment of the social support system. In this edition, we give special attention to assessing older adults for abuse as well as for the functioning of their social support situation. Personal finances may have an impact on health, nutrition, and residence. Although clinician inquiry in the area of economic status may not be detailed, the physician should be aware that there are older persons who fail to take prescribed medication or who alter the dosage schedule because of financial considerations. Although the economic situation of older Americans has improved considerably in recent decades, medication costs have risen significantly and are often not covered by insurance.

## Advance Directives

Older adults are encouraged to plan for uncertainty with regard to their medical care,[31] but few do. Advance directives are legally binding documents that allow individuals to project their wishes about medical treatment into a future period of incapacity. All hospitals, nursing facilities, and home health agencies in the United States must inform patients about their right to make advance directives. Discussion of advance directive options between the well patient and the doctor may someday become an ordinary part of office practice in the care of the older population, with informed patients having the opportunity to state their wishes, preferences, and values that are relevant to their future medical care. A revised chapter on eliciting the values of patients discusses a systematic method for addressing issues related to planning for care in the face of incapacity.

## Physical Examination

The history and physical examination should be tailored to the older patient with a focus on the discovery of remedial problems. Hearing and vision impairment, restricted mobility, and slowed response time must be considered in the history and physical examination of older persons. The presenting complaint may involve the most vulnerable organ system rather than the organ system expected. For example, congestive heart failure may present as delirium. Consequences of medical diagnoses on each of the domains of multidimensional assessment should be considered in every older patient. How might an additional medication for diabetes affect this patient's mental and functional status? On the other hand, the multidimensional status of the older person should be considered in a larger context when recommending treatment. What value does this patient place on dying at home? Integrating these aspects of assessment and treatment remains a worthwhile goal and a clinical challenge.

**Pain Assessment**

Knowing how to assess pain in older persons in clinical settings is essential to avoid unnecessary suffering and functional impairment, to monitor the response to therapy, and to achieve freedom from significant pain, which is an important component of quality of life. In a chapter on pain assessment, a general approach is recommended that applies when patients with dementia have deteriorated in functioning or appear to be uncomfortable or irritable but cannot express exactly what is wrong. The adequate assessment of pain is pertinent to the care of ambulatory older persons as well as older adults in specialized settings, such as the nursing home or hospice.

**Health Promotion and Disease Prevention**

The aspects of mental status, functional status, social situation, values history, and medical considerations act as a focus of preventive activities and as a guide for highlighting preventive activities that are appropriate for the individual patient. An individualized plan for health promotion and disability prevention grounded in evidence-based guidelines should be based on a multidimensional assessment because older persons vary greatly in their medical and functional status. Although age-related changes are frequently associated with physical and physiologic decline, health care professionals who treat older adults must avoid the temptation of thinking that older persons are beyond efforts at improving wellness or preventing illness.

**New Content**

In addition to the new content incorporated in the standard domains discussed previously, the new edition includes practical discussion of several new content areas such as enhancing adherence, assessment in the home and in the context of hospitalization, and working in assessment teams. Strategies to enhance adherence to medical treatment have the potential to have a great impact on care and are often not explicitly discussed. The settings of assessment include primary care where the demands of time and competing demands create a challenge for providing care that addresses all pertinent domains. Geriatric assessment occurring in teams may be required for older adults with complex presentations across medical, social, and other domains. Creating and working in teams bring their own challenges and opportunities.

## CONCLUSION

Professionals who care for older adults can benefit from reading this book from cover to cover; however, clinicians can also turn to specific chapters to find keys for assessing particular domains. The discussions of the elements of geriatric assessment found here can help in planning the evaluations included in the care of older persons. Technical jargon has been avoided to maximize usefulness for clinicians, but readers with more specialized needs can find additional information on geriatric assessment and instruments in other sources.[32–35]

Assessment findings must be linked to adequate treatment plans. Although this requires clinical training and experience, a systematic approach to assessment helps the clinician cover the important issues over time. Because values and circumstances vary from individual to individual and from family to family, specific recommendations based on a given constellation of findings from geriatric assessment cannot be provided. Nevertheless, the domains of assessment must be united in a coordinated whole by the practitioner for the proper assessment of the older patient, whether in the office, the home, the hospital, the assisted-living facility, the hospice, or the nursing home. With a view to the 21st century, the authors and contributors hope that practitioners will glean from this book assessment instruments and ideas that are useful in the routine assessment of older patients, thereby contributing to their effective and systematic care.

**REFERENCES**

1. US Bureau of the Census. *Population Projections of the United States by Age, Sex, Race, and Hispanic Origin: 1995 to 2050.* Washington, DC: US Government Printing Office; 1996. Current Population Reports, Series P25–1130.

2. Suzman RM, Willis DP, Manton KG. *The Oldest Old.* New York: Oxford University Press; 1992.

3. Dychtwald K, Flower J. *Age Wave: The Challenges and Opportunities of an Aging America.* Los Angeles: Jeremy P. Tarcher; 1989.

4. Lavizzo-Mourey R, Mackenzie ER. Cultural competence: Essential measurements of quality for managed care organizations. *Ann Intern Med.* 1996;124:919–921.

5. Macfadyen D. International demographic trends. In: Kane RL, Evans JG, Macfadyen D, eds. *Improving the Health of Older People: A World View.* New York: Oxford University Press; 1990:19–29.

6. Herzog AR, Kahn RL, Morgan JN, Jackson JS, Antonucci TC. Age differences in productive activities. *J Gerontol Soc Sci.* 1989;44:129–138.

7. Herzog AR, Morgan JN. Formal volunteer work among older Americans. In: Bass S, Caro F, Chen YP, eds. *Achieving a Productive Aging Society.* Westport, CT: Greenwood Press; 1993.

8. Erikson EH. *Childhood and Society.* New York: WW Norton and Company; 1963.

9. Erikson EH, Erikson JM, Kivnick HQ. *Vital Involvement in Old Age: The Experience of Old Age in Our Time.* New York: WW Norton and Company; 1986.

10. Rebok GW, Gallo JJ. Successful aging: Optimizing strategies for primary care geriatrics. In: Gallo JJ, Busby-Whitehead J, Rabins PV, Silliman R, Murphy J, eds. *Reichel's Care of the Elderly: Clinical Aspects of Aging,* 5th ed. Baltimore: Lippincott Williams & Wilkins; 1999:622–630.

11. Baltes PB. The many faces of human ageing: Toward a psychological culture of old age. *Psychol Med.* 1991;21:837–854.

12. Baltes PB, Baltes MM. *Successful Aging: Perspectives from the Behavioral Sciences.* New York: Cambridge University Press; 1990.

13. Toffler A. *The Third Wave.* New York: Bantam Books; 1980.

14. Toffler A. *Future Shock.* New York: Bantam Books; 1970.

15. American Geriatrics Society Public Policy Committee. Comprehensive geriatric assessment. *J Am Geriatr Soc.* 1989;37:473–474.

16. Folstein MF, Folstein SE, McHugh PR. Mini-Mental State: A practical method for grading the cognitive state of patients for the clinician. *J Psychiatr Res.* 1975;12:189–198.

17. Fillenbaum G. Screening the elderly: A brief instrumental activities of daily living measure. *J Am Geriatr Soc.* 1985;33:698–706.

18. Applegate WB, Blass JP, Williams TF. Instruments for the functional assessment of older patients. *N Engl J Med.* 1990;322:1207–1214.

19. Lachs MS, Feinstein AR, Cooney LM, et al. A simple procedure for general screening for functional disability in elderly persons. *Ann Intern Med.* 1990;112:699–706.

20. Beck JC, Freedman ML, Warshaw GA. Geriatric assessment: Focus on function. *Primary Care.* 1994;28:10–32.

21. Robinson BE, Lund CA, Keller D, et al. Validation of the Functional Assessment Inventory against a multidisciplinary home care team. *J Am Geriatr Soc.* 1986;34:851–854.

22. Pinholt EM, Kroenke K, Hanley JF, et al. Functional assessment of the elderly: A comparison of standard instruments with clinical judgment. *Arch Intern Med.* 1987;147:484–488.

23. Miller DK, Morley JE, Rubenstein LZ, Pietruszka FM, Strome LS. Formal geriatric assessment instruments and the care of older general medical outpatients. *J Am Geriatr Soc.* 1990;38:645–651.

24. Siu AL, Beers MH, Morgenstern H. The geriatric "medical and public health" imperative revisited. *J Am Geriatr Soc.* 1993;41:78–84.

25. Boult C, Boult L, Murphy C, Ebbitt B, Luptak M, Kane RL. A controlled trial of outpatient geriatric evaluation and management. *J Am Geriatr Soc.* 1994;42:465–470.

26. Boult C, Boult L, Morishita L, Smith SL, Kane RL. Outpatient geriatric evaluation and management. *J Am Geriatr Soc.* 1998;46:296–302.

27. Silverman M, Musa D, Martin DC, Lave JR, Adams J, Ricci EM. Evaluation of outpatient geriatric assessment: A randomized multi-site trial. *J Am Geriatr Soc.* 1995;43: 733–740.

28. Reuben DB, Frank JC, Hirsch SH, McGuigan KA, Maly RC. A randomized clinical trial of outpatient comprehensive geriatric assessment coupled with an intervention to increase adherence to recommendations. *J Am Geriatr Soc.* 1999;47:269–276.

29. Valenstein M, Kales H, Mellow A, et al. Psychiatric diagnosis and intervention in older and younger patients in a primary care clinic: Effect of a screening and diagnostic instrument. *J Am Geriatr Soc.* 1998;46:1499–1505.

30. Maly RC, Hirsch SH, Reuben DB. The performance of simple instruments in detecting geriatric conditions and selecting community-dwelling older people for geriatric assessment. *Age Ageing.* 1997;26:223–231.

31. Doukas D, Reichel W. *Planning for Uncertainty: A Guide to Living Wills and Other Advance Directives for Health Care.* Baltimore: Johns Hopkins University Press; 1993.

32. Rubenstein LZ, Wieland D, Bernabei R. *Geriatric Assessment Technology: The State of the Art.* New York: Springer Publishing; 1995.

33. McDowell I, Newell C. *Measuring Health: A Guide to Rating Scales and Questionnaires,* 2nd ed. New York: Oxford University Press; 1996.

34. Lezak MD. *Neuropsychological Assessment,* 3rd ed. New York: Oxford University Press; 1995.

35. Bialk BS, Vosburg FL. *Geropsychology Assessment Resource Guide.* Springfield, VA: National Technical Information Service, US Dept of Commerce; 1993. PB 93–213684.

# 2

# Emergency Assessment of the Older Adult

Chad VanDerHeyden and Arthur B. Sanders

## EMERGENCY CARE

*A 77-year-old female presents to an emergency department by ambulance. She complains of increasing weakness, and the medics indicate that it is difficult to obtain historical information because of apparent confusion. The paramedics also noted unilateral facial drooping. She was recently discharged from another hospital but is not certain which one or why she was admitted.*

Emergency medicine is a key element in the medical care of older persons in the United States. Shah et al. found that 18% of Medicare patients used the emergency department (ED) at least once in 1993.[1] The ED visit rate expressed as visits per 100 persons per year is a way to look at ED use within a population. Data from the 2002 National Ambulatory Medical Care Survey showed that persons 75 years old and older had a mean of 61 ED visits per 100 persons per year. This compares with a national mean of 39 ED visits per 100 persons per year.[2]

Not only does the ED visit rate for older patients exceed the average, it is rapidly increasing. Between 1992 and 1999, ED visits per 100 persons per year increased by 18% for patients 65 years old and older. The proportion of ED patients that are older is increasing. Persons over 65 years old represented 14.1% of ED patients in 1992 and 15.2% in 1999, representing an 8% increase.[3] A differential increase in visit rate by race has been shown such that the ED visit rate of older African-Americans has increased by 59% (from 45.4 to 72.2 visits per 100 patients per year) compared with a 13% increase in white seniors.[3]

In general, older persons require more ED resources than younger patients. Strange and Chen analyzed ED use by older and younger patients in 70 hospitals throughout the United States.[4] Older patients comprised 16% of ED visits in 1995 with 46% being admitted to an acute care hospital and 6% admitted to an intensive care unit. Older patients were seven times more likely to be admitted to the hospital, five times more likely to use ambulance services, and five times more likely to need comprehensive ED care compared with younger patients.[4] These data were consistent with another study by Singal et al. that showed that older patients required more ED and hospital resources, including laboratory tests, radiographs, ED throughput time, and ED charges, compared with younger patients.[5] In the Medicare database study, Shah et al. found that those persons using the ED were, on average, older, less educated, and living alone and had worse reported health and higher co-morbidity scores.[1] These studies indicate that older patients seeking care in EDs are often ill, have extensive workups, and are frequently admitted to acute care hospitals.

Visits to EDs in the United States have increased dramatically over the past decade. Ten percent of ambulatory medical care occurs in EDs. The National Ambulatory Medical Care Survey reported that ED visits increased by 23% from 90 million to 110 million between 1992 and 2002, an increase of almost 2 million visits per year. Patients 65 years old and older represented 16.5 million of the 110.2 million total ED visits in 2002. At the same time, the number of hospital EDs have decreased by 15%, further straining the emergency medical services (EMS) system.[2] Reeder et al. compared retrospective data between 1992 and 2000 at a single rural 750-bed hospital and found that ED visits increased by 28.6% while the population grew by only 16.1%. More strikingly, the increase was 40% in patients over 60 years old.[6] The increase is due to many factors in our health care system; however, the growing number of older persons in the United States who require significant emergency medical, ambulance, and acute hospital care is one important factor. The rapid increase in ED patient volume results in ED overcrowding and in a fraying of the ED as a safety net for our health care system. As the older portion of the US population increases, the stress on the emergency medical care system will become acutely worse. Over the next 35 years, patients over 65 years old may come to represent over one quarter of all ED visits. This represents a significant challenge to emergency medicine, acute care hospitals, and the prehospital EMS system. Emergency medicine is facing a crisis of overcrowding with limited resources and very little planning for the future needs of an aging population.

## PREHOSPITAL EMS SYSTEM

The prehospital EMS system includes the ambulance dispatch, the first responder, and the ambulance transport system. EMS plays a major role in the emergency care of geriatric patients. Older patients represent approximately one third of all EMS transports. Studies have demonstrated that seniors use EMS at up to four times the rate of younger adults.[4,5] Shah et al. surveyed 930 older ED patients and found that 30% arrived by ambulance. Reasons given for EMS transport included immobility (33%) and illness (22%).[7]

EMS systems developed over the past 30 years to extend the treatment of ill or injured patients before arrival in the hospital. Studies in the medical literature and experience with the use of medics during the Vietnam War have demonstrated that time is a crucial factor in the treatment of many emergency conditions such as cardiac arrest and multisystem trauma. The goal of an EMS system is to decrease the time between the point at which a possibly emergent condition is recognized and the point at which evaluation and intervention can begin. For example, the best chance for resuscitating patients who suffer cardiac arrest is through early cardiopulmonary resuscitation (CPR) and defibrillation in the community as part of the chain of survival in a coordinated EMS system. This is accomplished with the dispatch of the appropriate level of prehospital care (911 call system), CPR training in the community or telephonic CPR instruction by the dispatch professional, onscene management under protocol or medical direction, and ground or air ambulance transportation to the appropriate ED. Great variability exists in the way EMS systems operate throughout the United States. In some communities, EMS systems are based within the fire departments, and medics are also firefighters. In other cities, there are independent EMS agencies, whereas some communities have volunteer EMS providers.

Multiple levels of EMS services and providers also exist. Ambulance crews typically include one of the following: an emergency medical technician (EMT) Basic who has received approximately 110 hours of training and is certified by the state to perform basic interventions such as CPR, bag-valve-mask–assisted ventilation, splinting, and extrication; an EMT Intermediate who has received 200–400 hours of training and can perform some of the skills of a paramedic; and a paramedic who has completed approximately 1,000 hours of training and can obtain intravenous access, deliver medications, including narcotics, intubate, defibrillate, and interpret electrocardiograms (EKGs) in addition to all of the skills performed by EMTs. Flight crews also may include a highly trained registered nurse as well as a paramedic. EMS systems are not static and respond to changes in technology. For example, the development of automatic external defibrillators has led to a reassessment of the role of basic EMTs where many now carry automatic external defibrillators and deliver early defibrillation to patients in cardiac arrest.

After an ambulance has been called and the patient has been evaluated, several factors dictate where that patient will be transported. These include the acuity of the patient's condition, the hospital capability (trauma center, etc.), patient preference, and hospital availability (in overcrowded, divert situations). Community regulations developed by local EMS agencies, state laws, and protocols govern the activities of the EMS system and providers. Thus, the patient in the vignette can end up at Hospital B when she has received almost all of her care at Hospital A. It is for this reason that a written summary of the patient's medical history is crucial to emergency health care providers.

EMS health care professionals can play an important role in the assessment of the older adult. The medics and first responders have the unique opportunity of seeing the patient in his or her home environment. Home and family observations by EMS providers can be an important part of assessing the patient's functional status and can determine whether hospital admission is necessary. Gerson et al. demonstrated that EMS providers can be trained to look for and report signs of abuse or neglect of older persons.[8] EMS providers are skilled at gathering available information such as picking up medicine bottles, medication lists, and advance directives. This is especially important when involved in the care of any patient who has difficulty communicating. Medics can begin key diagnostic testing, including fingerstick blood glucose determination, pulse oximetry, and 12-lead EKGs and monitoring. Medics work under the authority of the emergency physician, take orders, and report their findings to the ED. Many communities have a system of prehospital advance directives in which the patient or his or her surrogate and primary care physician completes a prehospital advance directive form stating his or her preferences to limit his or her medical care, such as "do not attempt resuscitation." Medics will honor these directives, including do not attempt resuscitation orders, if properly completed.

Because prehospital care is so important to the care of older persons, health are providers should become familiar with the EMS system in their communities and advocate the need for a strong EMS system to meet the needs of a growing geriatric population in the United States.

*The case shows the dilemma of trying to evaluate a complicated older patient with very limited information. The patient's medical records and previous treatments have been at another hospital. Medical records may not be accessible for hours, if at all. The patient is unable to give a coherent and reliable history because of her acute or chronic medical condition. Information transfer is a key element in the emergency assessment of older patients who often have significant co-morbid diseases. What are the patient's underlying medical conditions? What medications is she on? Is her acute complaint an exacerbation of an underlying condition or a new disease? Even gathering the chief complaint may be a challenge in the assessment of some older patients. In order to care for this patient adequately, the emergency physician must have a system for rapidly identifying and addressing treatable conditions that pose an immediate threat to life or quality of life (e.g., loss of limbs or vision).*

## ED ENVIRONMENT

The ED environment is uncomfortable for older persons. It is a high-stress environment where patients often do not receive the amenities and special aids that are available in a clinic setting. Patients may be moved from room to room and sometimes placed in a hallway bed awaiting test results. Little privacy is available, and provider time is often limited and spent dealing with multiple patients who are ill. The ED beds are uncomfortable. The lighting and noise may be bothersome, especially to an anxious patient who is worried or who is in pain. Some EDs have made modifications that provide some amenities for older patients, such as more comfortable beds, indirect lighting, and more comfortable rooms.

**EMERGENCY MEDICINE MODEL OF CARE**

The emergency medical model of patient care differs from the medical model used in a clinic or office setting (Figure 2–1). Care begins in the prehospital arena with protocols or telephonic medical direction to prehospital emergency care professionals. After the patient arrives in the ED, an initial assessment occurs with stabilization if necessary. What are the true emergencies that must be considered for this patient's complaint? Does the patient need immediate treatment or monitoring? After these issues are addressed, the emergency physician proceeds to a focused history and physical exam based on the patient's chief complaint. The differential diagnosis is focused on the following questions:[9]

1. Is a life- or limb-threatening process causing this complaint?
2. Is there an urgent disease process that needs prompt attention?
3. What common conditions can cause the patient's symptoms?

Making a diagnosis is much less important than ruling out immediate threats to life or limb. For instance, if a patient presents with a chief complaint of "chest pain" in the absence of trauma, most emergency physicians will try to exclude true medical emergencies such as acute myocardial infarction, pulmonary embolism, pneumothorax, aortic dissection, and ruptured esophagus. In the limited time available in an emergency setting, the physician's history, physical, diagnostic testing, and even treatment will be directed toward sufficiently excluding the life-threatening conditions. Empirical treatment may occur while diagnostic testing is ongoing (e.g., nitroglycerin for chest pain). Once the life-threatening conditions are reasonably addressed, the emergency physician focuses on the *most likely* conditions, such as pneumonia, gastroesophageal reflux, and musculoskeletal pain. It is not unusual for the patient to leave the ED without a diagnosis and require follow-up and further evaluation in the outpatient primary care setting. If the patient appears ill, in-patient evaluation will be necessary even if the diagnosis is uncertain at the time of admission.

The efficiency and accuracy of this complaint-focused rapid evaluation practiced in the emergency setting are affected by the age of the patient. The older is the patient, the greater is the concern for life-threatening possibilities. A healthy 20 year old who presents with low back pain may have few serious diseases related to that complaint;

however, an 80 year old with new low back pain prompts concern about emergency conditions such as abdominal aortic aneurysm, necessitating a more comprehensive workup. Studies demonstrate that older persons receive more comprehensive ED evaluations, including diagnostic imaging and laboratory tests, and spend more time in the ED compared with younger adult patients.[4,5] The result is longer ED stays and a higher ED resource use than suggested by visit frequency alone.

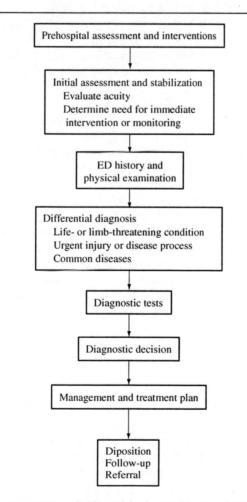

**Figure 2–1** The emergency medical model of care: Process of care in the emergency medical services system from prehospital to ED discharge.[9]

Diagnostic tests follow depending on what is available in the ED. For example, CT scans of the head are readily available to evaluate a patient for an acute bleed. However, an MRI of the head is generally not available to assess for subtle masses, etc. Many patients may not receive a final diagnosis for their complaint. The emergency physician will make a decision about whether the patient needs to be admitted to the hospital for further workup or can be followed in the clinic setting for further evaluation of his or her complaint. Once again, communication with a primary care physician or geriatrician is key to appropriate patient care. For example, a patient who presents with frequent falls will be assessed for injury from the fall and acute medical conditions that may cause the fall, such myocardial infarction or stroke. However, a more extensive fall assessment will be deferred to a clinic setting.

*The complaint-driven evaluation is never more obfuscated than in the patient who has dementia or delirium or who is noncommunicative. These conditions occur with increased frequency in the older population. Without family or caretakers present to discuss the reason for the ED visit and to establish a baseline for comparison, the emergency physician is left with a very difficult evaluation. Such was the case in the case vignette. The paramedics called ahead with a report of new-onset facial droop. The stroke team was activated. A computed tomography scanner was placed on standby, and registered nurses were allocated to the patient's room for more rapid evaluation. After the dust had settled and more time was available to request medical records, it became evident that this deficit had, in fact, been present for a number of years. Unfortunately, the evaluation of her new problem (hepatic encephalopathy) was delayed by a tangential evaluation, and valuable resources were inefficiently allocated.*

## PRINCIPLES OF GERIATRIC EMERGENCY MEDICINE

Emergency physicians are sensitive to the special needs of older patients and realize that the typical emergency medicine model of care must be augmented for older patients. To that end, an interdisciplinary task force has developed a list of principles of geriatric care (Table 2–1).[9]

Older patients often present with vague symptoms such as general weakness or not feeling well. These ambiguous complaints are more

**Table 2–1** Principles of Geriatric Emergency Medicine[9]

1. The patient's presentation is frequently complex.
2. Common diseases present atypically in this age group.
3. The confounding effects of co-morbid diseases must be considered.
4. Polypharmacy is common and may be a factor in presentation, diagnosis, and management.
5. Recognition of the possibility for cognitive impairment is important.
6. Some diagnostic tests may have different normal values.
7. The likelihood of decreased functional reserve must be anticipated.
8. Social support systems may not be adequate, and patients may need to rely on caregivers.
9. A knowledge of baseline functional status is essential for evaluating new complaints.
10. Health problems must be evaluated for associated psychosocial adjustment.
11. The emergency department encounter is an opportunity to assess important conditions in the patient's personal life.

difficult to classify and present a challenge to generating a manageable differential diagnosis. Common diseases present atypically in older persons. Acute conditions such as myocardial infarction and appendicitis may present without chest or abdominal pain. Many older persons have co-morbid diseases that must be taken into account in the ED evaluation. The emergency physician must decide whether the new complaint is an exacerbation of an underlying disease or a new disease process. For example, the patient who presents with a history of congestive heart failure and shortness of breath is assessed as to whether his or her symptoms are an exacerbation of his or her congestive heart failure or a new myocardial infarction, pneumonia, pulmonary embolus, etc. Many older persons are taking multiple medications. Emergency physicians must determine whether the complaint is due to an adverse drug event; a drug interaction with another drug, food, or disease; or a new disease. Studies have shown that 10% to 15% of older ED patients are on medications that may be inappropriate in older persons.[10] The patient who presents with weakness for 2 weeks may be having an adverse drug event. However, this diagnosis would not be immediately known until the symptoms are assessed over time when the drug is stopped. Close communication with the primary care physician or geriatrician is important to assess adverse drug events adequately.

Studies have shown that approximately 25% of older patients have cognitive deficits when screening is done in the ED.[11-14] Approximately 10% of older patients met criteria for possible delirium. It is unknown whether these cognitive deficits persist or are a factor of the stressful ED environment. Cognitive impairment is important because it affects the reliability of the patient history as well as the ability of the patient to be discharged from the ED. Diagnostic tests may have different values for older adults compared with younger patients. Laboratories often do not report reference ranges for older adults. Older patients have less functional reserve than younger adults. Thus, when stressed, they may quickly deteriorate physiologically. Older trauma patients may be in occult shock without manifesting classic symptoms until it becomes very difficult to resuscitate them.

An assessment of social support systems is important for older patients. An independently living 80-year-old patient who has a simple injury such as a sprained ankle may need significant social support to maintain independent living. Knowledge of the patient's baseline functional status is key for the emergency health care provider to assess the chief complaint. An acute change in functional status is an important clue to the possibility of serious illness such as sepsis, metabolic abnormalities, subdural hematoma, acute coronary syndrome, or adverse drug event. An accurate history of functional activities is key to understanding whether a major workup for acute functional decline is indicated. An example of a form for transfer of patients from a skilled nursing facility is presented in Figure 2–2 with lists of baseline function, cognitive status, advance directives, medications, and reason for transfer.

Psychosocial and emotional problems are common in older ED patients. When older ED patients were screened for depression in the ED, 25% to 30% had positive screens and needed more extensive evaluations.[15,16] Alcoholism, older person abuse, and other psychosocial issues are also common among older ED patients. When evaluating an older patient for another complaint such as a fall, emergency health care professionals must be aware of psychosocial implications. Many of these patients will be referred to their primary care physician or a geriatrician for definitive evaluation. Finally, in studies of older ED patients, many indicators of basic primary care were identified. In one study of 252 patients in five hospital EDs, 54% lacked flu vaccination, and 36% had symptoms of depression.[17] Falls, alcoholism, malnutrition, and incontinence are potential issues that can be identified by a dedicated EMS program. The ED, in conjunction with a geriatric or primary care network, may help to identify patients who are "at risk" and could benefit from geriatric assessment.

**Nursing Home to Hospital Transfer Form**
Name _____ Gender_____ DOB_____
Transferring facility _____ Religion _____
Dates of stay_____ Phone _____
SS#_____ Medicare #_____ Insurance #_____
Responsible relative/guardian_____
Address_____ Phone_____

Physician_____ Phone_____Nurse_____Phone_____
Other physician _____
Date/time of transfer_____ Recent vital signs_____
Reason for transfer_____
Physician orders on transfer_____
Hospitals/facilities discharged within 60 days_____
Advance directives_____
Critical care plan_____
Allergies_____ Immunizations_____
Medications_____
Other treatments (PT, resp, diet, etc.)_____
Past medical history_____
Primary diagnosis _____
Secondary diagnosis _____
Surgical history_____
Tobacco/alcohol _____

**BASELINE INFORMATION**
Ambulation _____
**Activities of Daily Living**
Bathing_____                    Transfer_____
Dressing_____                   Continence_____
Toileting _____                  Feeding_____
**Disabilities**
Amputation _____                Contracture_____
Paralysis_____                   Decubitus ulcer_____
**Impairments**
Speech _____                    Vision _____
Hearing _____                   Sensation_____
**Usual Mental Status**
Alert_____            Oriented _____         Wanders_____
Combative_____       Confused _____         Withdrawn _____
Other_____
Mini-mental status _____
Appliances/supports (e.g., wheelchair, cane, walker, prosthesis)_____
Other information to emergency providers _____
_____

**Figure 2–2** Nursing home to hospital transfer form: Sample information transfer form for geriatric patients being referred for ED treatment.[9]

## SUMMARY

Approximately one of five older adults will visit an ED each year. This chapter reviewed the general principles of emergency and prehospital care. The emergency medical model of care presents challenges in trying to provide high-quality care for older patients. Primary care physicians and geriatricians must work closely with emergency physicians to optimize the emergency care of older patients. This includes advocating for a strong EMS system that will be able to meet the future needs of a growing older population. Emergency physicians and geriatricians can also work on clinical protocols that address key syndromes for patients presenting to EDs such as frequent falls, abuse of older persons, adverse medication events, functional decline, and psychosocial issues. Communication among health care providers plays a vital role in the delivery of emergency care to this population. Primary care physicians can ensure the presence of a written medical summary, including the date, medications, baseline functional and cognitive status, prior medical history, surgeries, and contact information. Discussion of a prehospital advance directive is important in appropriate patients. Close communication among emergency, geriatric, pharmacy, and primary care providers is an invaluable asset when caring for the older adult in an emergency setting.

### REFERENCES

1. Shah MN, Rathouz PJ, Chin MH. Emergency department utilization by noninstitutionalized elders. *Acad Emerg Med.* 2001;8(3):267–273.

2. McCaig LF, Burt CW. *National Hospital Ambulatory Medical Care Survey: 2002 Emergency Department Summary.* Advance Data from Vital and Health Statistics; No. 340, 1.7MB. Hyattsville, MD: National Center for Health Statistics; 2004.

3. Burt CW, McCaig LF. Trends in hospital emergency department utilization: United States, 1992–99. National Center for Health Statistics. *Vital Health Stat.* 2001:13(150).

4. Strange GS, Chen EH. Use of emergency departments by elder patients: A five-year follow-up study. *Acad Emerg Med.* 1998:5:1157–1162.

5. Singal BM, Hedges JR, Rousseau EW, et al. Geriatric patient emergency visits part I: Comparison of visits by geriatric and younger patients. *Ann Emerg Med.* 1992;21:802–807.

6. Reeder TJ, Tucker JL, Cascio ES, Czaplijski TJ, Benson NH, Meggs WJ. Trends in emergency department utilization: Effect of changing demographics [abstract]. *Acad Emerg Med.* 2001;8:577.

7. Shah MN, Glushak C, Karrison TG, et al. Predictors of emergency medical services utilization by elders. *Acad Emerg Med.* 2003;10:52–58.

8. Gerson L, Schelble DT, Wilson JE. Using paramedics to identify at-risk elderly. *Ann Emerg Med.* 1992;21:688–691.

9. Sanders AB, ed. *Emergency Care of the Elder Person*. St. Louis: Beverly Cracom Publication; 1996.

10. Chin MH, Wang LC, Jin L, et al. Appropriateness of medication selection for older persons in an urban academic emergency department. *Acad Emerg Med*. 1999;6:1232–1241.

11. Lewis LM, Miller DK, Morley, et al. Unrecognized delirium in ED geriatric patients. *Am J Emerg Med*. 1995;13:142–145.

12. Gerson LW, Counsell SR, Fontanarosa PB, Smucker WD. Case finding for cognitive impairment in elderly emergency department patients. *Ann Emerg Med*. 1994;23:813–817.

13. Hustey FM, Meldon SW. The prevalence and documentation of impaired mental status in elderly emergency department patients. *Ann Emerg Med*. 2002;39:248–253.

14. Naughton BJ, Moran MB, Kadah H, et al. Delirium and other cognitive impairment in older adults in an emergency department. *Ann Emerg Med*. 1995;25:751–755.

15. Meldon SW, Emerman CL, Schubert DSP. Recognition of depression in geriatric ED patients by emergency physicians. *Ann Emerg Med*. 1997;30:442–447.

16. Meldon SW, Emerman CL, Schubert DSP, Moffa DA, Etheart RG. Depression in geriatric ED patients: Prevalence and recognition. *Ann Emerg Med*. 1997;30:141–145.

17. Gerson LW, Rousseau EW, Hogan TM, Bernstein E, Kalbfleisch N. Multicenter study of case finding in elderly emergency department patients. *Acad Emerg Med*. 1995;2:729–734.

# 3

# *Ethnicity and Geriatric Assessment*

Charles P. Mouton and Yolanda B. Esparza

The proportion of the US population that is over 65 years old is increasing rapidly. At the same time, the number of older adults from minority groups, such as Hispanics, African Americans, and Asian Americans, continues to rise.[1] For these reasons, it is fitting to begin a book on geriatric assessment by highlighting the need for cultural competence in the assessment of older persons.[2] Cultural competence in health care consists of at least three components: (1) knowing the prevalence, incidence, and risk factors (epidemiology) for diseases in different ethnic groups; (2) understanding how the response to medications and other treatments varies with ethnicity; and (3) eliciting the culturally held beliefs and attitudes toward illness, treatment, and the health care system. Cultural competence in assessment includes sensitivity to changes in meaning and circumstances that were not intended by the developers of a test. All of these areas cannot be covered in this short chapter, but instead, some clinical considerations in the assessment of older adults from diverse ethnic groups are highlighted, setting the stage for the detailed discussions of specific domains that follow in subsequent chapters.

A description of the epidemiology of medical conditions across different ethnic groups would take an entire chapter;[3] however, in many cases, solid information about the prevalence, incidence, and risk factors for even some common disorders of late life is lacking.[4] For example, there are few credible community-based estimates of the prevalence of Alzheimer's disease in ethnic minorities. Estimates of the prevalence of dementia and Alzheimer's disease in minorities from the few studies that have been done reveal substantial disease burden on the African American and Hispanic communities, with rates of Alzheimer's disease in minorities several times higher than in whites.[5,6] Although further study is needed on Alzheimer's disease in ethnic minorities for its own sake, such research could also shed light on why the association of apolipoprotein E with Alzheimer's appears to be attenuated in African Americans.[6,7] Similarly, little scientific evidence exists about how medications vary in their effect among ethnic minorities, especially for older adults. Examples of possible differences in response to medications according to ethnicity include the effects of antihypertensives[8] and antidepressants.[9,10]

This chapter focuses on culturally competent assessment in relationship to physical function, cognitive impairment, depression, social and economic issues, and ethics in medical decision making. First, some general comments are offered regarding (1) the heterogeneity of ethnic groups; (2) the reliability, validity, and use of assessment instruments for persons of a different cultural background from which the instruments were developed and tested; (3) enhancing communication between professional caregivers and older adults of diverse ethnic backgrounds; and (4) eliciting beliefs and attitudes about illness.

## HETEROGENEITY WITHIN OLDER ETHNIC MINORITIES

Clinicians must confront and question their casual conceptions of race and ethnicity. The human genome project demonstrates that there is more genetic heterogeneity within racial or ethnic groups than between them. Thus, racial categories probably better represent the historical differences in economic opportunity and wealth accumulation than actual biologic differences. When socioeconomic factors are considered, apparent differences between older persons from minority groups and other older persons disappear or narrow for many important outcomes. Differences in health and habits ascribed to race often reflect social rather than genetic differences.[11,12] Older adults are a diverse group, even within ethnic categories. It is just as important to understand this heterogeneity within ethnic groups as it is to understand the differences between ethnic groups.[13] For example, some

African Americans were brought to the United States against their will from Africa; others have migrated from the Caribbean. Hispanic Americans form a heterogeneous group, having cultural origins in Mexico, Puerto Rico, South and Central America, Cuba, and other Spanish-speaking countries. Asian Americans from China, Japan, Korea, and Southeast Asia have differing health practices and beliefs. Native American older adults derive from over 500 tribes, speaking over 150 languages. Because of this heterogeneity within cultural groups, clinicians should not lose sight of the need to evaluate each older person as an individual who has a cultural and personal contextual background that suffuses into every aspect of assessment and care. Clinicians should interpret the information in this chapter as general guidelines in assessment of older persons from minority groups, rather than as firm rules to follow when assessing older adults from specific ethnic groups.

## RELIABILITY, VALIDITY, AND USE OF INSTRUMENTS FOR ETHNIC MINORITIES

Any assessment procedure is subject to error. Error in measurement can arise because the instrument is inconsistent (poor reliability) or because the instrument does not measure what the clinician thinks it is measuring (poor validity). Neighbors and Lumpkin[14] questioned the assumption that the same construct is measured when instruments developed among whites are applied to African Americans or other minority ethnic groups. Differing idioms and colloquialisms can cause a translated instrument to have different meanings from those intended by the original developers. Even within ethnic groups, older persons who are recent immigrants may interpret items differently from older persons who have lived in the United States for some time.

At a more subtle level, some constructs may be so different across cultures as to be quite different or even irrelevant. Depressive disorder provides an example of cultural heterogeneity in expression that has drawn attention from anthropologists and medical researchers concerned with its detection and treatment.[15] Some cultures do not have concepts that are equivalent to the Western notion of depression. The Hopi Indians of Arizona, for example, describe an illness similar to major depression but without dysphoria.[16] The Flathead people of Montana express depression as a social phenomenon of loneliness—the feeling that no one cares for you.[17] Neurasthenic patients in

China deny dysphoria but do exhibit the other symptoms of depression, such as psychomotor retardation and somatic complaints.[18] Older African Americans tend to deny sadness but are more likely to report thoughts of death than older whites.[19]

In the domain of functional assessment, the willingness of older persons from certain groups to report difficulty taking care of themselves may be powerfully related to fear of admitting their dependence on others. Observed differences in functional status across ethnic groups may represent true differences but could represent measurement error from the instrument used in the assessment of physical function. Physical function assessment generally employs self-reporting instruments that rely on the subjective response of patients. Performance-based measures provide more objective measures of function but are harder to carry out in the clinical setting and may not always relate directly to performance at home.[20,21] The choice of method generally relates to the clinician's time constraints, training, and need for the most reliable and valid information. A number of instruments are illustrated and discussed in this book, but unfortunately, most of the instruments have not been specifically assessed for their performance in older minorities. An exception is the SF–36, whose reliability or reproducibility has been found to be as high in minority groups as in whites,[22] and which appears to be valid for assessment of functional status in Hispanic Americans.[23]

Finally, literacy and the level of educational attainment may be important considerations in assessing older adults, especially ethnic minorities who historically have had less opportunity to advance in school. Older women, in particular, grew up in a period when it was uncommon for girls to finish high school and attend college. The association of ethnic grouping with functional decline and other important health outcomes may have more to do with the level of educational attainment than race. At the age of 65 years, persons with 12 or more years of schooling have an active life expectancy (i.e., life spent without reported functional disability) that is 2 to 4 years longer than older adults with less education, regardless of ethnicity.[24] Closely tied to educational level attained is literacy, or the ability to understand and use written information. In one study of 144 African Americans over the age of 65 years living in New York City, half had a reading level that was below the eighth grade,[25] suggesting that materials designed for older persons must be evaluated for reading level. It remains to be seen whether improved educational opportunities for persons from ethnic minorities will result in older persons with diminished rates of functional impairment when compared with the current cohort of older persons. In clinical work, care should be taken to consider the educational level of clients who may not be accustomed to the type of questions that are asked in many functional and cognitive tests.

Clinicians need not develop their own instruments for assessment of depression, function, or other domains in order to assess properly older adults from different ethnic groups. Instead, in interpreting results from assessment, they should be aware that the reliability and validity of instruments developed, for example, among urban hospitalized patients in the Northeastern United States, may not be applicable to a border community in rural South Texas. The selection of instruments and other aspects of assessment should be tailored to the known demographic profile of the practice in which the questionnaires are to be used. As researchers and clinicians become more aware of the cultural context of assessment, it is hoped that more information will be available to make good decisions about geriatric assessment procedures that are most appropriate to different ethnic groups.

## ENHANCING COMMUNICATION WITH ETHNICALLY DIVERSE OLDER ADULTS

The assessment of older adults who do not speak or read English well and who have different worldviews and goals than those of the health care professional can be a difficult and arduous task. Good communication skills are required for interactions with all older adults. However, social distance, racism, unconscious fears, and similar concerns on the part of patients and professionals may contribute to additional problems in assessment and diagnosis of older adults from varying ethnic groups.[26] Early attention to building rapport will go a long way to facilitating communication. In many cultures, such as among Chinese and Mexican Americans, rapport begins through exchange of pleasantries or chitchat before beginning the business of medical history taking and physical examination.[27,28] Older Hispanic Americans often expect health care personnel to be warm and personal and express a strong need to be treated with dignity.[29] As a sign of respect, older persons should be addressed by their last names. Gesturing should be avoided because seemingly benign body or hand movements may have adverse connotations in other cultures. Clinicians should take care to evaluate whether questions or instructions have been understood, because some persons will nod "yes" while not really comprehending. Because outright questioning of authority is taboo in some cultures, physicians should encourage the patient to ask questions. He or she should tell the patient that even though some things are not normally discussed, it is necessary to do so in order to plan the best care.

## ELICITING BELIEFS AND ATTITUDES ABOUT ILLNESS

When caring for older adults, the clinician should make an attempt to elicit beliefs and attitudes about illness. Eliciting beliefs and attitudes about illness that may be rather different from one's own means maintaining an accepting attitude and putting the family and patient at ease that their ideas are valued in developing the care plan. The clinician should ask the patient what he or she thinks is wrong or causing the problem, whether there may be some ways to get better that doctors may not know about, what the patient has done to help the problem, and whether anyone else has been asked to help with the problem. To draw out beliefs about illness, the physician should ask the patient what worries him or her most about the illness and why the patient thinks that he or she is ill now.

Getting into the "assumptive world"[30] of the patient is time well spent. First, doing so provides useful information about over-the-counter medications or home remedies that might interfere with prescribed medicines. For example, older persons within traveling distance of Mexico obtain pharmacologically active compounds that are not always equivalent to medications bought in the United States.[31] In addition, traditional folk remedies play a central role in health care for older Mexican Americans and Asian Americans.[32] In many cases, standard prescriptions may be more acceptable if traditional remedies can continue to be taken. Second, assessing cultural beliefs about illness includes asking about diet. Dietary prescriptions are often a component of traditional healing practices in Native Americans.[33] Third, failure to elicit ideas about illness can result in poor communication, a lack of adherence to prescribed therapy, or refusal to undergo tests or therapeutic procedures. For example, the idea that illness is punishment for past deeds may inhibit participation in preventive or therapeutic procedures.[34] Also, eliciting the patient's ideas about illness and incorporating those into the treatment plan can help to build a bridge of trust between clinicians and older minority patients. Finally, asking and listening about the cultural beliefs of the patient help to establish rapport and show respect for the older person and can be one of the most interesting aspects of caring for older adults.

## SELECTED DOMAINS OF GERIATRIC ASSESSMENT

Subsequent sections of this chapter highlight specific considerations in the multidimensional evaluation of older persons from ethnic minority groups. Features of assessment relevant to ethnicity are covered. Readers should refer to other chapters for further information regarding assessments.

### Functional Assessment

The functional ability of older African Americans declines more rapidly than other races. In the North Carolina Established Populations for Epidemiologic Studies of the Elderly, 9.6% of African Americans older than 65 years reported difficulty with two or more activities of daily living, and 19% reported two or more difficulties with instrumental activities of daily living.[35,36] Older African Americans were 40% more likely to have trouble getting around and 50% more likely to be confined to their homes than whites,[37] and the gap between African Americans and whites appears to be widening.[38] However, in advanced age (the 9th and 10th decades of life), older African Americans appear to function better than whites probably because only the most hardy individuals survive.[35] Hispanic Americans also have significant burden of functional impairment as assessed by activities of daily living and instrumental activities of daily living.[39] Markides et al.[40] reported that functional impairment among Hispanic Americans was related to specific medical conditions such as diabetes mellitus, stroke, myocardial infarction, arthritis, and hip fracture. Functional impairment caused by these medical conditions was greater in older Hispanic Americans than in whites.[40-43] Among Asian Americans, comparative data on functional impairment and disability are insufficient to draw firm conclusions. Asian Americans of high socioeconomic status or who came from earlier immigrant groups probably have rates of disability that are similar to whites.[44]

### Cognitive Assessment

One purpose of evaluating cognitive status in older persons is to detect and manage dementia and delirium. Assessing older adults from ethnic minorities for cognitive impairment, dementia, and delirium presents a number of challenges, including finding suitable translators when command of English is poor, understanding the variable beliefs related to cognitive loss with age in different cultures, approaching the decision to institutionalize, and incorporating the ethical issues pertaining to medical decision making.[45] In this section, two commonly used instruments to assess cognitive status with respect to ethnicity are discussed: (1) the Folstein Mini-Mental State Examination (MMSE) and (2) the Short Portable Mental Status Questionnaire (SPMSQ).

African Americans and persons with less than 8 years of formal education tend to be falsely identified as possibly cognitively impaired when using the MMSE.[46–48] Typically, a cutoff score is employed as a way to standardize assessment and determine when cognitive impairment is significant. Among older African Americans, Hispanic Americans, and persons with educational attainment less than high school, a lower threshold score for determination of cognitive impairment has been recommended (less than 18 of a possible 30 points) to improve sensitivity (82%) and specificity (99%) for the diagnosis of dementia.[49,50] In other words, a standard cutoff of 23 or less to determine cognitive impairment tends to overestimate the number of African Americans and Hispanic Americans with true impairment of cognitive function. Increasing functional difficulty over time with decreasing MMSE scores was not found among African-American women, suggesting that the MMSE may not be a valid predictor of subsequent functional decline; this result is consistent with the idea that the MMSE may misidentify older African Americans as cognitively impaired.[51] The Hispanic Established Populations for Epidemiologic Studies in the Elderly indicated that when the standard MMSE threshold score of 23 was used, 22.3% of Mexican-American older adults were classified as cognitively impaired, but this high rate of cognitive impairment may reflect lower educational attainment.[52] The National Institute on Aging has begun to address this issue with the development of instruments for Spanish-speaking patients in the Alzheimer's Disease Cooperative Study. In addition to African Americans and Hispanic Americans, Asian-American older adults also show decline in the MMSE score for lower education and older age.[53] The SPMSQ has been specifically validated in older African-American and Hispanic-American samples with excellent sensitivity and specificity.[47,54,55] The clock-drawing task is another tool in the assessment of cognitive function. Clock drawing seems to be less sensitive to culturally based bias.

## Depression Assessment

Although the prevalence and incidence rates of depression in African Americans appear to be lower than in whites,[56] it is not clear the extent to which this relates to a tendency of older African Americans to report somatic symptoms related to depression but not sadness.[19] In clinical samples, as many as 11% to 33% of older African-American patients were found to be depressed.[57] Little is known about depression rates in older Hispanic Americans, who also present significant methodologic problems when measuring depression.[58] The lifetime prevalence of major depression among Mexican-American adults in California was reported to be 7.8%, but this study did not include adults over the age of 54 years.[59] In other studies using symptom scales, rates of depression in Mexican Americans were reported to be as high as 20% to 30%.[60–62] Suicide rates among older persons tend to be highest in white men and lowest in African-American women. Older Chinese women have a suicide rate that is estimated to be up to seven times higher than in white women.[44,63] Japanese women also have higher suicide rates than white women.[44] Rates of suicide among older adults are also very high in Eastern European countries.[64–66]

Because recognition of depression is problematic, standardized assessment instruments have been developed. In most cases, little information is available on how these instruments perform in older ethnic minority groups. Here, two instruments with regard to ethnicity are discussed: (1) the Centers for Epidemiologic Studies Depression Scale (CES-D) and (2) the Geriatric Depression Scale (GDS). The CES-D is a 20-item questionnaire that is designed to measure depressive symptoms in multiethnic, community-based samples.[67] Reliability estimates for the CES-D are high, ranging from 0.84 to 0.92. Samples of African Americans and other diverse groups have shown that the CES-D can usefully measure depression.[68] The CES-D has a sensitivity of 75% in older African Americans and 94% in older whites.[47,69,70] Recent tests of a new 10-item CES-D seem to have the same reliability and validity as the 20-item version. The GDS has good sensitivity and specificity in most samples, although it appears to have poorer performance among African Americans than among whites.[68–71] Among Hispanic Americans, the GDS was also less sensitive to significant depression.[72,73]

## Social and Economic Issues in Assessment

Frequently, it is the family who brings the older patient to see the doctor. Therefore, social environment plays an important part in the health of older adults. The quality and density of the social environment are critical factors in maintenance of independent living at home. Adequate social support and interaction are significant predictors of morbidity and mortality in older adults.[74,75] Many cultures have strong traditions of care for older family members. For example, among Hispanic Americans, the concept is called *familismo;* for Japanese families, filial piety and family obligation are called *koko*.[29,34] Resistance to accepting help from nonfamily members may reflect an unwillingness to transfer these family obligations to health care professionals. Families of older adults from ethnic minorities may have a great need to participate in the care of their older relatives. African-American caregivers report performing more caregiving activities and caring for persons with greater functional and cognitive impairment than did whites; however, white caregivers reported significantly more burden.[76] In addition to social support from the family, the church and other nonfamily caregivers are important sources of social and emotional support for older African Americans.[77,78]

At the same time, health care professionals should realize that caring family members may shield their relative from intrusive questions or procedures or may cover up deficiencies in the older patient's performance. Family members must be made aware that adequate assessment of older adults requires that they must act as clear translators of questions and answers, not only of assessment instruments, but also in relationship to recommended treatment. Family members may be able to suggest ways that the medical treatment can be integrated with the cultural beliefs and practices of the older person.

Minority older adults tend to show greater levels of financial strain than other races.[79,80] Older minorities face "double jeopardy"; that is, the combined effect of age and minority status leads to greater illness burden and greater strain on financial resources.[81-85] Also, the lack of wealth accumulation leads to greater financial strain across generations. Physicians need to consider the financial constraints of older minority patients when developing recommendations for treatment. Although direct questioning about finances may be offensive to some older adults, presenting the possibility of a less expensive but equally effective treatment shows a depth of understanding that is often appreciated by older persons.

## Ethics in Medical Decision Making

Advance care planning and end-of-life discussions are important components of geriatric assessment. Discussions with older minorities about treatment in the event of serious or terminal illness are often more complex than with middle-class whites because ethnic, religious, and cultural differences are added to the mix. For example, the core value of personal autonomy may not be as tightly held for some minority groups. Mexican-American and Korean older adults rely more heavily on family and physician input for end-of-life decisions than might be typical for whites. For such persons, physicians will have difficulty if they try to elicit a totally autonomous decision from the patient. In addition, older minorities are more likely than whites to prefer an aggressive treatment approach, often for fear of abandonment. Even when older persons from minority groups prefer a palliative approach to care, they are less likely to have communicated this to their physicians. Trust and comfort with a personal physician may be two of the most important requirements that will enhance end-of-life discussions.

## CONCLUSION

Geriatric assessment is an important component of clinical practice. Assessment can be carried out in a single visit or over a number of visits. Because older ethnic minorities are bound to make up a large proportion of patients in primary care, clinicians should pay special attention to the cultural factors that modify aspects of assessment, including the suitability of specific instruments. Combined with sensitivity to cultural issues and clinical judgment, the health and function of all older adults can be enhanced through careful considerations of the domains of geriatric assessment.

**REFERENCES**

1. Agree EM, Freedman VA. Implications of population aging for geriatric health. In: Gallo JJ, Busby-Whitehead J, Rabins PV, Silliman R, Murphy J, eds. *Reichel's Care of the Elderly: Clinical Aspects of Aging,* 5th ed. Baltimore: Lippincott Williams & Wilkins; 1999:659–669.

2. Lavizzo-Mourey R, Mackenzie ER. Cultural competence: Essential measurements of quality for managed care organizations. *Ann Intern Med.* 1996;124:919–921.

3. Mouton CP, Espino DV. Ethnic diversity of the aged. In: Gallo JJ, Busby-Whitehead J, Rabins PV, Silliman R, Murphy J, eds. *Reichel's Care of the Elderly: Clinical Aspects of Aging,* 5th ed. Baltimore: Lippincott Williams & Wilkins; 1999:595–608.

4. Gallo JJ, Lebowitz BD. The epidemiology of common late-life mental disorders in the community: Themes for a new century. *Psychiatr Serv.* 1999 Sep;50(9):1158–1166. Review.

5. Hendrie HC, Osuntokun BO, Hall KS, et al. Prevalence of Alzheimer's disease and dementia in two communities: Nigerian African and African Americans. *Am J Psychiatry.* 1995;152:1485–1492.

6. Teng MX, Stern Y, Marder K, et al. The APOE-epsilon-4 allele and the risk of Alzheimer's disease among African Americans, Whites, and Hispanics. *JAMA*. 1998;279: 751–755.

7. Maestre G, Ottman R, Stern Y, et al. Apolipoprotein E and Alzheimer's disease: Ethnic variation in genotype risks. *Ann Neurol*. 1995;37:254–259.

8. Prisant LM, Mensah GA. Use of beta-adrenergic receptor blockers in blacks. *J Clin Pharmacol*. 1996;36:867–873.

9. Pi EH, Wang AL, Gray GE. Asian/non-Asian transcultural tricyclic antidepressant psychopharmacology: A review. *Prog Neuropsychopharmacol Biol Psychiatry*. 1993;17: 691–702.

10. Sramek JJ, Pi EH. Ethnicity and antidepressant response. *Mount Sinai J Med*. 1996;63:320–325.

11. Cooper R, David R. The biological concept of race and its application to public health and epidemiology. *J Health Polit Policy Law*. 1986;11:97–116.

12. Lillie-Blanton M, Anthony JC, Schuster CR. Probing the meaning of racial/ethnic group comparisons in crack cocaine smoking. *JAMA*. 1993;269:993–997.

13. Whitfield KE. Studying cognition in older African-Americans: Some conceptual considerations. *J Aging Ethnicity*. 1996;1:41–52.

14. Neighbors HW, Lumpkin S. The epidemiology of mental disorder in the black population. In: Ruiz DS, ed. *Handbook of Mental Health and Mental Disorder Among Black-Americans*. Westport, CT: Greenwood Press; 1990:55–70.

15. Kleinman A, Good B. *Culture and Depression: Studies in the Anthropology and Cross-Cultural Psychiatry of Affect and Disorder*. Los Angeles: University of California Press; 1985.

16. Manson SM, Shore JH, Bloom JD. The depressive experience in American Indian communities: A challenge for psychiatric theory and diagnosis. In: Kleinman A, Good B, eds. *Culture and Depression: Studies in the Anthropology and Cross-Cultural Psychiatry of Affect and Disorder*. Los Angeles: University of California Press; 1985:331–368.

17. O'Nell TD. *Disciplined Hearts: History, Identity, and Depression in an American Indian Community*. Los Angeles: University of California Press; 1996.

18. Kleinman A. *Patients and Healers in the Context of Culture: An Exploration of the Borderland Between Anthropology, Medicine, and Psychiatry*. Los Angeles: University of California Press; 1980.

19. Gallo JJ, Cooper-Patrick L, Lesikar S. Depressive symptoms of Whites and African Americans aged 60 years and older. *J Gerontol Psychol Sci*. 1998;53B:277–286.

20. Guralnik JM, Reuben DB, Buchner DM, Ferrucci L. Performance measures of physical function in comprehensive geriatric assessment. In: Rubenstein LZ, Wieland D, Bernabei R, eds. *Geriatric Assessment Technology: The State of the Art*. New York: Springer Publishing; 1995:59–74.

21. Guralnik JM, Branch LG, Cummings SR, Curb JD. Physical performance measures in aging research. *J Gerontol*. 1989;44:M141–M146.

22. Ware JE, Kosinski M, Keller SD. A 12-item short-form health survey: Construction of scales and preliminary tests of reliability and validity. *Med Care*. 1996;34:220–223.

23. Arocho R, McMillan CA, Sutton-Wallace P. Construct validation of the USA-Spanish version of the SF–36 health survey in a Cuban-American population with benign prostatic hyperplasia. *Quality Life Res*. 1998;7:121–126.

24. Guralnik JM, Land KC, Blazer DG, Fillenbaum GG, Branch LG. Educational status and active life expectancy among older blacks and whites. *N Engl J Med.* 1993;329: 110–116.

25. Albert SM, Teresi JA. Reading ability, education, and cognitive status assessment among older adults in Harlem, New York City. *Am J Public Health.* 1999;89:95–97.

26. Brangman SA. African-American elders: Implications for health care providers. *Clin Geriatr Med.* 1995;11:15–23.

27. Gallagher-Thompson D, Talamantes M, Ramirez R, Valverde I. Service delivery issues and recommendations for working with Mexican American family caregivers. In: Yeo G, Gallagher-Thompson D, eds. *Ethnicity and the Dementias.* Washington, DC: Taylor & Francis Publishers; 1996:137–152.

28. Elliott KS, Di Minno M, Lam D, Tu AM. Working with Chinese families in the context of dementia. In: Yeo G, Gallagher-Thompson D, eds. *Ethnicity and the Dementias.* Washington, DC: Taylor & Francis Publishers; 1996:89–108.

29. Villa ML, Cuellar J, Gamel N, Yeo G. *Aging and Health: Hispanic-American Elders,* 2nd ed. Palo Alto, CA: Stanford Geriatric Education Center; 1993.

30. Frank JD, Frank JB. *Persuasion and Healing: A Comparative Study of Psychotherapy.* Baltimore: Johns Hopkins University Press; 1991.

31. Greene VL, Monahans DJ. Comparative utilization of community-based long-term care services by Hispanic and Anglo elderly in a case management system. *J Gerontol.* 1984;39:730–735.

32. Espino DV. Medication usage in elderly Hispanics: What we need to know. In: Sotomayor M, Ascencio NR, eds. *Proceedings on Improving Drug Use Among Hispanic Elderly.* Washington, DC: National Hispanic Council on Aging; 1988:7–11.

33. McCabe M, Cuellar J. *Aging and Health: American Indian/Alaska Native Elders,* 2nd ed. Palo Alto, CA: Stanford Geriatric Education Center; 1994.

34. McBride M, Morioka-Douglas N, Yeo G. *Aging and Health: Asian/Pacific Island American Elders,* 2nd ed. Palo Alto: Stanford Geriatric Education Center; 1996.

35. Miles TP, Bernard MA. Morbidity, disability, and the health status of Black American elderly: A new look at the oldest-old. *J Am Geriatr Soc.* 1992;40:1047–1054.

36. Foley DJ, Fillenbaum G, Service C. Physical functioning. In: Cornoni-Huntley JC, Ostfeld AM, Taylor JO, et al., eds. *Established Populations for the Epidemiologic Studies of the Elderly: Resource Data Book.* Washington, DC: National Institute on Aging, National Institute of Health, U.S. Public Health Service; 1990:34–50. Publication no. 90–495.

37. Edmonds MK. Physical health. In: Jackson JS, Chatters LM, Taylor RJ, eds. *Aging in Black America.* Newbury Park, CA: Sage Publications; 1993:151–167.

38. Clark DO. US trends in disability and institutionalization among older blacks and whites. *Am J Public Health.* 1997;87:438–440.

39. Andrews J. *Poverty and Poor Health among Elderly Hispanic Americans.* Baltimore: Commonwealth Fund Commission; 1989.

40. Markides KS, Stroup-Benham CA, Goodwin JS, Perkowski LC, Lichtenstein M, Ray LA. The effect of medical conditions on the functional limitations of Mexican-American elderly. *Ann Epidemiol.* 1996;6:386–391.

41. Espino DV, Neufeld RR, Mulvhill MK, Libow LS. Hispanic and non-Hispanic elderly on admission to the nursing home: A pilot study. *Gerontologist.* 1988;28:821–824.

42. Chiodo LK, Karren DW, Gerety MB, Mulrow CD, Cornell JF. Functional status of Mexican-American nursing home residents. *J Am Geriatr Soc.* 1994;42:293–296.

43. Rudkin L, Markides KS, Espino DV. Functional limitations in elderly Mexican-Americans. *Top Geriatr Rehabil.* 1997;12:38–46.

44. Lum OM. Health status of Asians and Pacific Islanders. *Clin Geriatr Med.* 1995; 11:53–69.

45. Yeo G, Gallagher-Thompson D (eds). *Ethnicity and the Dementias.* Washington, DC: Taylor & Francis Publishers; 1996.

46. Anthony JC, LeResche L, Niaz U, Von Korff M, Folstein MF. Limits of the 'Mini-Mental State' as a screening test for dementia and delirium among hospital patients. *Psychol Med.* 1982;12:397–408.

47. Baker FM. Issues in assessing dementia in African American elders. In: Yeo G, Gallagher-Thompson D, eds. *Ethnicity and the Dementias.* Washington, DC: Taylor & Francis Publishers; 1996:59–76.

48. Bohrstedt M, Fox PJ, Kohatsu ND. Correlates of Mini-Mental State examination scores among elderly demented patients: The influence of race-ethnicity. *J Clin Epidemiol.* 1994;47:1381–1387.

49. Tangalos EG, Smith GE, Ivnik RJ, et al. The Mini-Mental State examination in general medical practice: Clinical utility and acceptance. *Mayo Clin Proc.* 1996;71:829–837.

50. Crum RM, Anthony JC, Bassett SS, Folstein MF. Population-based norms for the Mini-Mental State examination by age and educational level. *JAMA.* 1993;269:2386–2391.

51. Leveille SG, Guralnik JM, Ferrucci L, Corti MC, Kasper J, Fried LP. Black/white differences in the relationship between MMSE scores and disability: The Women's Health and Aging Study. *J Gerontol Series B Psychol Sci Soc Sci.* 1998;53:201–208.

52. Royall DR, Espino DV, Polk MJ, Palmer RF, Markides KS. Prevalence and patterns of executive impairment in community dwelling Mexican Americans: Results from the Hispanic EPESE study. *Int J Geriatr Psychiatry.* 2004;19(10):926–934

53. Ishizaki J, Meguro K, Ambo H, et al. A normative, community-based study Mini-Mental State in elderly adults: The effect of age and educational level. *J Gerontol Soc Sci.* 1998;53:359–363.

54. Pfeiffer E. A short portable mental status questionnaire for the assessment of organic brain deficit in elderly patients. *J Am Geriatr Soc.* 1975;23:433–441.

55. Fillenbaum GG, Heyman A, Williams K, Prosnit B, Burchett B. Sensitivity and specificity of standardized screening tests for cognitive impairment and dementia among elder black and white community residents. *J Clin Epidemiol.* 1990;43: 651–658.

56. Gallo JJ, Royall DR, Anthony JC. Risk factors for the onset of major depression in middle age and late life. *Soc Psychiatry Psychiatr Epidemiol.* 1993;28:101–108.

57. Rosenthal MP, Goldfarb NJ, Carlson BL, et al. Assessment of depression in a family practice. *J Fam Pract.* 1987;25:143–148.

58. Wagner FA, Gallo JJ, Delva J. Depresión en la edad avanzada: ¿Problema oculto de salud pœblica para México? *Salud Publica Mexico.* 1999;41:189–202.

59. Vega WA, Kolody B, Aguilar-Gaxiola S, Alderete E, Catalano R, Caraveo-Anduaga J. Lifetime prevalence of DSM-III-R psychiatric disorders among urban and rural Mexican Americans in California. *Arch Gen Psychiatry.* 1998;55:771–778.

60. Kemp BS, Staples FR, Lopez-Aqueres W. Epidemiology of depression and dysphoria in the elderly Hispanic population. *J Am Geriatr Soc.* 1987;35:920–926.

61. Munoz E. Care for the Hispanic poor: A growing segment of American society. *JAMA.* 1988;260:2711–2712.

62. Black SA, Markides KS, Miller TQ. Correlates of depressive symptomatology among older community-dwelling Mexican Americans: The Hispanic EPESE. *J Gerontol Series B Psychol Sci Soc Sci.* 1998;53:S198–S208.

63. Liu WT, Yu E. Asian/Pacific American elderly: Mortality differentials, health status, and the use of health services. *J Appl Gerontol.* 1985;4:35–64.

64. Corin E. From a cultural stance: Suicide and aging in a changing world. *Int Psychogeriatr.* 1995;7:335–355.

65. La Vecchia C, Lucchini F, Levi F. Worldwide trends in suicide mortality, 1955–1989. *Acta Psychiatr Scand.* 1994;90:53–64.

66. Sartorius N. Recent changes in suicide rates in selected Eastern European and other European countries. *Int Psychogeriatr.* 1995;7:301–308.

67. Radloff LS. The CES-D Scale: A self-report depression scale for research in the general population. *Appl Psychol Meas.* 1977;1:385–401.

68. Mouton CP, Johnson MS, Cole DR. Ethical considerations with African American elders. *Clin Geriatr Med.* 1995;11:113–129.

69. Baker FM, Wiley C, Velli SA, Johnson JT. Reliability of the Geriatric Depression Scale and the Center for Epidemiologic Studies of Depression Scale in the elderly [abstract]. Annual Meeting of the American Psychiatric Association, September 24, 1994.

70. Baker FM, Parker DA, Wiley C, Velli SA, Johnson JT. Depressive symptoms in African American medical patients. *Int J Geriatr Psychiatry.* 1995;10:9–14.

71. Baker FM. A contrast: Geriatric depression versus depression in younger age groups. *J Natl Med Assoc.* 1991;83:340–344.

72. Baker FM, Espino DV, Robinson BH, et al. Assessing depressive symptoms in African-American and Mexican-American elders. *Clin Gerontol.* 1993;14:15–21.

73. Baker FM, Espino DV. A Spanish version of the geriatric depression scale in Mexican-American elders. *Int J Geriatr Psychiatry.* 1997;12:21–25.

74. Seeman TE, Kaplan GA, Knudsen L, Cohen R, Guralnik J. Social network ties and mortality among the elderly in the Alameda County study. *Am J Epidemiol.* 1987; 126:714–723.

75. Blazer DG. Social support and mortality in an elderly community population. *Am J Epidemiol.* 1982;115:684–694.

76. Fredman L, Daly MP, Lazur AM. Burden among white and black caregivers to elderly adults. *J Gerontol Series B Psychol Sci Soc Sci.* 1995;50:S110–S118.

77. Chadiha L, Morrow-Howell N, Darkwa OK, Berg-Weger M. Support systems of African American family caregivers of elders with dementing illness. *Afr Am Res Perspect.* 1998;4:104–114.

78. Chatters LM, Taylor RJ. Religious involvement among African Americans. *Afr Am Res Perspect.* 1998;4:83–93.

79. Jackson JS, Chatters LM, Taylor RJ. *Aging in African-American America.* Newbury Park, CA: Sage Publications; 1993.

80. The Commonwealth Fund. *National Comparative Survey of Minority Health Care.* New York: The Commonwealth Fund; 1995.

81. Cantor M. The informal support system of New York's inner-city elderly: Is ethnicity a factor? In: Gelfand DE, Kutsik AJ, eds. *Ethnicity and Aging: Theory, Research, and Policy.* New York: Springer Publishing; 1979:153–175.

82. Reed W. Health care needs and services. In: Harel Z, McKinney EA, Williams M, eds. *African-American Aged: Understanding Diversity and Service Needs.* Newbury Park, CA: Sage Publications; 1990.

83. Dowd JJ, Bengston VL. Aging in minority populations: An examination of the double jeopardy hypothesis. *J Gerontol.* 1978;33:427–436.

84. Jackson M, Kolody B, Wood JL. To be old and African-American: The case for the double jeopardy on income and health. In: Manuel RC, ed. *Minority Aging: Sociological and Social Psychological Issues.* Westport, CT: Greenwood Press; 1982.

85. Ferraro KF. Double jeopardy to health for African-American older adults? *J Gerontol.* 1987;42:528–533.

# 4

## *The Older Adult Driver*

David B. Carr and George W. Rebok

### OLDER DRIVERS

*An 84-year-old male is brought in by the family for further evaluation of cognitive decline. The daughter relates a 2-year history of short-term memory loss, with repetition, difficulty in naming, impaired ability to recall recent events, and geographic disorientation. Regarding the latter, he had been lost on two occasions while driving in familiar areas. The daughter is concerned about his safety behind the wheel given a recent accident. The patient has no insight into his deficits. He has a history of osteoarthritis, coronary artery disease, and hypertension. His medications include amlodipine and atenolol. On review of systems, he complains of neck and lower back pain, daytime somnolence, and dizziness. His examination is nonfocal, but he does have severe limited neck range of motion. His rapid pace walk reveals that he covers 20 feet in 12 seconds. His psychometric test profile reveals an abnormal clock-drawing task and a Trails B test of 200 seconds.*

This gentleman probably has dementia of the Alzheimer's type, which puts him at increased risk for a motor vehicle crash. His psychometric profile also places him at increased risk, along with various co-morbidities. The recommendation to stop driving was resisted. The family agreed to an on-the-road test by a driving rehabilitation specialist. It became obvious in traffic that the patient could not drive safely, as he had no regard or attention for other vehicles. The occupational therapist recommended no further driving. In the office follow-up visit with the physician, the recommendation to stop driving was given verbally and in writing to the patient and daughter. An alternate means of transportation was discussed. The daughter was available for assisting with the majority of his trips. The car was removed from the premises. The patient eventually moved into an assisted living environment.

The automobile is the most important source of transportation for older adults. The ability to drive or be driven is crucial for older persons to maintain an important link with society. Functional assessment, which can include driving ability, is a key component for clinicians involved in providing geriatric care. Clinicians should determine whether their patients are currently driving, provide information on healthy driving behaviors, assess medical conditions or physiologic variables that place their patients at increased risk for a motor vehicle injury or driving cessation, and intervene and treat medical illnesses that can impair driving skills.

Some clinicians may be reluctant to address driving habits. However, one could argue that impaired driving skills should not be viewed any differently from the prevention, detection, and improvement of impaired mobility such as walking, which can also result in a fall or other injury. Epidemiologic studies have identified risk factors for driving cessation and motor vehicle crash or injury in older adults.[1] There is still a need to validate current risk factors and to determine whether modification of the risk factors is a benefit to the patient or society. While awaiting further investigation in this area, the clinician should not delay in assessing or assisting older adults in an attempt to maintain or improve driving skills. When driving retirement occurs, clinicians who care for older adults should be ready to assist with suggestions for acceptable alternate modes of transportation.

## BEHAVIORS AND CHARACTERISTICS OF OLDER DRIVERS

There will be a rapid increase in the number of older drivers on the road in the next few decades. This can be attributed to the aging of our driving population in the United States and especially to an increase in the number of older adult female drivers.[2] It appears that each new cohort of older drivers is increasing its average miles driven per year but still drive fewer miles per year than other age groups.[3] Older drivers report less driving at night or during adverse weather conditions and avoid rush hour or congested thoroughfares. Although female older drivers may drive fewer days and are more likely to stop driving than men, some data suggest that this gender gap is narrowing.[4] Most importantly, functionally impaired older adults appear to restrict their exposure even further.[5,6] Unfortunately, the percentage of the population that is actively driving decreases with each decade.[7]

The traffic violation rate per licensed driver is increased for both the younger and older driver.[8] Older adults tend to be ticketed for making improper left-hand turns, failure to yield, or missing stop or traffic signs.[9] These violations tend to reflect problems with attention and complex traffic situations. Older drivers have been noted to take longer to complete turns in intersections.[10] In contrast, younger people tend to have higher rates of violations for speeding, reckless driving, and driving while intoxicated. Older adult drivers (over 65 years old) account for a very small percentage of the motor vehicle crashes and injuries in comparison to other age groups because of fewer numbers of licensed drivers and reduced exposure. However, public safety concerns about the driving performance of this group have been raised by many studies that reveal an increased crash rate per mile driven for drivers aged 70 years or more, but this finding may be affected by the type of roadway. This crash rate has been attributed to age-related changes in driving skills such as visual search and reaction time,[11] in addition to the presence of medical diseases.[12] The actual contribution of each of these factors to this increase in crash rate is unknown. In addition, older adults have increased vulnerability in crashes that result in more serious injuries to themselves, occupants, and other cars when compared with other age groups.[13,14] This is probably related more to fragility than to an increased involvement in crashes.[15]

Dementia may be one of the major medical illnesses that contributes to the increased crash rate in older adults.[16] This may not be surprising given the prevalence of dementia of the Alzheimer's type, which doubles every 5 years over the age of 65 years.[17] One study that administered cognitive tests to older adults during driver license renewal revealed that a significant number of drivers over the age of 80 demonstrated some degrees of cognitive impairment.[18] Studies in tertiary referral centers have revealed an increased crash rate in drivers with dementia of the Alzheimer's type in comparison with controls, although there have been exceptions. Larger population-based studies that are able to identify cognitively impaired drivers by brief cognitive screens have found modest increases in crash rates in older adult drivers.[19] However, it is often difficult to find associations between cognitive and visual impairment and crashes because of the infrequent occurrence of these events, along with the reduction in the number of trips made over time.

## OLDER DRIVERS AT RISK FOR A MOTOR VEHICLE CRASH

Common diseases in older drivers that have been noted to affect driving ability include, but are not limited to, visual impairment,[20,21] diabetes mellitus,[22] seizure disorders,[23] Alzheimer's disease,[24] cerebrovascular accidents,[25] depression,[26] cardiovascular disease,[27,28] sleep disorders,[29] arthritis and related musculoskeletal disorders,[30] and alcohol and drug use.[31] More studies are needed to examine the effect of multiple illnesses on the driving task.

Diseases should be graded as to their severity and ability to impact on driving errors or the human factors. For instance, diabetes has a potential to affect the three important domains of driving: (1) perception (e.g., from retinopathy or cataract), (2) cognition (e.g., from hypoglycemia), and (3) motor response (e.g., from neuropathy). Thus, a clinician may have to make a determination as to the severity of the disease and the impact on the intrinsic factors and weigh these findings within the context of a patient who may have co-morbidities. Doing so becomes more difficult in older drivers when one may be dealing with multiple mild to moderate diseases (e.g., visual impairment, mild cognitive impairment, and arthritis).

Diseases or syndromes that can impair consciousness, such as angina, arrhythmias, diabetes, seizures, syncope, transient ischemic attacks, cerebrovascular accidents, and arthritis, should be assessed for severity to determine whether the disease has a potential to impact driving. Polypharmacy is not uncommon in older adults. Many common medication classes have been studied and noted to either increase the crash risk or to impair driving skills when assessed by simulators or road tests. These include, but are not limited to, narcotics and benzodiazepines,[32] antihistamines, antidepressants, antipsychotics, hypnotics, alcohol, and muscle relaxants. One study that focused on older drivers noted that long-acting benzodiazepines are associated with increased crash rates.[33] Another report suggests that a significant number of older adults may be driving while intoxicated or under the influence of other medications.[34,35]

Another approach to index crash risk in older adults is to perform functional or physiologic measures.[36] With increasing age and the presence of age-related diseases, studies have documented a decline in vision,[37] hearing,[38] and reaction time.[39] Impairments in executive function appear to correlate strongly with older adults with a history of motor vehicle crashes.[40] A decline has been noted in the functional visual field or "useful field of view" with age, and this measure has also been correlated with crash data in an older driver sample that was screened to be at high risk for a crash.[41] A brief computerized version of the useful field of vision is available to clinicians. However, its utility as an office screen or assessment tool awaits further studies to determine its sensitivity, specificity, and positive predictive value in additional settings such as outpatient medical clinics or other high-risk cohorts of older drivers.

There is a growing consensus among clinicians and experts in the field that many conditions and decrements in driving behaviors and physiologic variables can impact driving and can easily be assessed by clinicians.[42-45] The interested clinician is referred to the website—Counseling and Assessment of Older Driving—which describes the ADReS (Assessment of Driving Related Skills) battery, which has the potential to risk stratify older adults.[46] Clinicians can check static visual acuity with the Snellen chart; hearing with the whisper test or hand held audiometry; attention and reaction time with Trails A or B; visual spatial skills with the clock-drawing task; and judgment, insight, muscle strength, and joint range of motion with a physical exam. Impairments in any of these variables should be assessed for their etiologies, and a treatment plan should be developed. Referral to a subspecialist may be in order. The ability of psychometric tests to predict risk for crashes may diminish over time[47] and may need to be repeated for those older adults who continue to drive after a driving assessment. The American Medical Association (AMA) website on driving[46] also describes a useful algorithm for assessing older adult drivers and is shown in Figure 4–1.

Although physicians may have some reluctance in addressing driving issues in the office because of perceived liability risk and concern over patient acceptance, many recognize the importance of assessing driving skills.[48] Clinicians should also incorporate an injury control approach into their health maintenance practice for older adults. Important driving issues that the clinician should discuss with the older

**Physician's Plan for Older Drivers' Safety (PPODS)**
**Is the patient at risk for medically impaired driving?**
*Perform initial screen—*

- Observe the patient
- Be alert to red flags
  - Medical conditions
  - Medications and polypharmacy
  - Review of systems
  - Patient's or family member's concern

*If screen is positive—*

- Ask health risk assessment/social history questions
- Gather additional information

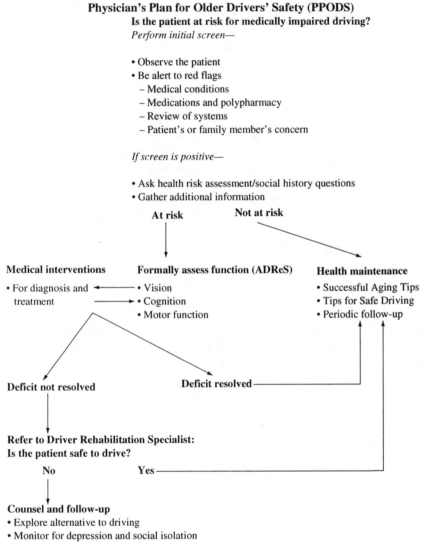

**At risk**        **Not at risk**

**Medical interventions**    **Formally assess function (ADReS)**    **Health maintenance**

- For diagnosis and          - Vision                               - Successful Aging Tips
  treatment                  - Cognition                            - Tips for Safe Driving
                             - Motor function                        - Periodic follow-up

**Deficit not resolved**              **Deficit resolved**

**Refer to Driver Rehabilitation Specialist:**
**Is the patient safe to drive?**

No                    Yes

**Counsel and follow-up**
- Explore alternative to driving
- Monitor for depression and social isolation
- Adhere to state reporting regulations

**Figure 4–1** PPODS Chart. *Source:* Wang CC, Kosinski CJ, Schwartzberg JG, Shanklin AV. *Physician's Guide to Assessing and Counseling Older Drivers.* Washington, DC: National Highway Traffic Administration; 2003. American Medical Association.

driver include using a seat belt, limiting alcohol consumption, refraining from using a cellular phone while driving, obeying the speed limit, and enrolling in refresher courses, such as the Driving Safety Program by the American Association of Retired Persons.

## DRIVING RETIREMENT

Recent studies would indicate that older adults tend to drive fewer miles when affected by illness that can impair their perception and cognition.[49] The clinician may at times have to recommend that his or her patient stop driving, especially when a significant medical condition is involved. Many older drivers have been driving longer than their physicians have been practicing medicine. Hence, it is important for health professionals to discuss these issues in a sensitive manner. The physician can play an important role in enforcing driving cessation by encouraging the patient's acceptance of the situation. The physician should also suggest alternative transportation resources. These discussions should be documented in the patient's chart. It should be noted that older adults are often advised to stop driving becasue of health reasons but often continue to drive despite this advice, especially in rural areas.

Public transportation systems[50] may have reduced fares for senior citizens. Because of restricted sites and the physical or cognitive limitations in the older driver, these services are typically underused. State- or local-sponsored services may provide door-to-door transportation for older adults in large vans, many of which are equipped with lifts. Local communities, societies, retirement centers, or local church groups may use funds or volunteers to provide services to physicians' offices, grocery stores, and meetings.

Patients may refuse to stop driving despite advice from a family member or a clinician. The patient may request a referral for another opinion. This should be reserved for only questionable cases because some evaluations (private or state) may be cursory or superficial. The clinician may consider writing a letter to the state department of motor vehicles (DMV). The ethics and legal ramifications of this letter are discussed in the last section of this chapter.

Special mention is made of the older adult driver who does not have insight into his or her own illness, such as when he or she is suffering from Alzheimer's disease. Unfortunately, primary care physicians may not recognize that their older adult patients who drive have significant cognitive impairment.[51] The spouse, family, physician, occupational therapist, and DMV may need to work together to keep those individuals judged to be unsafe from driving. In situations in which the patient does not have insight into his or her driving limitations, these efforts may include involving the police or DMV to confiscate the driver's license or involving family members to remove access to car keys, move the automobile off the premises, change door locks, file down the ignition keys, or disable the battery cable. An elegant and useful guide from the Hartford Insurance company should be available in physicians' offices to address this important issue and may be helpful to the driver with cognitive impairment and his or her spouse.[52] Copies can be sent free of charge, and the order form is available on the website. A list of helpful resources to patients, clinicians, and caregivers is provided in Table 4-1.

## ASSESSING DRIVING SKILLS

Many health professionals and organizations may assist in the education, training, or assessment of the older driver. These include, but are not limited to, subspecialists in the field of medicine (e.g., neurology and cardiology), neuropsychologists, occupational therapists, physical therapists, courses such as the Driver Safety Program from the American Association of Retired Persons, the medical advisory board of the state or driver improvement office, and insurance companies. A driving simulator may also play a role in assessing driving abilities,[53] and some studies have indicated correlation with crash risk[54] but may not be available in many centers.

Road performance tests are yet another method for evaluating driving skills. Road tests have some limitations because they are often scored subjectively, the road conditions may vary, and the tests may be performed in a car on a driving course that is unfamiliar to the subject. However, road tests have been advocated by several authors as the preferred method to assess driving competency,[55] and impairment in these tests has been correlated with an increase in future crash risk.[56] Occupational therapists, often based at rehabilitation centers, may have specific training and experience in evaluating drivers with medical impairments. The therapist may be able to assist in modifications to the vehicle that could enable its safe and timely operation.

The physical therapist can be an indispensable member of the driving rehabilitation team. Large studies on older adult drivers in the community indicate that back pain, arthritis,[57] and the use of pain medications[58] are associated with increased crash rates. Thus, limitations in muscle strength caused by pain or disuse or restrictions in

**Table 4–1** Physician and Caregiver Resources for Older Drivers

**Clinicians**

American Occupational Therapy Association (AOTA)
www.aota.org/olderdriver

The Association for Driver Rehabilitation Specialists (ADRS)
www.aded.net

National Highway Traffic Safety Administration (NHTSA)
www.nhtsa.dot.gov

American Medical Association (AMA): Physician's Guide to Assessing and Counseling
  Older Drivers
www.ama-assn.org/go/olderdrivers

Mayo Clinic Health Information
www.mayo.edu/geriatrics-rst/driving.html

Administration on Aging (AOA)
www.granddriver.info

Insurance Institute for Highway Safety (IIHS)
www.iihs.org/safety_facts/state_laws/older_drivers_htm

DriveABLE
www.driveable.com

**Educational Material and Courses for Older Drivers**

AARP Driver Safety Program
www.aarp.org

Automobile Association of America (AAA)
www.csaa.com/home

AARP: Driving Safety Program
www.aarp.org/families/driver_safety

Family and Friends Concerned About an Older Driver
www.ntis.gov

Family Conversations with Older Drivers
www.thehartford.com

At the Crossroads: A Guide to Alzheimer's Disease, Dementia, and Driving
www.thehartford.com

**Alternative Transportation Options**

AOA Edlercare
www.eldercare.gov

AAA Foundation for Traffic Safety
www.seniordrivers.org

American Public Transportation Association
www.apta.com

Community Transportation Association
www.ctaa.org

Local Agency on Aging

range of motion of joints such as the hands, feet, and neck may play an important role in driving impairment. Interventions to improve muscle strength and joint function have the potential to improve driving skills.

Even if medically impaired patients pass a road test, a question of how closely to monitor the patient over time will always exist. Repeat road tests can be expensive, but when drivers with Alzheimer's disease who pass road tests are followed longitudinally, skills can be expected to decline in the presence of chronic disease.

## ETHICAL, LEGAL, AND PUBLIC POLICY ISSUES

Patients and families do not always comply or agree with clinicians' recommendations to stop driving. Physicians may simply decide to document this refusal in the chart, as long as the opinion is given to someone who has decision-making capacity. However, this situation may justify a letter to the state's DMV. The courts often require physicians as one of the key players in keeping unsafe drivers off the road.[59] This breach of confidentiality may be appropriate when performed in the best interest of the community.[60] Obviously, the state DMV will ultimately have the final decision as to whether someone can remain licensed to drive. Most states will follow the advice of the physician or occupational therapist. Appeal processes exist for these situations, however. The decision to report patients to the DMV varies depending on personal practices and state requirements. Because the common law and statutes vary among states, legal counsel should be obtained to help guide the evaluation process and determine the regulations that should apply for practices in each state. Some states such as California require physicians to report specific medical conditions such as dementia of the Alzheimer's type.

## FUTURE RESEARCH NEEDS AND CONCLUSIONS

Current research and studies on older drivers have focused on methods to identify the medically impaired driver who is at risk for a motor vehicle crash or at risk for driving cessation. A comprehensive, step-by-step approach appears to be the most appropriate method to assess older adult drivers when safety issues or functional impairment have been raised or identified. Physicians should take an active role in assessing risk for injury while driving. Referral to other professionals or organizations may be helpful in the evaluation and treatment process as well as in the maintenance of the driving skills of older adults. When driving retirement occurs, clinicians should monitor for social isolation and depression and discuss transportation options when appropriate. Programs that are available in Canada such as Drive-ABLE[61] are already available in some states and may be useful to assess medical conditions or chronic medication use in older drivers.

Public policy efforts focused on the routine assessment of senior drivers during license renewal are already occurring in some states. In fact, questionnaires have indicated that older adults are willing to undergo some tests to promote safer driving for the public but do not reach consensus on which measures should be instituted.[62] The efficacy of routine screening measures during license renewal such as vision tests and road tests are in question because in-person license renewal appears to be the only measure in the United States noted to be associated with a decrease crash risk in older adults.[63] However, road tests administered in other countries may be more efficacious and should be studied.[64] More work is needed on the utility of educational programs that have the potential to improve driving skills.[65–67] Research on the type of screening and the utility and feasibility of the screening measures during license renewal to decrease the crash rate is still needed.

### REFERENCES

1. Marottoli RA, Richardson ED, Stowe MH, et al. Development of a test battery to identify older drivers at risk for self-reported adverse driving events. *J Am Geriatr Soc.* 1998;46:562–568.

2. Retchin SM, Anapolle J. An overview of the older driver. *Clin Geriatr Med.* 1993;9:279–296.

3. O'Neil, D. The older driver. *Rev Clin Gerontol.* 1996;6:295–302.

4. Bauer MJ, Adler G, Kuskowski MA, Rottunda S. The influence of age and gender on the driving patterns of older adults. *J Women Aging.* 2003;15:3–16.

5. Ball K, Owsley C, Stalvey B, et al. Driving avoidance and functional impairment in older drivers. *Accid Anal Prev.* 1998;30:313–322.

6. West CG, Gildengorin G, Haegerstrom-Portnoy G, et al. Vision and driving self-restriction in older adults. *J Am Geriatr Soc.* 2003;51:1348–1355.

7. Foley DJ, Wallace RB, Eberhard J. Risk factors for motor vehicle crashes among older drivers in a rural community. *J Am Geriatr Soc.* 1995;43:776–781.

8. Graca JL. Driving and aging. *Clin Geriatr Med.* 1986;2:577.

9. Retting RA, Weinstein HB, Solomon MG. Analysis of motor-vehicle crashes at stop signs in four US cities. *J Safety Res.* 2003;34:485–489.

10. Cox AB, Cox DJ. Compensatory driving strategy of older people may increase driving risk. *J Am Geriatr Soc.* 1998;46:1058–1059.

11. Reuben D. Assessment of older drivers. *Clin Geriatr Med.* 1993;9:445–459.

12. Waller J. Cardiovascular disease, aging, and traffic accidents. *J Chronic Dis.* 1967;20:615–620.

13. Morris A, Welsh R, Frampton R, et al. An overview of requirements for the crash protection of older drivers. *Annual Proceedings/Association for the Advancement of Automotive Medicine.* 2002;46:141–156.

14. Braver ER, Trempel RE. Are older drivers actually at higher risk of involvement in collisions resulting in deaths or non-fatal injuries among their passengers and other road users? *Injury Prev.* 2004;10:27–32.

15. Li G, Braver ER, Chen LH. Fragility versus excessive crash involvement as determinants of high death rates per vehicle-mile of travel among older drivers. *Accid Anal Prev.* 2003;35:227–235.

16. Odenheimer G. Dementia and the older driver. *Clin Geriatr Med.* 1993;9:349–364.

17. Cummings JL. Alzheimer's disease. *N Engl J Med.* 2004;351:56–67.

18. Stutts JC, Stewart JR, Martell CM. Cognitive test performance and crash risk in an older driver population. *Accid Anal Prev.* 1998;30:337–346.

19. Foley DJ, Wallace RB, Eberhard J. Risk factors for motor vehicle crashes among older drivers in a rural community. *J Am Geriatr Soc.* 1995;43:776–781.

20. Shinar D, Schieber F. Visual requirements for safety and mobility of older drivers. *Hum Factors.* 1991;33:505–519.

21. Coeckelbergh TR, Brouwer WH, Cornelissen FW, et al. The effect of the visual field defects on driving performance: A driving simulator study. *Arch Ophthalmol* 2002;120:1509–1516.

22. Koepsell TD, Wolf ME, McCloskey L, et al. Medical conditions and motor vehicle collision injuries in older adults. *J Am Geriatr Soc.* 1994;42:695–700.

23. Hansotia P, Broste SK. The effect of epilepsy or diabetes mellitus on the risk of automobile accidents. *N Engl J Med.* 1991;324:22–26.

24. Drachman DA, Swearer JM. Driving and Alzheimer's disease: The risk of crashes. *Neurology.* 1993;42:2448–2456.

25. Wilson T, Smith T. Driving after stroke. *Int Rehabil Med.* 1983;5:170–177.

26. Doege TC, Engelberg AL, eds. *Medical Conditions Affecting Drivers.* Chicago: American Medical Association; 1986.

27. Gallo JJ, Rebok GW, Lesikar SE. The driving habits of adults aged 60 years and older. *J Am Geriatr Soc.* 1999;47:335–341.

28. Ahlgren E, Lundqvist A, Nordlund A, et al. Neurocognitive impairment and driving performance after coronary artery bypass surgery. *Euro J of Cardiothorac Surg.* 2003;23:334–340.

29. Findley LJ, Unverzagt ME, Suratt PM. Automobile accidents involving patients with obstructive sleep apnea. *Am Rev Respir Dis.* 1988;138:337–340.

30. Roberts WN, Roberts P. Evaluation of the elderly driver with arthritis. *Clin Geriatr Med.* 1993;9:311–322.

31. Ray WA, Gurwitz J, Decker MD, Kennedy DL. Medications and the safety of the older driver: Is there a basis for concern? *Hum Factors.* 1992;34:33–47.

32. Drummer OH, Gerostamoulos J, Batziris H, et al. The involvement of drugs in drivers of motor vehicles killed in Australian road traffic crashes. *Accid Anal Prev.* 2004;36:239–248.

33. Hemmelgarn B, Suissa S, Huang A, et al. Benzodiazepine use and the risk of motor vehicle crash in the elderly. *JAMA*. 1997;278:27–31.

34. Higgins JP, Wright SW, Wrenn KD. Alcohol, the elderly, and motor vehicle crashes. *Am J Emerg Med*. 1996;14:265–267.

35. Johansson K, Bryding G, Dahl ML, et al. Traffic dangerous drugs are often found in fatally injured older male drivers. *J Am Geriatr Soc*. 1997;45:1029–1031.

36. Wallace RB, Retchin SM. A geriatric and gerontologic perspective on the effects of medical conditions on older drivers: Discussion of Waller. *Hum Factors*. 1992;34:17–24.

37. Kline DW, Schieber F. Vision and aging. In: Birren JE, Schaie KW, eds. *Handbook of the Psychology of Aging*, 3rd ed. New York: Van Nostrand Reinhold; 1990:296-331.

38. Olsho L, Harkins S, Lenhardt M. Aging and the auditory system. In: Birren JE, Schaie KW, eds. *Handbook of the Psychology of Aging*, 2nd ed. New York: Van Nostrand Reinhold; 1985:332–377.

39. Salthouse T. Speed of behavior and its implications for cognition. In: Birren JE, Schaie KW, eds. *Handbook of the Psychology of Aging*, 2nd ed. New York: Van Nostrand Reinhold; 1985:400–426.

40. Daigneault G, Joly P, and Frigon JY. Executive functions in the evaluation of accident risk of older drivers. *J Clin Exp Neuropsychol*. 2002;24:221–238.

41. Owsley C, Ball K, McGwin G, et al. Visual processing impairment and risk of motor vehicle crash among older adults. *JAMA*. 1998;279:1083–1088.

42. De Raedt R, Ponjaert-Kristoffersen I. Short cognitive/neuropsychologist test battery for first-tier fitness-to-drive assessment of older adults. *Clin Neuropsychol*. 2001;15: 329–336.

43. Messinger-Rapport BJ. How to assess and counsel the older driver. *Cleve Clin J Med*. 2002;69:184–190.

44. Lesikar SE, Gallo JJ, Rebok GW, Keyl PM. Prospective study of brief neuropsychological measures to assess crash risk in older primary care patients. *J Am Board Fam Pract*. 2002;15:11–19.

45. Kantor B, Mauger L, Richardson VE, Unroe KT. An analysis of an older driver evaluation program. *J Am Geriatr Soc*. 2004;52:1326–1330.

46. American Medical Association (2005). Physician's guide to assessing and counseling older drivers. Accessed June 7, 2005 from http://www.ama-assn.org/ama/pub/category/10791.html.

47. Staplin L, Gish KW, Wagner EK. MaryPODS revisited: Updated crash analysis and implications for screening program implementation. *J Safety Res*. 2003;34:389–397.

48. Bogner HR, Straton JB, Gallo JJ, et al. The role of the physicians in assessing older drivers: Barriers, opportunities, and strategies. *J Am Board Fam Pract*. 2004;17:38–43.

49. Fisk GD, Owsley C, and Mennemeier M. Vision, attention, and self-reported driving behaviors in community-dwelling stroke survivors. *Arch Physical Med Rehab*. 2002;83:469–477.

50. Roper TA, Mulley GP. Caring for older people: Public transport. *BMJ*. 1996;313: 415–418.

51. Valcour VG, Masaki KH, Blanchette PL. Self-reported driving, cognitive status, and physician awareness of cognitive impairment. *J Am Geriatr Soc*. 2002;50:1265–1267.

52. The Hartford Financial Services Group (2000). At the crossroads: A guide to Alzheimer's disease, dementia, and driving. Accessed June 7, 2005 from http://www.thehartford.com/alzheimers/brochure.html.

53. Rebok GW, Keyl PM. Driving simulation and older adults. In: Burdick DC, Kwon S, eds. *Gerotechnology: Research and Practice in Technology and Aging.* New York: Springer; 2004:191–208.

54. Lee HC, Lee AH, Cameron D, Li-Tsang C. Using a driving simulator to identify older drivers at inflated risk of motor vehicle crashes. *J Safety Res.* 2003;34:453–459.

55. Stutts JC, Wilkins JW. On-road driving evaluations: A potential tool for helping older adults drive safely longer. *J Safety Res.* 2003;34:431–439.

56. Keall MD, Frith WJ. Association between older driver characteristics, on-road driving test performance, and crash liability. *Traffic Injury Prevention.* 2004;5:112–116.

57. Foley DJ, Wallace RB, Eberhard J. Risk factors for motor vehicle crashes among older drivers in a rural community. *J Am Geriatr Soc.* 1995;43:776–781.

58. Tuokko H, Beattie BC, Tallman K, et al. Predictors of motor vehicle crashes in a dementia clinic population: The role of gender and arthritis. *J Am Geriatr Soc.* 1995;43:1444–1445.

59. Gray C, Sullivan P. MDs still the key to eliminating unfit drivers, jury decides. *CMAJ.* 2002;166:1196.

60. Gracal L. Driving and aging. *Clin Geriatr Med.* 1986;2:586.

61. Anonymous. DriveABLE: New clinical tool measures driving competency. *Can Fam Phys.* 2000;46:142–143.

62. Parker D, McDonald L, Rabbitt P, Sutcliffe P. Older drivers and road safety: The acceptability of a range of intervention measures. *Accid Anal Prev.* 2003;35:805–810.

63. Grabowski DC, Campbell CM, Morrisey MA. Elderly licensure laws and motor vehicle fatalities. *JAMA.* 2004;291:2840–2846.

64. Keall MD, Frith WJ. Association between older driver characteristics, on-road driving test performance, and crash liability. *Traffic Injury Prev.* 2004;5:112–116.

65. Eby DW, Molnar LJ, Shope JT, et al. Improving older driver knowledge and self-awareness through self-assessment: The driving decisions workbook. *J Safety Res.* 2003;34:371–381.

66. Owsley C, McGwin G, Phillipps JM, et al. Impact of an educational program on the safety of high-risk, visually impaired, older drivers. *Am J Prev Med.* 2004;26:222–229.

67. Ball KK, Wadley VG, Edwards JD. Advances in technology used to assess and retrain older drivers. *Gerontechnology.* 2002:251–261.

# 5

# *Enhancing Advance Directive Discussions Using the Values History*

David J. Doukas, Laurence B. McCullough, and Monica Crane

eriatric assessment requires an examination of the present and preparation for the future. Patients need to consider their long-term care options, as well as health directives for a broad array of interventions. This consideration is hinged on the input of physicians. Physicians are responsible for addressing future health concerns as part of their fiduciary responsibility for managing their patients' medical ailments, taking ownership of the task of initiating discussions on advance directives. Unfortunately, many physicians have been reticent in discussing advance directives or reluctant to respect them when the appropriate time comes.[1,2] Physicians are reluctant to discuss advance directives because of their own discomfort, as well as a perception that they will burden their patients and families by the discussion.[1] Further shortcomings in advance directives were reflected in the SUPPORT study.[2] This multicenter trial found that despite discussions on end-of-life treatments that were integrated into the medical care of hospitalized patients, stated preferences are not routinely translated into physician's orders.

Both living wills and the durable powers of attorney for health care (DPA/HC) address preferences for future health care. The Patient Self-Determination Act of 1990 intended to enhance use of these instruments by requiring health care institutions that receive Medicare and

Medicaid funds to ask patients if an advance directive has been signed. Although studies revealed that signing rates increased, the universal execution of the advance directive did not.[3] Advance directives have a sound ethical foundation, but often they fail to assess or acknowledge people's values in their formulation, execution, and implementation. People view their lives and health care as part of their remembrances of loved ones lost and how their own mortality can be influenced through the use of advance directives.

Doukas and McCullough proposed in the late 1980s to make this process more systematic using an instrument that both assesses and acknowledges the values of patients in end-of-life health care planning, the Values History.[4-7] The Values History enhances autonomy through an intake of patient values and health care preferences that are to be carried out when decision making by the patient is no longer possible. The Values History facilitates communication by asking the patient to identify values and preferences before the patient can no longer speak for himself or herself. As such, the Values History is a valuable adjunct in fulfilling the ethical foundation of the Patient Self-Determination Act to inform patients about their right to refuse medical therapy (including the use of advance directives).[8] These values and preferences are to be discussed first in the outpatient setting, with additional Values History discussions occurring with changes of health status. This approach decreases the probability of encountering uncertainty about the person's preferences for end-of-life care. Addressing values and preferences when discussing advance directives is an essential aspect of geriatric care. The patient must be informed about not only advance directives, but also the importance of their values and preferences. These enable the physician and family to implement them. The Values History eases this process by addressing relevant values that underlie the informed consent process for these directives.

## THE LIVING WILL

The living will is a written statement (or oral declaration as allowed in applicable law) that documents a person's competent decision to withhold or withdraw artificial means of health care in circumstances of terminal illness (and, in many states, irreversible comatose and vegetative states) when the person can no longer make decisions. The living will allows the person to decide in advance which life-prolonging therapies in the treatment of a terminal disease process and its complications should not be administered. The individual is free to revoke the living will—even when he or she is later incapacitated. The instrument cannot be revoked or interfered with by third parties (i.e., physicians or family), provided that it has been executed according to the procedures defined in applicable law. Veterans Health Affairs accepts living wills on the basis of Veterans Health Affairs policy.

Sometimes the language of the living will is unclear about which particular medical procedures are to be refused. This lack of precision can lead to misinterpretation of what the person has refused.[9] Physician interpretation of the person's intent as well as his or her assessment of the probability of recovery can shade the likelihood of advance directive implementation.[9] Furthermore, many states have a specific format for the living will, designated by statute; however, the Cruzan case's findings make that point tenuous.[10–12]

Living wills are legally sanctioned instruments that allow the competent person to exercise autonomous control over future medical care in anticipation of future incapacity. The ethics and law of informed consent doctrine require that patients be informed about medically reasonable therapies and the alternative of no intervention at all. Informed consent doctrine requires that patients have the right to accept or refuse any therapy, and this right to accept or decline potentially life-sustaining medical therapies can be indicated in a living will. Thus, end-of-life treatment options should be discussed by doctors with their patients, especially with older adults who may be faced with end-of-life decisions. Living wills should be based on the patient's values regarding terminal treatment and care. However, living wills typically do not address those fundamental values that help them articulate explicit end-of-life preferences. In order to understand the patient's reasoning and motivation in executing a living will, more information is required than the instrument itself typically includes.

## THE DPA/HC

The DPA/HC is a legal document that transfers the power of medical decision making from the patient to an agent, who can be a relative or other trusted individual when the patient lacks decision-making capacity. This agent is assigned to make health care decisions when that person is incapacitated. The so-called durability conveys that the power begins with and continues through the patient's incapacity. The agent should not be the physician, as there is the potential of conflict of interest in the decision-making process. The DPA/HC takes effect at incapacity, not only in the narrow end-of-life confines of the living will. Veterans Health Affairs and nearly all states provide for the DPA/HC. The duty of the DPA/HC agent on the patient's incapacity is to consider the medically reasonable options and then select the option(s) that most closely adhere to the previously discussed or written preferences of the individual. This process is called the substituted judgment standard. If the patient's preferences are not known, decisions should be based on the patient's best interests, that is, the best interest standard. The DPA/HC is more flexible than the living will. Although the living will avoids the potential burden of placing decision making on another's shoulders, the DPA/HC may be a better approach because it can accommodate a wider spectrum of future medical conditions and possible medical responses. Also, patients may feel more confident in designating a DPA/HC to voice and enforce their interests than in signing specific medical treatments or refusals. The main objection to the DPA/HC is whether the agent has a sufficient understanding of all of the patient's many health care preferences.[13] Often patients are reluctant to discuss their values, much less their specific preferences about terminal care with their agent.

## THE FAMILY COVENANT

The use of the family covenant has been advocated by one of the authors (D.J.D.) and John Hardwig in end-of-life treatment advance planning.[14] The family covenant is a means by which a patient can select whom within the family and other intimates should be allowed to be included in the information sharing and decision-making processes in treatment selection both before and after incapacity. The determination of who is to be included in this process is entirely vested in the patient and should best reflect those persons of family and/or acquaintance who can reflect reliably the values and treatment preferences of the patient. This model transcends the narrow scope of DPA/HC documents with an appreciation that families often are very relevant in these decisions. Nevertheless, a physician cannot assume that each person in the patient's surroundings has a reliable understanding of the values of the patient. Thus, this model begins with an agreement that endures over time concerning to whom information should flow. The passage of time allows for the accumulation of trust, thus strengthening the relationship and allowing for ongoing discussion, deliberation, and decision making. The family covenant can then be used as a method to discuss advance directives and other relevant advance care planning options, such as those discussed previously.

## THE VALUES HISTORY

The Values History (Appendix A) was first published in the literature a decade and a half ago to identify better end-of-life health care values and treatment preferences based on those values.[6] The Values History complements the living will and DPA/HC rather than replaces them. The Values History first asks the individual to identify his or her values and beliefs regarding terminal care, followed by considering end-of-life treatment decisions in advance, given these values. By first articulating end-of-life values, the patient's perspective is better understood by the patient, his or her family, and his or her physician. The intended effect is to enhance communication as well as the implementation of the treatment preferences when appropriate.

### The Preamble

The preamble articulates the premise of the Values History: to supplement the person's advance directive(s). These values and preferences guide physicians when an individual without decision-making capacity is terminally ill, irreversibly comatose, in a persistent vegetative state, or otherwise a qualified patient under applicable advance directive law and the withholding or withdrawing of life-sustaining measures is being contemplated. As with other advance directive instruments, the Values History is changeable and revocable as long as the person is able to voice his or her preferences.

### The Values Section

The person first identifies life values relevant to the treatment decisions that must be made. The foundation to this section is a thought-provoking query as to whether the length of life or the quality of life is more important to the patient. Identifying those values *most* important to him or her from a list of 13 common end-of-life values then follows this first choice, as it may have great bearing on considering these values. Other values can be added to this list, as it is not intended to be comprehensive, just a starting point for facilitating communication. These identified values can then help the individual formulate his or her treatment preferences toward end-of-life medical care.

## The Preferences Section

The Preferences Section contains a list of medical interventions, with acute-care decisions first and then chronic-care treatment options. Many preference statements introduce the concept of a "trial of intervention," either limited by time or benefit. This approach allows for a therapy to be used for a designated period of time or in order to ascertain whether medical benefit is present and continued after a therapy is initiated.

Discussing cardiopulmonary resuscitation (CPR) is fundamental in considering end-of-life care, as withholding or stopping resuscitation in dire circumstances will usually result in death. Many physicians, hospitals, and importantly, patients presume that this medical therapy will be provided. Code status is of particular importance in chronic and critical illness where such decisions are increasingly relevant. Such orders can also be used in out-of-hospital do not resuscitate orders, as allowed in many states for patients in home and hospice care. Respirator and endotracheal intubation discussions help to clarify the unifying concept of advanced cardiac life support (ACLS) resuscitation—if ACLS protocols are to be used, they must be used with established standards. "Partial codes" are not condoned in one's treatment preferences, as they may set up false hopes for treatment benefit where there is none.

Each subsequent chronic care directive is based in the context of future long-term recuperative or vegetative care. The chronic care treatment options include total parenteral nutrition, intravenous hydration/medication, all medications for the treatment of illnesses by other routes (e.g., oral or by intramuscular injection), enteral feeding tubes, and dialysis. The physician should make clear that pain medications will always be prescribed as needed.

Preferences then follow addressing autopsy, proxy negation, and organ donation. The investigation of the causes of death may be very important for some, such that the option of autopsy helps to understand genetic familial disease risks better. The person is given an opportunity to add any other medical preferences not otherwise addressed. The unique and singularly helpful Proxy Negation directive allows the individual to name those who are to be excluded from the person's health care decision making in the future. This preference is useful when family members have a different philosophy or religious belief regarding medical care or who have a conflict of interest. The last directive encourages the person to consider a Gift of Life by filling out a Uniform Donor Card (specific to the reader's state), allowing for the postmortem use of organs in transplantation, medical therapy, and medical research or education. Families are encouraged to respect this personal decision, as well as that of autopsy.

## Clinical Use of the Values History

All competent geriatric patients should be offered the Living Will, the DPA/HC, and the Values History. All three should therefore be part of geriatric assessment. In the primary care office, preliminary questioning on end-of-life care should be initiated by the physician. This discussion usefully begins with the DPA/HC designation, as it is often an easier task to identify a proxy decision maker. This point is where the family covenant can be introduced in order to identify boundaries set by the patient on who should be included in discussions on medical care and treatment decision. Often, this point in time is also when the identification of the Proxy Negation is relevant. The next step would be to discuss the living will in the context of future terminal illness or irreversible incapacity. When the patient signs (i.e., executes) his or her living will and/or DPA/HC, this should be documented within the medical record, with copies also placed in the medical record, and an appropriate note discussing the conversations that led to these decisions, as well as patient-expressed delineations of how the family can or should have a place in their future health care. The physician's next step would be to introduce the Values Section of the Values History.

Subsequently, the physician should discuss the preferences listed in the Values History. These discussions should be rooted in the context of the person's own medical problems. For example, the physician should explain the lack of benefit of CPR to someone with conditions that generally reduce the chances of successful CPR. Generally, the acute-care treatment options (e.g., CPR, intubation, and ventilation) should also be discussed early with signature of the Values History to demonstrate their consent to the document. The remainder of the Values History can be discussed during follow-up visits as part of other health maintenance exams, with documentation of subsequent decisions as they are articulated. Each treatment preference should be individually signed and dated as agreed to over time. The physician should document these treatment preferences in the medical record for that date. Treatment preferences are to be rooted in the patient's values from the Values Section, as well as other relevant concerns that are likely to arise in discussion.

Values-based discussion allows for a more meaningful understanding of the individual's reasoning while also probing possible inconsistent values. Also, any impediments to a person's ability to formulate an informed consent may be gleaned. The physician could thereby help the person therapeutically to restore his or her decision-making capacity. Throughout this evolving advance directive informed consent process, the law and ethics of informed consent require the physician to presume that persons are able to consent to these decisions unless unable to do so. The burden of proof is on the physician to establish and document in the medical record that the individual is unable to make these decisions.

The Values History preserves respect for the patient by allowing the DPA/HC agent as well as other identified family covenant members to use the patient's values and preferences in the event of future incapacity. The patient should understand that the basis for this respect is best secured in advance to help his or her significant others help him or her in the future. If the individual has no advance directive or proxy, the physician should inform him or her that signing them would best ensure that his or her wishes would be carried out. Five states (i.e., California, Delaware, Michigan, Missouri, and New York) have had case law arise in which "clear and convincing" standards of evidence (i.e., explicit written or oral declarations) were required before withholding or withdrawing life-prolonging care. Every patient must understand that making no decision *is a decision*—in that treatment against his or her own values may be imposed if no advance directive is executed.

## CASE VIGNETTE

*Mr. Bob Jones comes into Dr. Zelda Smith's office for an extended appointment for assessment of his abilities now that he is widowed and living alone at the age of 78 years. Dr. Jones asks Mr. Smith whether he has an advance directive. He replies, "Yes, I have a living will, and one of those Health Care Proxies (a DPA/HC),*

*and my son John is the proxy." Dr. Smith asks what John under-
stands about Mr. Jones' end-of-life values and preferences. He
replies, "John will know what to do," but that indicates that he
has never had any specific conversations on end-of-life treatment
as both he and his son have been a bit reticent about talking about
it. He also states that he has an estranged daughter, Betty, with
whom he has had no contact for 9 years, and they have sharply
different views on health, life, and religion.*

*Dr. Smith uses this opportunity to initiate a conversation about
advance directive values, with an emphasis on asking why Mr.
Jones had executed his advance directives. His responses regarding
the trauma of seeing his wife die then stimulates a discussion on
his own quality of life and other associated values. Dr. Smith discusses the Values History with Mr. Jones, who then completes the
Values Section and addresses several acute care preferences by ini-
tialing each and signing the form. Over the next two physician appointments, John joins Dr. Smith and Mr. Jones in discussing the
remainder of the Preferences Section. Mr. Jones also lists Betty in
the Proxy Negation so that she will not attempt to usurp John's role
at some later date. All parties recognize how this discussion will
help in the future, and the completed copy of the form is placed in
is medical chart, with Mr. Jones keeping the original and his son
having a copy. This duplication allows for ready use in case of hospitalization and to assist the proxy to help with decision making,
which in turn, will help Dr. Smith with the writing of orders in the
hospital.*

## Barriers in Using the Values History

Potential barriers may arise in using the Values History. First, as
noted previously, the physician may delay advance directive discussions to the person until the "right time."[1] This delay of informed
consent can thereby prohibit decisions about future health care. Both
the physician and the patient can lose a valuable opportunity to discuss values regarding end-of-life care if the patient becomes ill and decisions need to be made in the absence of helpful discourse on values
and preferences. Patient ambivalence or wariness in discussing advance directives can be a barrier to the Values History. Physicians
should attempt continued sensitive discussion, particularly regarding

what may happen if no advance directive is ever signed, as noted previously. Family members can impede the Values History's implementation if no attempt is made to engage them. A family member may disagree with a patient's refusal of medical therapies and attempt to circumvent the refusal. In such circumstances, it is helpful to acknowledge the family member's concerns and values and to inform him or her that advance directives are intended to safeguard the patient's autonomy and dignity. The family covenant helps to identify proactively the relevant family members in medical decision making, as well as who should not be part of these discussions or subsequent decisions. Such information, when documented in the medical records, can help the patient and physician identify who has "standing" to speak for the patient when incapacity comes.

**Legal Considerations**

All states now have an advance directive statute (either living will, DPA/HC, or both). Almost all of these statutes allow for directives to be appended to them.[10] If a state does not have a statute with this stipulation, it is still prudent to append the Values History to an advance directive, as competent values and preferences will enhance the legal evidence and moral clarity supporting the document. Organ donation statutes vary according to jurisdiction, such that seeking the applicable Organ Donor Card for the Department of Motor Vehicles and attaching it to the Values History is strongly recommended.

**CONCLUSION**

The Values History is an important complement to formal advance directives that helps to understand the patient's living will and the DPA/HC better. The Values History supplements, rather than replaces, these advance directives. Thus, all parties can gain a deeper level of meaning of what the patient wants in the future. The greatest utility of the Values History is to facilitate discussion regarding basic health care values and value-based preferences. A longitudinal conversation best approximates the ethical preference that informed consent is a *process* rather than an event.[15] By using the Values History, the patient can best safeguard his or her own future autonomy and dignity by communicating core health values and translating these values into preferences that the physician can implement when appropriate.

## REFERENCES

1. Doukas D, Gorenflo D, Coughlin S. The living will: A national survey. *Fam Med.* 1991;123:354–356.

2. The SUPPORT Investigators. A controlled trial to improve outcomes for seriously ill hospitalized patients: The study to understand prognoses and preferences for outcomes and risks of treatment. *JAMA.* 1995;274:1591–1598.

3. Teno JM, Lynn J, Wenger N, et al. Advance directives for seriously ill hospitalized patients: Effectiveness with the patient self-determination act and the SUPPORT intervention. *J Am Geriatr Soc.* 1997;45:500–507.

4. Doukas D, McCullough L. Assessing the Values History of the aged patient regarding critical and chronic care. In: Gallo J, Reichel W, eds. *The Handbook of Geriatric Assessment,* 1st ed. Rockville, MD: Aspen Publishers; 1988:111–124.

5. Doukas D, Lipson S, McCullough L. Value History. In: Reichel W, ed. *Clinical Aspects of Aging,* 3rd ed. Baltimore: Williams & Wilkins; 1989:615–616.

6. Doukas D, McCullough L. The Values History: The evaluation of the patient's values and advance directives. *J Fam Pract.* 1991;3:145–153.

7. Doukas D, Reichel W. *Planning for Uncertainty: A Guide to Living Wills and Other Advance Directives for Health Care.* Baltimore: Johns Hopkins University Press; 1993.

8. Omnibus Budget Reconciliation Act, Public Law No. 101–508 §§4206, 4751 (1990).

9. Eisendrath S, Jonsen A. The living will: Help or hindrance? *JAMA.* 1983;249:2054–2058.

10. Society for the Right to Die. *The Physician and the Hopelessly Ill Patient: Legal, Medical, and Ethical Guidelines.* New York: The Society for the Right to Die; 1985.

11. Cruzan v Director, Missouri Department of Health, 467 US 261, 10 S Ct 2841 (1990).

12. Doukas DJ. After the Cruzan case: The primary care physician and the use of advance directives. *J Am Board Fam Pract.* 1992;5:201–205.

13. Wanzer S, Adelstein J, Cranford R, et al. The physician's responsibility toward hopelessly ill patients. *N Engl J Med.* 1984;310:955–959.

14. Doukas DJ, Hardwig J. Using the family covenant in planning end-of-life care: Obligations and promises of patients, families, and physicians. *J Am Geriatr Soc.* 2003; 51:1–4.

15. Doukas DJ. Ask them and they will tell you: Advance directives in patient care. *Am Fam Phys.* 1999;59:530–533.

# Appendix A
# The Values History

Patient name: _____

This Values History serves as a set of my specific value-based directives for various medical interventions. It is to be used in health care circumstances when I may be unable to voice my preferences. These directives shall be made a part of the medical record and used as supplementary to my living will and/or durable power of attorney for health care.

## I. VALUES SECTION

Values are things that are important to us in our lives and our relationships with others—especially loved ones. There are several values important in decisions about terminal treatment and care. This section of the Values History invites you to identify your most important values.

## A. Basic Life Values

Perhaps the most basic values in this context concern length of life versus quality of life. Which of the following two statements is the most important to you?

_____ 1. I want to live as long as possible, regardless of the quality of life that I experience.
_____ 2. I want to preserve a good quality of life, even if this means that I may not live as long.

## B. Quality-of-Life Values

There are many values that help us to define for ourselves the quality of life that we want to live. Review this list (and feel free to either

*Source:* Doukas D, McCullough L. The Values History: The Evaluation of the Patient's Values and Advance Directives, Vol. 31, No. 1, pp. 145–153. © 1991. Dowden Publishing Company, Inc. Reproduced with permission from *The Journal of Family Practice.*

elaborate on it or add to it), and circle those values that are most important to your definition of quality of life.

1. I want to maintain my capacity to think clearly.
2. I want to feel safe and secure.
3. I want to avoid unnecessary pain and suffering.
4. I want to be treated with respect.
5. I want to be treated with dignity when I can no longer speak for myself.
6. I do not want to be an unnecessary burden on my family.
7. I want to be able to make my own decisions.
8. I want to experience a comfortable dying process.
9. I want to be with my loved ones before I die.
10. I want to leave good memories of me to my loved ones.
11. I want to be treated in accord with my religious beliefs and traditions.
12. I want respect shown for my body after I die.
13. I want to help others by making a contribution to medical education and research.
14. Other values or clarification of values above:

_____

_____

_____

_____


## II. PREFERENCES SECTION

Some directives involve simple yes or no decisions. Others provide for the choice of a trial of intervention. Use the values identified above to explain why you made the choice you did. The information will be very useful to your family, health care surrogate (or proxy), and health care providers.

**Initials/Date**
____ ____ 1. I want to undergo cardiopulmonary resuscitation.
____ Yes
____ No
Why?

_____

_____

_____

_____

___ ___ 2. I want to be placed on a ventilator. (Please note: If you answer NO to CPR #1, then the default is NO on this item as well, as this option is part of the treatment of cardiopulmonary resuscitation.)

___ Yes

___ Trial for the time period of _____

___ Trial to determine effectiveness using reasonable medical judgment

___ No

Why?

_____

_____

_____

_____

___ ___ 3. I want to have an endotracheal tube used in order to perform items 1 and 2. (Please note: If you answer NO to CPR #1, then the default is NO on this item as well, as this option is part of the treatment of cardiopulmonary resuscitation.)

___ Yes

___ Trial for the time period of _____

___ Trial to determine effectiveness using reasonable medical judgment

___ No

Why?

_____

_____

_____

_____

___ ___ 4. I want to have total parenteral nutrition administered for my nutrition.

___ Yes

___ Trial for the time period of _____

___ Trial to determine effectiveness using reasonable medical judgment

___ No

Why?

_____

_____

_____

_____

_____ _____ 5. I want to have intravenous medication and hydration administered; regardless of my decision, I understand that intravenous hydration to alleviate discomfort or pain medication will not be withheld from me if I so request them.

_____ Yes

_____ Trial for the time period of _____

_____ Trial to determine effectiveness using reasonable medical judgment

_____ No

Why?

_____

_____

_____

_____

_____ _____ 6. I want to have all medications used for the treatment of my illness continued; regardless of my decision, I understand that pain medication will continue to be administered, including narcotic medications.

_____ Yes

_____ Trial for the time period of _____

_____ Trial to determine effectiveness using reasonable medical judgment

_____ No

Why?

_____

_____

_____

_____

_____ _____ 7. I want to have nasogastric, gastrostomy, or other enteral feeding tubes introduced and administered for my nutrition.

_____ Yes

_____ Trial for the time period of _____

_____ Trial to determine effectiveness using reasonable medical judgment

_____ No

Why?

_____

_____

_____

_____

_____ _____ 8. I want to be placed on a dialysis machine.
_____ Yes
_____ Trial for the time period of _____
_____ Trial to determine effectiveness using reasonable medical judgment
_____ No
Why?

_____

_____

_____

_____

_____ _____ 9. I want to have an autopsy done to determine the cause(s) of my death.
_____ Yes
_____ No
Why?

_____

_____

_____

_____ _____ 10. I want to be admitted to the intensive care unit if necessary. (Please note: If you answer NO to CPR #1, then the default in some hospitals is NO on this item as well, as refusing cardiopulmonary resuscitation means you also refuse intensive care unit treatment.)
_____ Yes
_____ No
Why?

_____

_____

_____

_____ _____ 11. If I become a patient in a long-term care facility or if I receive care at home and experience a life-threatening change in health status, I want 911 called in case of a medical emergency. (Add your state-required "At Home DNR order" here, if applicable.)
_____ Yes
_____ No

Why?

_____

_____

_____

_____

____ ____ 12. Other directives:

_____

_____

_____

_____

I consent to these directives after receiving honest disclosure of their implications, risks, and benefits by my physician, free from constraints and being of sound mind.

_____
Signature                                    Date

_____
Witness

_____
Witness

____ ____ 13. Proxy negation:
I request that the following persons NOT be allowed to make decisions on my behalf in the event of my disability or incapacity:

_____

_____

_____

_____

_____
Signature                                    Date

_____
Witness

_____
Witness

____ ____ 14. Organ donation:
Specific state version inserted/attached here

# 6

# *Recognizing Mistreatment in Older Adults*

Carla VandeWeerd, Adolfo Firpo, Terry Fulmer, Gregory J. Paveza, and Marguarette M. Bolton

Elder mistreatment (EM) is a multifaceted clinical syndrome that affects thousands of older adults each year. EM was previously characterized primarily as assault of an older person, but it is now clear that EM includes subcategories of actions and outcomes that harm the well-being of the older person. In addition to physical abuse, the subcategories of EM are sexual abuse, psychologic abuse, financial abuse, and neglect, each of which result in decreased quality of life and increased mortality for those who experience it. Best practice demands a thorough EM assessment for all older adults as part of any geriatric health assessment. There are now several good screening and assessment instruments in the literature,[1-3] and to ensure that a geriatric health assessment is complete and carefully documented, one of these screening and assessment instruments should be used. Progress in our understanding of risk for EM and appropriate care planning depends on a systematic assessment and documentation of the older adult.

## THE SCOPE AND CONSEQUENCES OF EM

EM, as defined by the National Research Council,[3] is as follows: "Elder Mistreatment refers to (a) intentional actions that cause harm or create a serious risk of harm (whether or not harm is intended) to a vulnerable elder by a caregiver or other person who stands in a trust relationship to an elder or (b) failures by a caregiver to satisfy the elder's basic needs or to protect the elder from harm." It represents a serious issue affecting thousands of older adults. In the most commonly cited population-based study of older adults, Pillemer and Finkelhor[4] found an overall prevalence of EM to be 32 older persons per 1,000 for an annual prevalence of 700,000 to 1.2 million cases of EM in the United States. The recently completed National Elder Abuse Incidence Study[5] also examined the overall incidence of EM and found that approximately 551,000 persons were identified as abused or neglected in 1996 and acknowledges that this number may be as high as 800,000.

There is a shared belief among experts in the field that the consequences of EM are substantial. EM results in emotional difficulties such as decreased self-esteem,[6-10] depression,[11,12] and feelings of inadequacy and self-contempt.[8,9] It has been shown to result in family distress, impaired life functioning,[12] and cognitive difficulties.[6] It has also been linked to health problems such as immunologic dysfunction,[6,10-13] and increased mortality.[14]

EM research has been refined over the past decade, and emphasis has been placed on understanding the subcategories of this phenomenon. Researchers have begun to study individual or "component" forms of EM and to identify specific risk factors for individual mistreatment forms. Five categories of EM are generally distinguished:[7,15-18] (1) physical abuse or aggression, (2) financial or material abuse, (3) psychologic abuse or chronic verbal aggression, and (4) neglect, by self or caregiver (this chapter addresses only neglect by the caregiver), and (5) sexual abuse. Using specific subtypes of EM may have differing risk profiles and may require differing forms of intervention.

## EM ASSESSMENT

EM assessment is a complex process because the clinical syndrome is still evolving in the research literature. No straightforward tests can define EM quantitatively. An astute clinician must use an interdisciplinary approach to come to a decision as to whether EM is suspected and what actions should be taken. This is difficult. Approaches to assessment are further complicated by differences in state laws[19-21] and the complex nature of familial relationships, which often discourage the reporting of mistreatment, and alter the standards of acceptable behavior.

Conceptual frameworks have been found to be useful for constructing approaches to EM assessment. One such approach, the risk and vulnerability model, developed by Rose and Killien,[22] and first applied to EM in 1994 by Frost and Willette,[23] has been used to guide assessment approaches (Figure 6–1).[24] Risk refers to hazards or stressors in the external environment to the older person that can contribute to the likelihood of mistreatment, such as having a caregiver who is emotionally unstable, whereas vulnerability refers to characteristics within an older person, such as decreased cognitive status, that may influence the likelihood of mistreatment. Such a framework helps guide clinical thinking when approaching the EM assessment. Others have used a public health/epidemiologic model, using constructs from national data sets, including demographics and health constructs such as depressions, functional capacity, social support, and cognitive capacity to frame the approach.[4,16,25] In a field this young,

CONSTRUCTS

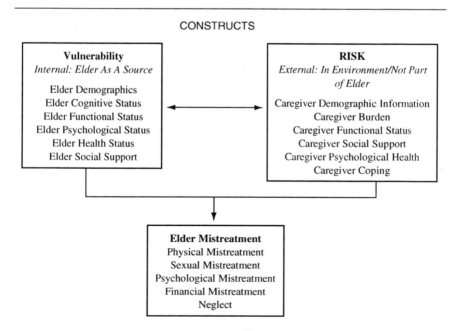

**Figure 6–1:** A risk vulnerability model of EM.[24]

each approach adds valuable new insights into how to best shape an EM assessment.

Assessment indices for the individual forms of mistreatment have begun to evolve, and assessment protocols and screening tools have been developed to aid practitioners in their recognition of the subtypes of EM.[2,3]

In the clinical setting, under no circumstances is the caregiver to be present during the older person's assessment for any kind of possible EM. In order to assist in the examination, translation services should be provided for those older persons who are not fluent in English and cannot communicate effectively during their examination and history taking. The translator must be a paid interpreter without any relationship to the older person or caregiver. If a suitable translator is not available, a follow-up visit must be arranged when such services can be provided. Ideally, the interpreter should be competent in the older person's native language, familiar with the older person's cultural background, and skilled in interpersonal relationships with older persons.

Ambivalent feelings toward caregivers or family members expressed or inferred from the older adult's answers and behavior during the interview should be construed as indicators of mistreatment and should be kept in the mind of the examiner throughout the interview and physical examination and probed repeatedly with delicacy and gentleness. It is most difficult to obtain an explicit accusation of any form of mistreatment from an older person that feels vulnerable or at the mercy of the caregiver and who is without reliable and trustworthy alternatives to the limited support he or she is provided with.

Assessment of older persons showing confusion or signs of dementia should be assessed with the assistance of a professional clinical staff skilled in handling older persons with decreased mental capacity. The gender of the clinician and/or assisting staff may be an important consideration for effective and efficient assessment.

## PHYSICAL ABUSE ASSESSMENT

### Overview

Physical abuse results from any action of a caregiver that leads to physical harm or injury of an older adult whose care is entrusted to him or her. A widely accepted definition of physical abuse is the infliction of physical pain or injury such as punching, slapping, pushing, or hitting an older adult.[3,26]

## Clinical Interview and History Taking

A reliable interview and examination for indicators of physical abuse require safeguarding the privacy of the older person, who should be approached and treated with respect and consideration throughout the entire process. The caregiver should never be allowed to be present during the assessment and should be requested to step out of the room or the examination area.[26]

If an older adult, in a clinical interview, makes a complaint of abusive behavior, it must be taken very seriously and must be referred to social services for follow-up. The history should reflect a description of the circumstances and situations in which abusive behavior was exhibited by the caregiver, including the immediate preceding activities in which the caregiver and older adult were engaged in before the physical abuse was inflicted. Timing of such events and the circumstances under which it occurred are extremely important and help direct the in-depth questioning about the clinical and social history of the older person during the examination process.

Narratives about a caregiver's abusive behaviors will most often occur when absolute privacy is provided to the older person and is isolated from the caregiver. The older adult must be kept in comfortable surroundings where support and reassurance of his or her privacy and confidentiality of the examination are made explicit to him or her. Reassurances of privacy and confidentiality must be repeatedly communicated to the older adult at various times during the assessment process and reinforced by the general environment, particularly the examiner's and staff's sensitive behaviors reflecting genuine concern and care for the well-being of the older person at all times.

## Physical Examination for Signs of Physical Abuse

Physical abuse often results in signs that are easy to find during the patient's physical examination. The difficulty with assessment is not to confuse physical signs of abuse with that of an accident or of clinical presentations.

Just as a patient's complaint of physical abuse by the caregiver mobilizes a focused search for supporting evidence during the history and physical examination, the process of assessment of findings disclosed by the patient's physical examination requires each finding to be considered in the context of the patient's complete personal, social, and medical history and all other findings of the physical exam.

The assessment of physical injuries requires a careful and conscientious search for features indicating that they were inflicted on the patient by another person, with intent, and that they were the result of repeated acts of physical abuse such as slapping, hitting, biting, burning, pushing, or other similar behavior.

### Possible Indicators of Physical Abuse in the Medical Record

Signs of physical injury observed during physical examination are recorded in the patient's medical record. For this reason, all assessments for EM, regardless of the results of the current physical examination and history of present illness, require a comprehensive review of the patient's past medical records. Ideally, recent and old medical records should be available, obtained, and systematically reviewed by highly trained clinical examiners such as physicians, pathologists, nurses (particularly advance practice nurses), social workers, and clinical pharmacists for indicators of any form of mistreatment, particularly physical abuse.

Current clinical experience and existing knowledge confirm that the most important indicators of physical abuse are obtained from the review of medical records such as past documented bone fractures and abnormal results of laboratory tests. Isolated findings by themselves are insufficient to support a conclusion of physical abuse and demand that each finding be analyzed in the context of the patient's overall situation and circumstance at the time of the finding. An assessment of physical abuse from the findings in the older adult's medical records is based on the validation and documentation of abusive events described by the patient during past medical history taking and the documentation of recurrent similar injuries along the patient's medical care trajectory, such as concurrent injuries, particularly fractures or skin burns at different stages of healing, or the presence of skin bruises at different stages of resolution (p. 269).[27] Each event and its circumstance provide a location in the time line of the older person's path of physical abuse and victimization by those trusted with his or her care.

The assessment of physical abuse from clinical laboratory data is extremely difficult. However, laboratory findings may help toward a better understanding of the events and circumstances of situations where injury to the older person occurs and the caregiver's explanation suggests nonintentionality to harm. Although experimental evidence is lacking, logic applied to the current understanding and knowledge of the effects of blood anticoagulating agents and the underlying physiology of atrophic skin of advanced age suggest that extensive bruising of the skin may be enhanced in patients on oral anticoagulant therapy. In addition to laboratory tests for levels of anticoagulants, it is important to keep in mind that disorders of blood coagulation can occur in older patients, and most of them are detected by routine testing and should be generally requested during a patient's medical evaluation.

## Risk Factors for Physical Abuse

The literature[26,28,29] indicates that risk factors of suspected and documented cases of physical abuse are older adult isolation; diminished mental capacity of the older person, as in dementia and Alzheimer's disease; and or difficulty with activities of daily living (ADL) and instrumental ADL. These factors establish and modulate the tension in the existing and evolving relationship between the caregiver and the older person. Factors believed to influence the behavior of the caregiver toward mistreatment of the older adult include personal family stress, the use or abuse of alcohol or drugs, and untreated psychiatric problems.[26]

## Scope of Physical Abuse

Physical abuse has been documented in all ethnic, racial, social, economic, and educational levels and in all social environments, including urban and rural areas in all settings from the homes of older persons living alone, family member or paid caregivers, daycare centers, community centers, nursing homes, extended living facilities, clinics, and hospitals.[26] In this regard, the documentation in the literature is extensive and is supported with solid and reliable empirical data.[24,25,28-32] What is lacking is the same level of empirical evidence demonstrating casual mechanisms and conditions under which caregivers become abusive of those they are charged to care for and the infliction of the kinds of injuries that are indicative of older person abuse.

## SEXUAL ABUSE ASSESSMENT

Sexual abuse results from behaviors by a caregiver that violate the limits of propriety and sensitivity of an older person regarding his or her intimacy and sexuality. Rape is at one end of the spectrum of sexual abuse and often involves violence and constitutes a special form of physical abuse.[33] Physical findings during the genital examination may lead the clinician to raise questions about possible sexual abuse, but unfortunately, genital examination of an older person is not usually performed as part of a routine physical examination.[34,35]

Less extreme forms of sexual abuse can be equally damaging to the older adult and can be expressed by abnormal behavior of the older adult and raise concerns of the examiner for sexual mistreatment as a possible problem. Acculturation and socialization define the limits of propriety of behaviors that bring the caregiver and the older person into close intimate contact, and the perceptions of an older person in activities such as toileting and dressing are highly influenced by their age and culture. Inappropriate touching of an older adult by a caregiver in ways that may be interpreted as sexual in nature by the older person is based on their cultural norms and beliefs. Generally, these are actions of the caregiver that have sexual connotations to the older person and make them feel uncomfortable and as violating their dignity and humiliating them. Such incidents often elicit significant anxiety in the older person along with embarrassment and shame that leads to withdrawal, avoidance, or refusal to receive assistance with ADLs. The nature of behaviors offensive to the sexual sensitivity of a person is highly influenced and often determined by his or her culture and belief structure.

## Clinical Interview and History Taking

In no other aspect of the assessment should the general principles of privacy, sensitivity, and behaviors indicative of caring and respect be more important than when attempting to identify indicators of sexual abuse. Sexuality is an extremely sensitive and private matter that demands respect and gentleness for effective assessment and is, perhaps, the most complex dimension of the assessment process. The cultural background of the older person will influence the ease of a sexually mistreated older person to describe behaviors perceived by them as sexual in nature to the examiner.

The gender of the examiner, his or her cultural beliefs about sexuality, and his or her perceptions of what constitute transgressions against one's own sexuality also play a role in the examiner's ability to expose and identify indicators of sexual abuse during the clinical interview and history taking.

Discovery of sexual mistreatment among the older population is also hindered by the perceptions and beliefs of the examiner, clinical staff, persons in the immediate social environment of the older person, and his or her relatives, friends, and acquaintances. Ageist attitudes of personnel involved in older adult assessment can become a major barrier to the capacity to disclose mistreatment of an older adult in general and of sexual abuse in particular.[36]

History taking should include questions about pain or soreness in the genital area or anus or pain or discomfort when walking or sitting. Ask about uncomfortable itching, a burning sensation, and a past history of sexually transmitted diseases, fungal infections, or trichomonads. Any positive answer should be followed by when and how these were discovered, diagnosed, and treated. Ask the older person if he or she was ever made to feel uncomfortable while being helped by the caregiver during toileting, dressing, or other intimate or highly personal activities. Did the patient ever feel that he or she was inappropriately touched or made to feel ashamed or humiliated? How did it happen? Was this discomfort communicated to the caregiver? What happened? How did the caregiver react and respond to the concerns and feelings of the older person?[26] Other questions that may lead to suspicion of sexual mistreatment include asking the older person whether he or she ever noticed that his or her undergarments were torn, stained with blood, or felt wet and sticky and could not remember how they became that way.

## Physical Examination for Signs of Sexual Abuse

Complete assessment should include at least the external examination of the sex organs and the anus by a competent, properly trained clinician. Bruising, blood, or lacerations are signs commonly indicative of sexual abuse and require a complete gynecologic and rectal examination by a physician for evidence of sexual intercourse and lesions of sexually transmitted diseases. The complete gynecologic examination should include samples for Papanicolaou vaginal and cervical smears and laboratory tests for sexually transmitted diseases.

The patient should be asked to walk across the room and to sit on a hard-surfaced chair, and under very close direct observation, the examiner must look for signs of difficulty, pain, discomfort, or sensitivity that is inconsistent with the physical examination. The undergarments should also be examined for tearing, blood, or body fluids, and the findings must be considered within the context of the overall examination and patient's medical and social history.

## Risk Factors for Sexual Abuse

The same risk factors described for physical abuse apply to sexual abuse and should be considered in the overall context of the older person's situation. The mechanisms by which these factors constitute elements of risk to older persons are the same. Excessive dependency on a caretaker, isolation of the older adult, untreated psychiatric problems in the family, the caregiver, or the older person have been commonly identified and felt to be related to sexual abuse of older persons in all settings.[24,36]

## PSYCHOLOGIC MISTREATMENT ASSESSMENT

Psychologic EM results from intentional or unintentional abusive behaviors of a caregiver that provoke fear, anguish, or anxiety in an older person and includes verbal abuse and humiliation.[26]

Common complaints of psychologically abused older persons include expressions of fear, difficulty sleeping, and excessive preoccupations, often over health, that are highlighted by imaginary illnesses or diseases unsupported by the medical history and examination. Some patients may complain of being unable to control some behaviors of which they are aware. Compulsive behaviors may be described by a relative, a caregiver, a provider, or an external observer but denied by the older person during the clinical examination. A history of any change in the level of tolerance of any kind of sensory stimulation, including exaggerated reactions to touch and mood, may also indicate psychologic abuse and can be detected during questioning about feelings of sadness with or without crying and the circumstances under which such feelings or emotions arise. Violence, aggression, obstinacy, and screams by an older person can all be expressions of psychologic abuse and should be considered indications for referral and further evaluation.

## Clinical Interview and History Taking

The older person may spontaneously express to the examiner feelings of fear, and such confidence requires careful inquiry into the nature of the patient's fear with particular attention to the situations and conditions under which it is experienced. Details about when, where, and how are important for assessment and should be explored during in-depth questioning of environmental factors that may influence the experience of fear, anguish, or anxiety over personal safety from harm from another person, or a situation perceived as of risk, or if the emotional distress is the result of internal turmoil caused by excessive preoccupation over the older person's life situation, loved ones, or other issues. Such concerns are not necessarily indicative of abuse, but the psychologic assessment must be analyzed along with the context of past history, the social situation, and living environment of the older person and the caregiver.

Careful observation, listening, and sensitive questioning during the interview are critical. Areas of questioning relevant to psychologic processes include sleep history, particularly changes in the usual patterns, repeatedly waking during the night, restlessness of sleep, and inability to have a restful sleep. History or increased sensitivity to normal or familiar stimuli in the environment of the older person, such as fear of the dark, being left alone, and being touched, should also be noted.

While the examination is in progress, obsessive thoughts can be discovered by general questions about the things that occupy the person's mind earlier in the day, yesterday, or during the week. General open questions can be as follows: What things make you worry? Have you been worrying about anything in particular now or over the past few days? Obsessions are not always easy to detect, but phobias or excessive fears triggered by specific objects can be detected. It should be noted when phobic reactions are observed and if the older person expresses fear or strong sensations of anxiety provoked by specific objects, animals, or insects and how they avoid such objects or situations.

Most older persons show high level of interest in their health status and become preoccupied by symptoms that are new or recurrent, especially when medication or treatment was expected to resolve or eliminate them and the symptoms still persist. All of these are normal concerns. Obsessive preoccupation over illness and diseases that have been ruled out by medical evaluation, particularly when these are replaced by new symptoms and complaints, constitutes hypochondria and may be a patient's subconscious response to psychologic distress and a call for help and medical attention.

## Physical Exam for Signs of Psychological Mistreatment

Physical signs that raise suspicion of possible psychologic abuse of an older person include sucking, biting, rocking, repetitive, or compulsive actions such as hand washing and exaggerated passive submissive behavior in the presence of, or avoiding contact with, the caregiver. In some cases, abusive or destructive behavior by the older person is an indicator of psychologic abuse and a reaction to anger or frustration experienced by the older person who is being psychologically maltreated by a caregiver.[3,26]

A review of the medical record for a past history of attempted suicide, medication overdose, episodes of depression, prolonged sadness or withdrawal, changes in mood and disposition from an established pattern indicative of changes in personality, loss or gain of weight, missing appointments, and other variations in established patterns of behavior must also be examined for underlying medical causes, and after medical reasons are discarded, these should become possible indicators of psychologic mistreatment.

### Risk Factors for Psychologic Mistreatment

Factors that place an older adult at risk for psychologic abuse are the same as in cases of physical abuse: isolation of the older person, unusual family stress, drug or alcohol addiction in the family, and untreated psychiatric problems of the caregiver. It also includes excessive dependency of the older person on the caregiver, which can be due to physical limitations of the older person as in marked decreased functional capacity to perform ADLs and instrumental ADLs or a psychologic dependency, which can be a sign of internal emotional factors of mental deficiency.[37–40]

### NEGLECT ASSESSMENT

Neglect results from the consistent failure of a caregiver to meet one or more needs that are considered basic and necessary to maintain optimal physical and mental function of an older person or to eliminate or reduce possible risk of harm or injury while providing care.[19,26,41] During the clinical interview and physical examination, older persons can exhibit signs or report symptoms of physical or psychologic neglect (p. 10).[26] Neglect of the caring responsibilities entrusted to a caregiver can be intentional or unintentional. Unintentional neglect by caregivers can be due to a lack of knowledge about how to provide the services needed by the older person to satisfy his or her basic needs, a lack of awareness about the existence of needs in older persons under their care, or a lack of resources necessary to satisfy the needs of the older persons (p.10).[26]

Physical neglect refers to the deprivation of basic goods and services to the older persons, such as food, water, maintenance care, and hygiene. Other goods that are basic to the older adult are eyeglasses, hearing aids, false teeth, walkers, or crutches. Failure to provide safety precautions while caring for an older adult also constitutes physical neglect. Psychologic neglect results from failure of a caregiver to provide social stimulation to a dependent older person. This includes prolonged isolation of the older person or failing to provide him or her with companionship, ignoring the older person when he or she tries to communicate, or giving the older person the "silent treatment." Changes in routine, news, or information are also important factors for the mental health and the general well-being of the older population and failure to provide them as part of caring for the older person also represents psychologic neglect (p. 11).[26]

## Clinical Interview and History Taking

Decreased functional capacity evidenced by difficulty with ADLs correlates inversely with vulnerability to older person neglect. The clinical interview should include questions about the functional capacity of older persons in performing ADLs independently and if in need of assistance the degree of help required and received from the caregiver. The caregiver should be accessible and reliable in his or her duties to provide support with the ADLs of an older person.[42]

During questioning, probe into more significant indicators of caregiver neglect by asking older persons whether they were ever left alone for prolonged periods of time or in situations in which they felt unsafe such as in a park, near a stairway, or uncomfortably close to a heating stove or in the sun. Has the older person ever been abandoned in an emergency room after being taken there by someone else? The latter is considered the most common form of abandonment and is an extreme form of older person neglect that is sometimes discussed and considered by some authors as a distinct type of EM.[26]

Poor nutrition can be expressed as anemia, complaints of tiredness, and constant fatigue; however, these are also common symptoms of cardiac disease, which should be initially considered and discarded. Interview questions for assessment of neglected nutrition focus on appetite, eating habits, and satisfaction with the quality and quantity of food. In the emergency room, support staff often become aware and comment about older persons who eat their food ravenously and sometimes even ask for more. These observations may be important and call for focused questioning about eating habits and the availability of and quality of food and meals provided.[42,43]

Failure to comply with medical care plans can be an important indicator of care neglect. The older person must be questioned in detail, but with sensitivity, about the reasons for missing appointments for follow-up visits, rehabilitation therapy, and any difficulty in following instructions about taking their medications or using medical appliances.

## Physical Examination for Signs of Neglect

Poor hygiene and dehydration are possibly the most common expressions of older person neglect seen at the emergency room[26] and must always be considered risk indicators of older person neglect. Dehydration must be recognized and treated immediately because it is commonly a compounding factor to the mental status of the older person[42,43] and complicates the interview. Malnutrition or low body weight should be interpreted in the context of a detailed history of changes in body weight, eating habits, and nutritional history. A recent loss of weight may indicate malignancy and requires careful history and examination to exclude such a diagnostic possibility.

The examination may disclose findings indicative of unattended health needs. The most common example offered in this category is that of decubitus ulcers arising from inadequate turning and changing in posture of an immobilized patient confined to a bed or wheelchair.[44,45] Another example is the presence of contractures as a residual of a cerebrovascular accident, which exceeded the anticipated degree of disability from the estimated magnitude of the cerebral injury and resulted from the lack of adequate physical and occupational rehabilitation during recovery from the acute illness.

Extreme withdrawal, infantile behaviors such as thumb sucking, indifference to the examination process, listlessness, or agitation indicating delirium may all indicate psychologic neglect or abuse and require a referral for comprehensive psychologic assessment and repeated follow-up visits. Assessment and a mental health management plan are required in these cases.[40,46,47]

## Risk Factors for Neglect

Excessive dependency of an older person on a caregiver is perhaps the most important and significant risk factor for older person neglect,[48–50] and it is influenced by multiple factors that may tip the delicate balance in which the caregiver–older person relationship exists. As the level of dependence increases, the demand for care from the caregiver also increases, and in order to maintain an adequate balance of need and care, these demands will require greater skills and capacity of the caregiver. A totally dependent bedridden older adult is more prone to becoming isolated because the caregiver must come to him or her every time and is at high risk of developing decubitus ulcers.

An older adult who is highly dependent on an adult child, with multiple additional responsibilities from his or her work and family, may become neglected despite the best efforts of the caregiver.[51–53] This is especially real when an additional unexpected or unusual stress emerges within the caregiver's family or employment. Addiction to alcohol or drugs of the caregiver, older person, or any family member introduces additional significant stresses to the relationship and is a well-recognized risk indicator of neglect and EM. Untreated psychiatric problems of the older person, caregiver, or any family member also pose additional and significant risk factors for neglect or any other form of mistreatment.[29]

## FINANCIAL ABUSE ASSESSMENT

Definitions of what constitutes financial abuse of an older adult vary from state to state, but generally, financial abuse refers to the inappropriate use of an older person's resources for personal gain.[3,26,54] Examples of financial abuse include denying an older person access to his or her money or preventing him or her from controlling his or her assets;[54,55] taking or misusing an older adult's money or property with or without their knowledge;[54,56] cashing an older adult's pension checks without permission;[54,57] providing true but misleading information that influences the older adult over the use or assignment of assets;[54,58] negligently mishandling assets, including misuse by a fiduciary or caregiver;[54,58] misusing ATM or credit cards;[54,59] forging or forcing an older adult's signature;[54,56,57] overcharging for services that are improperly done or not provided;[54,59] and getting an older adult to sign a deed, will, contract, or power of attorney through deception, coercion, or undue influence.[54,56,57]

Financial abuse accounts for approximately 12% of all cases reported to protective service agencies.[5] Although the exact impact of financial mistreatment can be difficult to assess, there is no doubt that losing assets accumulated over a lifetime, or the control of one's money and property, can be devastating and result in significant practical, physical, and mental health consequences,[58] with impacts as severe as though one were the victim of a violent crime.[60] Being financially exploited may result in an inability to purchase needed medical treatments, food, clothing, and shelter and to live one's life independently.[61,62] It also can result in decreased self-esteem, depression, fear, social isolation, and medical complications that can result in increased mortality and death.[54,63,64]

In the assessment of these cases, one must keep in mind the complicated nature of these transactions. It is often hard to determine whether an older adult willingly turned over his or her assets to the caregiver or was coerced in exchange for care, affection, and attention.[58] Was this a result of well-intentioned but bad advice or action? Was it intentional fraud and abusive conduct? A thorough history and physical assessment are therefore needed to determine whether an older adult has been the victim of financial mistreatment.[54]

## Clinical Interview and History Taking

It is often difficult for experienced professionals to determine whether financial mistreatment has occurred.[54,58] Careful observation, listening, and sensitive questioning during the interview are critical.[26,54] Older adults should be questioned about their financial circumstances so that an assessment regarding financial adequacy can be made. Do they have the ability to meet their financial obligations such as mortgage, medical care, food, clothing, and other expenses, and can it be done without help of a caregiver? Careful attention should be paid to the older adult who indicates shortage of funds, a lack of awareness of his or her financial circumstance, or who seems fearful or subdued during financial discussions. The clinical interview should include questions regarding changes in financial circumstance as evidenced through changes in behavior. Indicators of lifestyle changes such as a withdrawal from previously established habits such as vacations, shopping, eating out, or deprivation of previously enjoyed activities or services may be indicative of changes in standard of living and possible financial mistreatment. A thorough social history and cognitive assessment should be undertaken, and the level of suspicion for this type of abuse should also be increased for older persons with cognitive impairment or for those who appear socially isolated. These factors put the older person at risk, as they predispose the older person to be trusting of caregivers, relatives, and acquaintances.

## Physical Exam for Signs of Financial Abuse

Physical indicators of financial abuse need to be evaluated within the context of the clinical interview and history taking. These indicators may include evidence of emaciation such as loss of muscle tone, loose skin, decreased skin integrity, as evidenced by skin dryness or lesions, and poor personal hygiene such body odor, bad breath, tooth decay, brittle hair, and dirty clothes. An unkempt appearance, especially in a person previously meticulous, is indicative of an underlying stress or lifestyle change, and particular attention should be paid to integrating the clinical history to determine whether financial abuse may be the root cause of these changes. Reappearance of previously controlled conditions may also be indicative of financial abuse if sufficient funds to purchase medications or treatments are unavailable.[54]

## Risk Factors for Financial Abuse

Several characteristics have been identified as risk factors that may predispose an older adult to an increased likelihood of financial abuse. A lack of familiarity with financial matters;[56,61] having assets to be exploited;[54,61] social isolation, loneliness, and recent loss of loved ones;[56,61,64] having family members who have unmet financial need or substance abuse problems;[56] being dependent;[65] and being a victim of other forms of abuse[61] have been postulated to increase the likelihood of financial abuse.

## SCREENING TOOLS

It is essential to screen for EM and that it be part of the routine health assessment for all geriatric patients, particularly those who are unable to report it because of cognitive impairment or fear.[66] The American Medical Association[26] recommended screening of geriatric patients for abuse and neglect regardless of subjective complaint and if physical signs are present. Several tools exist for the screening of EM: the Indicators of Abuse Screen;[67] the Hwalek-Sengstock Elder Abuse Screening Test Revised;[68] the Conflict Tactic Scale;[69] and the Elder Abuse Assessment Inventory (EAI).[70] For a screening tool to be useful, it must be accurate, easy and efficient to use, and useful in a variety of clinical settings. The EAI (Figure 6–2) is useful across varied clinical settings, including the emergency department, is easy to ad-

| General Assessment | Very Good | Good | Poor | Very Poor | Unable to Assess |
|---|---|---|---|---|---|
| 1.  Clothing | 1 | 2 | 3 | 4 | 9999 |
| 2.  Hygiene | 1 | 2 | 3 | 4 | 9999 |
| 3.  Nutrition | 1 | 2 | 3 | 4 | 9999 |
| 4.  Skin integrity | 1 | 2 | 3 | 4 | 9999 |

| Neglect Assessment | No Evidence | Probably No Evidence | Probably Evidence | Evidence | Unable to Assess |
|---|---|---|---|---|---|
| 5.  Bruising | 1 | 2 | 3 | 4 | 9999 |
| 6.  Contractures | 1 | 2 | 3 | 4 | 9999 |
| 7.  Decubiti | 1 | 2 | 3 | 4 | 9999 |
| 8.  Dehydration | 1 | 2 | 3 | 4 | 9999 |
| 9.  Diarrhea | 1 | 2 | 3 | 4 | 9999 |
| 10.  Impaction | 1 | 2 | 3 | 4 | 9999 |
| 11.  Lacerations | 1 | 2 | 3 | 4 | 9999 |
| 12.  Malnutrition | 1 | 2 | 3 | 4 | 9999 |
| 13.  Urine burns/excoriations | 1 | 2 | 3 | 4 | 9999 |

| Usual Lifestyle | Totally Independent | Mostly Independent | Mostly Dependent | Totally Dependent | Unable to Assess |
|---|---|---|---|---|---|
| 14.  Administration of medications | 1 | 2 | 3 | 4 | 9999 |
| 15.  Ambulation | 1 | 2 | 3 | 4 | 9999 |
| 16.  Continence | 1 | 2 | 3 | 4 | 9999 |
| 17.  Feedings | 1 | 2 | 3 | 4 | 9999 |
| 18.  Maintenance of hygiene | 1 | 2 | 3 | 4 | 9999 |

**Figure 6–2** Clinical Screening for Elder Mistreatment: The Elder Abuse Assessment Inventory (EIA).[70,73]

| Usual Lifestyle | Totally Independent | Mostly Independent | Mostly Dependent | Totally Dependent | Unable to Assess |
|---|---|---|---|---|---|
| 19. Management of finances | 1 | 2 | 3 | 4 | 9999 |
| 20. Family support | 1 | 2 | 3 | 4 | 9999 |

| Social Assessment | Very Good Quality | Good Quality | Poor Quality | Very Poor Quality | Unable to Assess |
|---|---|---|---|---|---|
| 21. Financial situation | 1 | 2 | 3 | 4 | 9999 |
| 22. Interaction with family | 1 | 2 | 3 | 4 | 9999 |
| 23. Interaction with friends | 1 | 2 | 3 | 4 | 9999 |
| 24. Interaction with nursing home personnel | 1 | 2 | 3 | 4 | 9999 |
| 25. Living arrangement | 1 | 2 | 3 | 4 | 9999 |
| 26. Observed relationship with care provider | 1 | 2 | 3 | 4 | 9999 |
| 27. Participation in daily social activities | 1 | 2 | 3 | 4 | 9999 |
| 28. Support systems | 1 | 2 | 3 | 4 | 9999 |
| 29. Ability to express needs | 1 | 2 | 3 | 4 | 9999 |

| Medical Assessment | No Evidence | Probably No Evidence | Probably Evidence | Evidence | Unable to Assess |
|---|---|---|---|---|---|
| 30. Duplication of similar medications (e.g., multiple laxatives, sedatives) | 1 | 2 | 3 | 4 | 9999 |
| 31. Unusual doses of medication | 1 | 2 | 3 | 4 | 9999 |
| 32. Alcohol/substance abuse | 1 | 2 | 3 | 4 | 9999 |

**Figure 6–2** (continued)

*continues*

| | No Evidence | Probably No Evidence | Probably Evidence | Evidence | Unable to Assess |
|---|---|---|---|---|---|
| 33. Greater than 15% dehydration | 1 | 2 | 3 | 4 | 9999 |
| 34. Bruises and/or trauma beyond what is compatible with alleged trauma | 1 | 2 | 3 | 4 | 9999 |
| 35. Failure to respond to warning of obvious disease | 1 | 2 | 3 | 4 | 9999 |
| 36. Repetitive admissions due to probable failure of health care surveillance | 1 | 2 | 3 | 4 | 9999 |

| **Emotional/Psychologic Neglect** | No Evidence | Probably No Evidence | Probably Evidence | Evidence | Unable to Assess |
|---|---|---|---|---|---|
| 37. Older person states being left alone for long periods of time | 1 | 2 | 3 | 4 | 9999 |
| 38. Older person being being ignored or given the "silent treatment" | 1 | 2 | 3 | 4 | 9999 |
| 39. Older person states failure to receive companionship, news, changes in routine, and information | 1 | 2 | 3 | 4 | 9999 |
| 40. Subjective complaint of neglect | 1 | 2 | 3 | 4 | 9999 |

**Figure 6–2** (continued)

| Summary Assessments | No Evidence | Probably No Evidence | Probably Evidence | Evidence | Unable to Assess |
|---|---|---|---|---|---|
| 41. Evidence of neglect | 1 | 2 | 3 | 4 | 9999 |
| 42. Evidence of physical abuse | 1 | 2 | 3 | 4 | 9999 |
| 43. Evidence of psychologic abuse | 1 | 2 | 3 | 4 | 9999 |
| 44. Evidence of financial abuse | 1 | 2 | 3 | 4 | 9999 |

| Disposition | Yes | No |
|---|---|---|
| 45. Referral to social service | 1 | 0 |
| 46. Referral to other<br>If yes, please specify_____ | 1 | 0 |

**Figure 6–2** (continued)

minister, and offers an efficient method for organizing observations relevant to a mistreatment judgment.[71,72]

## CONCLUSION

Assessing EM is a complex phenomenon that is often influenced by contextual factors of the caregiving/care-receiving relationship. Effective assessment requires the integration of data from diverse sources, including oral history, physical examination, and a knowledge of predisposing risk factors. Multidisciplinary team assessment in which older adults are evaluated by a team of geriatric professionals, including nurses, social workers, pharmacists, and doctors, will likely have the most success recognizing and treating EM. Screening and assessment tools should be used as a standard protocol in the overall geriatric health assessment in order to organize and clarify the indictors of mistreatment.

## REFERENCES

1. Fulmer T, Guadagno L, Bitondo Dyer C, Connolly MT. Progress in elder abuse screening and assessment instruments. *J Am Geriatr Soc.* 2004;52:297–304.

2. Fulmer T. Elder mistreatment. *Annu Rev Nurs Res.* 2002;20:369–395.

3. National Research Council. *Elder Mistreatment: Abuse, Neglect, and Exploitation in an Aging America*. Panel to Review Risk and Prevalence of Elder Abuse and Neglect. Bonnie RJ, Wallace RB, eds. Committee on National Statistics and Committee on Law and Justice, Division of Behavioral and Social Sciences and Education. Washington, DC: The National Academies Press; 2003.

4. Pillemer KA, Finkelhor D. The prevalence of elder abuse: A random sample survey. *Gerontologist.* 1988;28:51–57.

5. The National Center on Elder Abuse at the American Public Human Services Association in Collaboration with Westat, Inc. Prepared for The Administration for Children and Families and the Administration on Aging the U.S. Department of Health and Human Services. The National Elder Abuse Incidence Study: Final report. Washington, DC: National Aging Information Center; 1998.

6. Barer B. The secret shame of the very old: "I've never told this to anyone else." *J Mental Health Aging.* 1997;3:365–375.

7. Comijs HC, Pot AM, Smit JH, Bouter LM, Jonker C. Elder abuse in the community: Prevalence and consequences. *J Am Geriatr Soc.* 1998;46:885–888.

8. Lewis M. *Shame: The exposed self.* New York: Free Press; 1992.

9. Metge J. *In and Out of Touch: Whakamaa in Cross Cultural Perspective.* Wellington, NZ: Victoria University Press; 1986.

10. Saverman B. *Formal Careers in Healthcare and the Social Services Witnessing the Abuse of Elderly in Their Homes.* Umea, Sweden: Umea University; 1994.

11. Light E, Lebowitz B. *Alzheimer's Disease Treatment and Family Stress: Directions for Research.* Rockville, MD: National Institute of Mental Health; 1994.

12. Zarit SH, Todd PA, Zarit JM. Subjective burden of husbands and wives as caregivers: A longitudinal study. *Gerontologist.* 1986;26:260–266.

13. George LK, Gwyther L. Caregiver well-being: A multidimensional examination of family caregivers of demented adults. *Gerontologist.* 1986;26:253–259.

14. Lachs MS, Williams CS, O'Brien S, Pillemer KA, Charlson ME. The mortality of elder mistreatment. *JAMA.* 1998;280:428–432.

15. Comijs HC, Jonker C, van Tilburg W, Smit JH. Hostility and coping capacity as risk factors of elder mistreatment. *Soc Psychiatry Psychiatr Epidemiol.* 1999;34:48–52.

16. Lachs MS, Williams C, O'Brien S, Hurst L, Horwitz R. Older adults: An 11-year longitudinal study of adult protective service use. *Arch Intern Med.* 1996;156:449–453.

17. Pillemer KA, Finkelhor D. Causes of elder abuse: Caregiver stress versus problem relatives. *Am J Orthopsychiatry.* 1989;59:179–187.

18. Poertner J. Estimation of the incidence of abused older persons. *J Gerontol Social Work.* 1986;9:3–15.

19. Capezuti E, Brush BL, Lawson WT. Reporting elder mistreatment. *J Gerontol Nursing.* 1997;23:24–32.

20. Jogerst GJ, Daly JM, Brinig MF, Dawson JD, Schmuch GA, Ingram JG. Domestic elder abuse and the law. *Am J Public Health.* 2003;93:2131–2136.

21. National Center on Elder Abuse. State elder abuse laws, 6 August, 2003. Available at http://www.elderabusecenter.org/default.cfm?p=statelaws.cfm#requirements (accessed 2 February, 2005).

22. Rose MH, Killien M. Risk and vulnerability: A case for differentiation. *ANS Adv Nurs Sci.* 1983;5:60–73.

23. Frost MH, Willette K. Risk for abuse/neglect: Documentation of assessment data and diagnoses. *J Gerontol Nursing.* 1994;20:37–45.

24. Fulmer T, Guadagno L, Bolton MM. Elder mistreatment in women. *J Obstet Gynecol Neonatal Nurs.* 2004;33:657–663.

25. Lachs MS, Williams C, O'Brien S, Hurst L, Horwitz RI. Risk factors for reported elder abuse and neglect: A nine-year observational cohort study. *Gerontologist.* 1997; 37:469–474.

26. American Medical Association. *Diagnostic and treatment guidelines on elder abuse and neglect.* Chicago: American Medical Association; 1992.

27. Quinn MJ, Tomita SK. *Elder Abuse and Neglect: Causes, Diagnosis, and Intervention Strategies.* New York: Springer Publishing Company; 1986.

28. Lachs MS, Fulmer T. Recognizing elder abuse and neglect. *Clin Geriatr Med.* 1993;9:665–681.

29. Reay AM, Browne KD. Risk factor characteristics in careers who physically abuse or neglect their elderly dependents. *Aging Mental Health.* 2001;5:56–62.

30. Paris B, Meier DE, Goldstein T, Weiss M, Fein ED. Elder abuse and neglect: How to recognize warning signs and intervene. *Geriatrics.* 1995;50:47–51; quiz 52–53.

31. Canadian Task Force on the Periodic Health Examination. Periodic health examination, Secondary prevention of elder abuse and mistreatment. *CMAJ.* 1994;151: 1413–1420.

32. Mosqueda L, Burnight K, Liao S, Kemp B. Advancing the field of elder mistreatment: A new model for integration of social and medical services. *Gerontologist.* 2004;44:703–708.

33. Kaplan SJ. Family violence. *New Dir Ment Health Serv.* 2000;86:49–62.

34. Jones J, Dougherty J, Schelble D, Cunningham W. Emergency department protocol for the diagnosis and evaluation of geriatric abuse. *Ann Emerg Med.* 1988;17: 1006–1015.

35. Clarke ME, Pierson W. Management of elder abuse in the emergency department. *Emergency Medicine Clinics of North America.* 1999;17:631–644, vi.

36. Vinton L. Working with abused older women from a feminist perspective. *J Women Aging.* 1999;11:85–100.

37. Katz S, Ford A, Moskowitz R, Jackson B, Jaffe M. Studies of illness in the aged: The index of ADL: A standardized measure of biological and psychosocial function. *JAMA.* 1963;185:914–919.

38. Moritz DJ, Kasl SV, Berkman L. Cognitive functioning and the incidence of limitations in activities of daily living in an elderly community sample. *Am J Epidemiol.* 1995;141:41–49.

39. Cefalu CA, Ettinger WH, Espeland M. A study of the characteristics of the dementia patients and caregivers in dementia-nonspecific adult day care programs. *J Am Geriatr Soc.* 1996;44:654–659.

40. Inouye SK, Bogardus ST Jr, Baker DI, Leo-Summers L, Cooney LM Jr. The Hospital Elder Life Program: A model of care to prevent cognitive and functional decline in older hospitalized patients: Hospital Elder Life Program. *J Am Geriatr Soc.* 2000;48:1697–1706.

41. Brownell P, Welty A, Brennan M. Elder Abuse and Neglect. In New York State Office for the Aging. Project 2015: The Future of Aging in New York State. Albany, NY: NY State Office for the Aging; 2001–2003.

42. Teresi J, Cross PS, Golden R. Some applications of latent trait analysis to the measurement of ADL. *J Gerontol B Psychol Sci Soc Sci.* 1989;44:s196–s204.

43. Harrell R, Toronjo CH, McLaughlin J, Pavlik VN, Hyman DJ, Dyer CB. How geriatricians identify elder abuse and neglect. *Am J Med Sci.* 2002;323:34–38.

44. Foreman MD, Theis SL, Anderson MA. Adverse events in the hospitalized elderly. *Clin Nurs Res.* 1993;2:360–370.

45. Wallace M, Fulmer T. Fulmer SPICES: An overall assessment tool of older adults. *The Alabama Nurse.* 2003;30:26.

46. Foreman MD, Zane D. Nursing strategies for acute confusion in elders. *Am J Nurs.* 1996;96:44–51.

47. McDougall G. A review of screening instruments for assessing cognition and mental status in older adults. *Nurse Practitioner.* 1990;15:18–28.

48. Fulmer T. The debate over dependency as a pre-disposing factor in elder abuse and neglect. *J Elder Abuse Neglect.* 1990;2:51–59.

49. Steinmetz SK. Elder abuse by adult offspring: The relationship of actual vs. perceived dependency. *J Health Hum Resour Admin.* 1990;12:434–463.

50. Quinn MJ. Undue influence and elder abuse: Recognition and intervention strategies. *Geriatrics.* 2002;23:11–16.

51. Norris FH, Kaniasty K. Received and perceived social support in times of stress: A test of the social support deterioration deterrence model. *J Pers Soc Psychol.* 1996;71:498–511.

52. Irvin BL, Acton GJ. Stress mediation in caregivers of cognitively impaired adults: Theoretical model testing. *Nurs Res.* 1996;45:160–166.

53. Suitor JJ, Pillemer KA. Sources of support and interpersonal stress in the networks of married caregiving daughters: Findings from a 2-year longitudinal study. *J Gerontol B Psychol Sci Soc Sci.* 1996;51:S297–S306.

54. Tueth MJ. Exposing financial exploitation of impaired elderly persons. *Am J Geriatr Psychiatry.* 2000;8:104–111.

55. The National Center on Elder Abuse. *Creating and Promoting an Elder Abuse Action Agenda.* Washington, DC: National Policy Summit on Elder Abuse; 2001.

56. National Committee for the Prevention of Elder Abuse. Elder Abuse: Financial Abuse; 2001. Available at http//:www.preventelderabuse.org/elderabuse/fin_abuse.html.

57. National Center on Elder Abuse. The Basics: What is Elder Abuse? What Are the Major Types of Elder Abuse? 2001. Available at http://www.elderabusecenter.org/basic (accessed 2 February, 2005).

58. Dessin C. Financial abuse of the elderly. *Idaho Law Review.* 2000;36:203–226.

59. Paveza G, Hughes-Harrison V, VandeWeerd C. *Financial Exploitation of Older Adults: The Development of a Typology of Victims and Perpetrators.* In Annual Meeting of the Gerontological Society of America, 1997; Cincinnati, Ohio.

60. Deem D. Notes from the field: Observations in working with the forgotten victims of personal financial crimes. *J Elder Abuse Neglect.* 2000;12:33–48.

61. Choi N, Kulick D, Mayer J. Financial exploitation of elders: Analysis of risk factors based on county adult protective services data. *J Elder Abuse Neglect.* 1999;10:39–62.

62. Cooker J, Little B. Investing in the future: Protecting the elderly from financial abuse. *FBI Law Enforcement Bulletin.* 1997;2:1–5.

63. Fielo SB. How does crime affect the elderly? *Geriatr Nurs.* 1987;8:80–83.

64. Podnieks E. National survey on abuse of the elderly in Canada. *J Elder Abuse Neglect.* 1992;4:5–58.

65. Quinn M. Undoing undue influence. *J Elder Abuse Neglect.* 2000;12:9–16.

66. Dyer C, Connolly M, McFeeley P. The clinical and medical forensics of elder abuse and neglect. In Panel to Review Risk and Prevalence of Elder Abuse and Neglect. Bonnie RJ, Wallace RB, eds. *Elder Mistreatment: Abuse, Neglect, and Exploitation in an Aging America.* Washington, DC: The National Academies Press; 2003.

67. Reis M, Nahmiash D. Validation of the indicators of abuse (IOA) screen. *Gerontologist.* 1998;38:471–480.

68. Hwalek M, Sengstock M. Assessing the probability of abuse of the elderly: Towards the development of a clinical screening instrument. *J Appl Gerontol.* 1986;5:153–173.

69. Straus MA, Gelles R, Steinmetz SK. *Behind Closed Doors: Violence in the American Family.* New York: Anchor Books; 1980.

70. Fulmer T, Street S, Carr K. Abuse of the elderly: Screening and detection. *J Emerg Nurs.* 1984;10:131–140.

71. Fulmer T, Paveza G, VandeWeerd C, et al. Neglect assessment in urban emergency departments and confirmation by an expert clinical team. *Journals of Gerontology, Medical Sciences* (in press).

72. Fulmer T, Paveza G, Abraham I, Fairchild S. Elder neglect assessment in the emergency department. *J Emerg Nurs.* 2000;26:436–443.

73. Fulmer T, Cahill VM. Assessing elder abuse: A study. *J Gerontol Nursing.* 1984; 10(12):16–20.

# Section II
# Domains of Assessment

# 7

# *Cognitive Assessment*

Joseph J. Gallo and Marsha N. Wittink

Many studies since Dr. Michael Shepherd and colleagues' seminal work, *Psychiatric Illness in General Practice*, published over 30 years ago,[1] have revealed that mental disorders were common in the primary care setting but that individuals with these disorders frequently went unrecognized, with adverse consequences for them, their family, and the health care system. In the United States, Regier et al. have called attention to the de facto mental health services system composed of the general medical services and have highlighted the need for understanding of how to integrate general medical care and mental health care.[2] Compared with younger persons, older adults were most likely to receive mental health care from the primary care sector, not from specialists in mental health.[3] The primary care setting remains particularly important for African Americans, who are more likely than white patients to obtain mental health care from a primary care provider.[4-7]

Mental state assessment is pivotal in evaluating the health of older persons. The accuracy of the medical and social history obtained from an older person will depend on adequate mental and affective functioning. Cognitive impairment predicts poor agreement between self-reported and observer-rated measures of functioning.[8] Assessment of mental status is encouraged in order to detect unsuspected mental impairment and to provide a basis for comparison in future encounters. Most practitioners who deal with older persons have had the experience of treating an older person who is seen by the casual observer to be able to carry on a reasonably coherent conversation, but in whom mental status testing reveals significant difficulties. The person may be able to perform well in a job that has been held for many years as long as the routine is not interrupted. In novel situations, the extent of the deficit may become painfully evident to family or coworkers. The family may not even be aware that behavioral changes are secondary to subtle intellectual deterioration.

Ample evidence reveals that cognitive impairment and psychiatric disorder are often not recognized by health care professionals. Fully one third of older patients admitted to a medical floor in one study of cognitive status in older adults had significant mental impairment.[9] Other investigators demonstrated that in a 250-bed hospital affiliated with Brown University only 14 of 65 patients (21%) with cognitive deficits detected on the screening examination had documentation by the patients' physicians that such deficits had been recognized. In only two cases was a mental status examination a part of the patient's record.[10] Other studies have documented the failure of physicians to perform mental status testing routinely on older patients. Significant proportions of demented older persons were not diagnosed by their physicians yet were identified by brief mental status screening examination as being impaired.[11,12] Among patients evaluated by a psychiatrist before discharge from medical or surgical wards, only 27% of patients with mental impairment were diagnosed before discharge; most were believed to have moderate to severe impairment. In outpatient practice, few patients with cognitive impairment are recognized without screening.[13-15] Even among persons with diagnosed dementia whose family members recognized memory problems, only half received a medical evaluation.[16,17] In primary care settings, 67% of persons with dementia remained undiagnosed in one study.[18] Physicians may also fail to recognize depression, alcohol abuse, and drug misuse in their patients.[19]

The recognition of mental impairment is of more than just academic importance. Patients with abnormal scores on the screening examination had a greater chance of having episodes of confusion during the hospitalization,[10] after discharge,[19] and postoperatively.[20] Cognitively impaired hospitalized patients are less stable with increased morbidity and mortality,[21,22] a risk of loss of independence,[19,22-24] postoperative complications,[20] and behavioral difficulties.[25]

The discovery of cognitive impairment should prompt a search for an etiology. The best hope of finding a reversible process may hinge on the clinician's early recognition. Behavioral or personality changes may be placed in context when mental impairment is found to be present. Drugs that impair cognition should be avoided if possible. Specific pharmacologic therapy may mandate early detection of dementia.[26] For these reasons, it seems compelling to insist that mental status testing be a part of routine procedure for all older patients, particularly at the time of nursing home or hospital admission.[10,15,27] In other cases, clinical cues or "triggers" should prompt an assessment that may begin with the use of assessment instruments discussed later in the chapter.

The Agency for Health Care Policy and Research (AHCPR) Guidelines on Early Identification of Alzheimer's Disease and Related Dementias presented a number of examples of clinical cues that should prompt an assessment of mental status, namely, difficulty learning and remembering new information, difficulty handling complex tasks, an inability to solve problems, trouble with spatial ability and orientation (e.g., driving), trouble finding the right words, and behavioral disturbances.[28] The guideline panel recommended that mental status testing be interpreted in the context of functional status. Situations in which there is inconsistent information on mental status and functional status (i.e., one, but not both, is impaired) call for further neuropsychologic assessment and possibly referral for diagnosis and evaluation of dementia. The components of mental status and functional status discussed in this and the next chapter, implemented with the instruments discussed, can assist in the evaluation of older adults when the clinical cues for dementia, delirium, depression, or other mental disturbances are present.

The failure of many physicians to perform mental status testing on older individuals is unfortunate. Frequently, it is the person's personal physician who is best able to judge his or her competence, not a consultant who does not have an ongoing relationship with the patient. A periodic assessment of mental status in the chart can be valuable in these circumstances, particularly if legal questions arise.[29] Mental status testing of asymptomatic older adults must be balanced by concerns about falsely labeling the patient as demented. Poor performance on a mental status assessment instrument can arise from many causes. Dementia is a syndrome, a constellation of symptoms and characteristics that require clinical evaluation (discussed in more detail later in the chapter).

## THE MENTAL STATUS EXAMINATION

The mental status examination samples behavior and mental capability over a range of intellectual functions (Exhibit 7–1). The shorter standardized examinations to detect cognitive impairment that are

**Exhibit 7-1** Components of the Mental Status Examination

Level of consciousness
Attention

Language
 Fluency
 Comprehension
 Repetition

Memory
 Short-term memory
 Remote memory

Proverb interpretation
Similarities
Calculations
Writing
Constructional ability

*Source:* Adapted with permission from RL Strub and FW Black. *The Mental Status Examination in Neurology,* pp 163–172, © 1980 FA Davis Company.

discussed later in this chapter attempt to crystallize the examination so that a range of intellectual functions is tested by one or two questions in each area. When the screening instrument detects impairment, further examination is warranted. In clinical settings, this usually means more detailed mental status testing to localize and define the problem. When further characterization of the intellectual functioning is required, neuropsychologic testing may be in order. This becomes particularly salient when the individual's cognitive strengths and weaknesses must be delineated to make decisions about supervision and rehabilitative services, in the differential diagnosis of dementia and depression, or after stroke.[30]

Some health care professionals take the mental status examination no further than asking a few questions about orientation, having the person perform calculations, and requiring that he or she remember three items. In some situations, however, a thorough assessment can be crucial in an appropriate diagnosis and hence management. The classic example is an individual with an intracranial hemorrhage who is not making any sense and is mistakenly thought to be psychotic or confused because a specific language disturbance is not recognized. Granted, not every patient needs to be examined in precisely the way described here, but the standard screening mental status instruments discussed later in this chapter are short enough to be used in their entirety to assist in identifying cognitive impairment.

The complete mental status examination encompasses an assessment of the level of consciousness, attention, language, memory, proverb interpretation, similarities (e.g., "how are an apple and an orange alike?"), calculations, writing, and constructional ability (e.g., copying complex figures). A detailed overview of the mental status examination is provided by Strub and Black in *The Mental Status Examination in Neurology.*[31]

## Higher Cognitive Functions

The interview should start with questions of significance to the patient, which also gauge his or her memory and may help allay anxiety. Introductory statements that indicate interest in the older patient as a person (e.g., occupation, children, grandchildren, and hobbies) also indicate the patient's current and previous level of mental and social functioning. General appearance and grooming, posture, behavior, speech, and word choice can speak volumes to the careful observer.[32] The examiner should be wary of hearing and visual deficits that may mimic cognitive impairment.

An older patient meeting the physician or nurse for the first time may be anxious about the encounter. He or she may be coming to the interview reluctantly or even coerced by family or neighbors. He or she may worry that the physician or nurse is testing to see whether he or she is "crazy." Even in a nonthreatening environment, the interview can cause anxiety, thereby resulting in apparent confusion, inaccurate or incomplete reporting of information, and poor performance on testing. There is fear of error, and the patient may become hesitant to perform requested tasks. Disturbances of memory and intelligence exhibited during the examination may be a reflection of psychic stress and depression rather than dementia. It is wise to intersperse questions that are stressful or that focus on disability with others that are not and to end the interview on a positive note.[33]

The higher cognitive functions that may be specifically tested include the patient's fund of information and ability to reason abstractly and perform calculations (Table 7–1). After some preliminary questions about personal history are discussed, the patient may be asked questions regarding current events in the news (e.g., "who is the president now?") or commonly known historical information (e.g., "when did World War II end?") to assess the fund of information. In

---

**Table 7–1** Higher Integrative Functions

| Location | Assessment |
| --- | --- |
| Frontal lobes | Points finger each time the examiner makes a fist and makes a fist when the examiner points |
| Temporal lobes | *Dominant:* standard aphasia testing (spontaneous speech, repetition, comprehension, writing, and naming)<br>*Nondominant:* interprets affect (names affects shown in photos of faces or conveyed in examiner's voice) |
| Parietal lobes | *Dominant:* names fingers, knows left and right, performs calculations on paper, reading<br>*Nondominant:* constructs copy of matchstick figure made by the examiner |
| Occipital lobes | Matches colors and objects if unable to name them |

*Source:* Adapted with permission from EC Shuttleworth, Memory Function and the Clinical Differentiation of Dementing Disorders, *Journal of the American Geriatric Society,* Vol. 30, pp. 365–366, © Lippincott Williams & Wilkins.

---

evaluating responses, it is critical to know the level of educational attainment and whether English is the patient's first language.

Assessment of insight and judgment has important implications for considering driving skills and independence. Accidents and burns may be more common among cognitively impaired persons with poor insight and judgment.[34] Observe the patient's responses to mental status testing and conversation to note whether statements belie a lack of insight into deficits.[34]

Proverb testing and similarities shed light on the patient's reasoning ability, intelligence, and judgment. The examiner needs to be careful that the patient is not repeating the meaning of a proverb from memory rather than reasoning what an abstract interpretation might be. The Cognitive Capacity Screen[9] and the Kokmen Short Test of Mental Status,[35] discussed later in the chapter, are examples of screening instruments that include a test of reasoning with similarities, a task requiring the subject to think in abstract categories to discover how two concepts are alike. An example of a similarity is this: "How are a poem and a novel alike?" It has been suggested that the use of similarities is better than the use of proverb testing for the assessment of abstraction ability.[36]

The ability to perform calculations may be tested with serial 7s (i.e., "take 7 away from 100 and keep subtracting 7 from the answer all the way down"), serial 3s (i.e., "take 3 away from 20 and keep subtracting 3 from the answer all the way down"), or simple math problems. Corrected mistakes should not be counted as errors. Calculation ability also requires substantial memory and concentration ability. Occasionally, patients who have difficulty with serial 7s will handle the subtractions flawlessly if the problem is expressed in dollar terms (i.e., "if you had $100 and took away $7, how much would you have left?").

## Memory

Of all of the components of the mental status examination, memory assessment most commonly engenders anxiety and understandably so. It sometimes puts the patient at ease when the examiner prefaces the evaluation, particularly when using a standard questionnaire, with an explanation such as the following: "I'm going to ask you some questions. Some are easy. Some may be hard. Please don't be offended because it's the same routine I use for everyone." The examiner should give positive reinforcement during the examination with expressions such as "that's OK" or "that's fine."

Memory can be thought of as comprising three components. First and most fleeting is immediate recall. This can be assessed with digit repetition. Normal older persons can correctly recall five to seven digits.[37,38] The second component of memory is short-term memory, ranging over a period of minutes to days. This is usually tested by asking the person to remember three to four objects or abstract terms and then requesting him or her to recall them 5 or 10 minutes later after an intervening conversation or other testing. Examples of words used are "apple, table, penny"[39] and "brown, honesty, tulip, eyedropper."[31] The memory of aphasic persons may be tested by asking them to recall where items have been hidden in the room. It has been suggested that older persons do not use mnemonics when given a memory task and that this in part accounts for their failure to recall items.[38] Also, there is some evidence for increased processing time in older persons, and this may interfere with learning.[40] A third component of memory is remote or long-term memory. In one study, older adults were able to recall 80% of a catechism that had been learned some 36 years before.[41]

In general, older persons' self-reports of memory difficulty correlate poorly with objective measures of memory function. Not uncommonly, persons who complain fervently of memory loss are depressed, whereas someone with Alzheimer's disease may be oblivious to profound memory deficit. Early in the course of the disease, however, Alzheimer's patients may complain of memory loss.[42] Normal middle-aged or older persons may complain of memory difficulties, but their memory symptoms fit what has been called benign senescent forgetfulness or, more recently, age-associated memory impairment[43,44] or aging-associated cognitive decline.[45,46] These patients may be aware of a problem and apologize. They may not recall details of an experience, but certainly remember the experience itself. The forgetfulness fluctuates so that details not recalled at one time may be remembered at another.

Patients with a more significant memory loss often have accompanying intellectual deficits. Kral referred to this as malignant memory loss because the patients in his original series with this type of memory decline had greater mortality than a group who did not.[44] Patients with malignant memory loss not only forget details of an event but may not recall the experience itself or may confabulate about forgotten details.[37,44]

New nomenclature is emerging to describe the memory decline that is associated with normal aging. It replaces the term "benign senescent forgetfulness." Some middle-aged and older persons exhibit memory dysfunction caused by age in the routine tasks of daily life, such as trouble remembering items on a shopping list or forgetting telephone numbers. To fulfill the criteria for age-associated memory impairment, the person must have objective evidence of impairment on a memory function test, such as the Wechsler Associate Learning Subtest, but also must have absence of dementia (the diagnosis of which would imply a more global intellectual impairment), as evidenced by the Folstein Mini-Mental State Examination (MMSE).[43,47] Subjects with a family history of Alzheimer's dementia who met criteria for age-associated memory impairment did not have evidence of altered glucose metabolism.[48] Criteria for aging-associated cognitive decline will stimulate further developments on subthreshold dementia.[48,49] The fourth edition of the *Diagnostic and Statistical Manual (DSM-IV)* includes research criteria for mild neurocognitive disorder characterized by memory and other cognitive impairment that is due to a general medical condition but does not meet full criteria for dementia.[50]

## Attention and Level of Consciousness

Before an examiner can test and comment on the higher intellectual functions of the brain, including memory, some assessment (even if informal) must be made of the patient's level of consciousness. Obviously, functions such as orientation and memory cannot be tested in a comatose patient.

Orientation to surroundings is a fundamental beginning to mental status testing, but unfortunately, in routine clinical situations, the mental status evaluation often ends there. Questions regarding orientation to time, place, person, and situation are basic. Most people continually orient themselves by means of daily routines, clocks and watches, calendars, news media, and social activities. Older persons, on the other hand, particularly those living alone or in nursing homes, may not experience these activities and, as a result, may have poor orientation to time and events.[33,51]

After it is determined by observation that the person is alert enough for mental status testing to proceed, his or her attentiveness is assessed. Assessing attentiveness is important because a person who is easily distracted and unable to attend to the examiner will have poor performance on mental status testing solely because of inattention. Special note must be taken of the person who is inappropriately distracted by environmental noise or talking in the hallway. In such a case, a specific examination for attention deficit indicative of delirium may be warranted. Tests of attention sometimes used include digit repetition and the "A" test of vigilance. The length of a string of digits able to be repeated immediately after presentation tends to remain stable with age. A normal 90-year-old person should be able to repeat four digits, perhaps even seven or eight, after the examiner.[37] In the "A" test, the patient is asked to tap the table when the letter "A" is heard while the examiner presents random letters at a rate of one letter per second. The examiner observes for errors of commission and omission.

Neglect is a form of inattention in which the individual does not attend stimuli presented from a particular side, and it occurs most commonly with nondominant hemisphere lesions (usually the right). The examiner needs to avoid interviewing such a person from the neglected side if communication is to be effective.

## Language

Language should be observed and tested in a comprehensive mental status examination.[52] Spontaneous speech is observed during the initial interview. Does the patient make errors in words or grammatical construction? Persons with dysarthria, who have difficulty in the mechanical production of language, use normal grammar. Do spoken words flow smoothly? Fluency is one of the features that is used to differentiate the aphasias.

A simplified approach to aphasia divides the spoken language functions to be tested into three areas: comprehension, fluency, and repetition. Comprehension can be tested by asking the patient yes or no questions. If there is doubt about the responses, the patient may be asked to point to objects in the room. The task may be made more difficult by having him or her try to point to objects in a particular sequence or after the examiner has provided a description of the item rather than the item's name.

Fluency is a characteristic of speech that describes the rate and rhythm of speech production and the ease in initiating speech. Patients may be asked to name objects and their parts, such as a wristwatch and its band, buckle, and face. Repetition is tested with easy expressions (e.g., "ball" or "airplane") progressing to more difficult ones (e.g., "Methodist Episcopal" or "around the rock the rugged rascal ran").

The aphasias can be organized around the three characteristics of comprehension, fluency, and repetition (Figure 7–1). The person in whom the entire language neural substrate is destroyed, for example, due to infarction and edema after a stroke, has a global aphasia and, indeed, may be mute. All three language parameters are impaired in such a case. After a period of recovery, some language function may return.

Wernicke's aphasia is characterized by impaired comprehension and repetition. Speech is fluent but marked by paraphasia (i.e., words or sounds that are replaced by other sounds, such as "wife" or "car" for "knife") and neologisms (i.e., nonsense words). Persons with this type of aphasia have severe difficulty with comprehension and may not even be aware that their own speech output is incoherent, which can be a considerable obstacle in rehabilitation. The person with Wernicke's aphasia may describe a picture of a boy reaching into a cookie jar this way: "It's a barl, a boil, oh, you know, getting the thing, the thing, it's just the top, boy, you know."

Persons with Wernicke's aphasia may improve significantly in their comprehension but continue to exhibit fluent speech with paraphasia. This condition is called conduction aphasia. The neurologic lesion in conduction aphasia may involve the arcuate fasciculus, the connection between the anterior (motor) and posterior (sensory) language areas. Persons with conduction aphasia usually do not demonstrate the amount of verbal output noted in those with Wernicke's

REPETITION

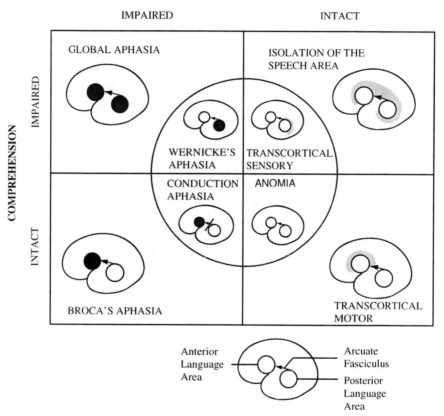

**Figure 7-1** Aphasia diagram: The three components of language function to be tested are comprehension, fluency, and repetition. Aphasias depicted within the central circle are the fluent aphasias. Source: Reprinted from J Gallo et al., *Mental Status Assessment, Handbook of Geriatric Assessment,* 2nd ed., p. 19, © 1994 Aspen Publishers, Inc.

aphasia. They may be able to read well for comprehension but cannot read aloud.

Persons with an initial Wernicke's aphasia may continue to improve beyond a conduction type of aphasia (i.e., they will have better comprehension) and ultimately be left with an anomic aphasia. With anomic aphasia, persons have difficulty finding words but show fluent speech, good repetition, and good comprehension.

Patients with relatively preserved comprehension, impaired repetition, and severely limited verbal output consisting of mostly nouns and verbs (i.e., telegraphic speech) have Broca's aphasia. Although repetition is impaired, it may be clearer than the person's spontaneous speech. Because his or her speech contains mostly nouns and verbs, he or she may have difficulty with the expression "no ifs, ands, or buts." Broca's aphasia involves an anterior brain lesion, and if the nearby motor strip is affected, a concomitant hemiplegia occurs. The person with Broca's aphasia may describe a picture of a boy reaching into a cookie jar this way: "Boy . . . yes, ah . . . jar, cookie."

Patients with global aphasia, Wernicke's aphasia, conduction aphasia, and Broca's aphasia have impaired repetition ability in common. There are rarer syndromes of aphasias, called transcortical aphasias, in which repetition function is remarkably preserved out of proportion to the disability in comprehension and fluency.

Isolation of the speech area is a transcortical aphasia that occurs when a zone of infarction extends around the boundaries of the speech areas so that they are isolated from the associative regions of the brain. This may occur in so-called watershed infarcts because of hypotension and resultant ischemia in the "watershed" zone between the areas of distribution of the anterior and middle cerebral arteries. Such a lesion can also be found after carbon monoxide poisoning or prolonged hypoxia. Persons with isolation of the speech area can repeat words and phrases perfectly, even words from foreign languages that they have never heard. Their spontaneous speech is sparse and nonfluent, and comprehension is impaired (see Figure 7–1).

Partial transcortical syndromes, isolating only part of the speech apparatus, are probably more common than complete isolation of the speech area. The anterior (i.e., transcortical motor) or posterior (i.e., transcortical sensory) language areas may be isolated from the associative cortices of the rest of the brain.

Comprehension is relatively preserved in persons with transcortical motor aphasia. Their speech is similar to that of someone with Broca's aphasia, which is an aphasia that also involves anterior portions of the cortex. Persons with transcortical sensory aphasia have fluent speech and impaired comprehension, similar to those with Wernicke's aphasia. Both transcortical sensory aphasia and Wernicke's aphasia involve posterior portions of the cortex. The spontaneous speech of the individual with transcortical sensory aphasia is filled with paraphasic errors (i.e., word substitutions), but repetition is preserved. Sorting out aphasia is easier when the three domains of fluency, comprehension, and repetition are kept in mind. Other language syndromes include reading difficulty only (i.e., alexia), alexia with writing difficulty (i.e., agraphia), and Gerstmann's syndrome (i.e., acalculia, agraphia, right/left disorientation, and finger agnosia or inability to name the fingers).

## Writing and Construction Ability

The components of the mental status examination discussed to this point can smoothly follow the history interview because it is primarily a verbal examination. At this point in the examination, the patient may be presented with a blank sheet of paper for subsequent tests.

The patient is asked to write his or her name at the top of the page. Although the signature is usually overlearned and can be intact even with writing difficulty for more complex tasks, this action acclimates the patient to the idea that he or she is going to be asked to do some writing, and the signature is a nonthreatening way to begin. Below the signature, the patient is asked to write a complete sentence, perhaps about the weather. While the person has the blank sheet of paper and pen in hand, construction ability may be tested. The ability to reproduce the line drawings of the examiner represents construction ability. This can be a very sensitive test of parietal lobe damage and is an early abnormality in dementia. Trouble with construction ability is not something most persons will complain of specifically, but testing constructional ability can be revealing. The testing begins with simple figures such as a triangle or square and progresses to more complex drawings such as a cube, house, or flowerpot. Mattis reminds us that testing the ability to copy figures is not specific to dementia because trouble with this test may reflect motor incoordination or apraxia.[36]

Asking the patient to draw a clock showing the numerals and time (e.g., "10 minutes past 11 o'clock") can act as a single item screen for cognitive impairment. The examiner draws a large circle on a blank sheet of paper and asks the patient to fill in the numbers as on a clock. This task is thought to be a sensitive test of parietal lobe dysfunction. Persons with primarily right or nondominant hemisphere dysfunction write the numbers correctly but plan poorly. Those with primarily left or dominant hemisphere dysfunction have trouble writing the numbers but execute the general plan of the clock correctly, perhaps placing lines where the numbers should be. Clock drawing has been used to screen for cognitive impairment[53] as well as to follow progression of diagnosed Alzheimer's disease.[54] Several scoring methods for the clock-drawing task are available.[53-57] The examination of higher integrative functions is summarized in Table 7–1.[58]

## DIFFERENTIAL DIAGNOSIS OF DEMENTIA

In considering the differential diagnosis of cognitive impairment, the primary distinction that must be made by the clinician is among dementia, delirium, or a specific neurologic deficit, such as aphasia or amnesia. At the outset, it must be emphasized that older adults may exhibit delirium superimposed on dementia. The aged central nervous system may be especially vulnerable to dysfunction brought about by metabolic disturbances. A decline in function of persons with dementia should prompt a search for potentially reversible conditions.

Dementia is a syndrome that is characterized by a loss of intellectual capacity involving not only memory but also cognition, language, visuospatial skills, and personality. All five components need not be impaired, but they frequently are to varying degrees. Dementia implies intellectual impairment in clear consciousness and may be progressive, stable, or remitting. The term "organic mental disorder" has been dropped in the *DSM-IV*.[50] Criteria for several subtypes of dementia are delineated in *DSM-IV*: dementia of the Alzheimer type, vascular dementia, dementia caused by human immunodeficiency virus, dementia caused by head trauma, dementia caused by Pick's disease, dementia caused by Creutzfeldt-Jakob disease, dementia caused by other general medical conditions, substance-induced persisting dementia, and dementia caused by multiple etiologies.

Delirium is marked by clouding of consciousness, usually of acute onset (i.e., in hours or days). Persons who are delirious may be agitated or lethargic, and levels of activity may vary throughout the day. Agitated delirium calls attention to the person, whereas that of those persons who are quietly delirious may go unrecognized and unattended. It cannot be overemphasized, however, that delirium is a syndrome, not a diagnosis. The recognition of delirium, like fever, requires further explanation.[59] A standardized schedule to detect delirium has been published,[60] but short instruments that assess cognitive function may serve this purpose as discussed later in this chapter.

After the clinician determines that global intellectual impairment is present and consistent with dementia, a consideration of the specific etiology is in order. Although the chance of finding a remedial condition seems remote, the list of diagnostic possibilities is so large and the scope of the problem in an aging society is so great that dementia and any concurrent conditions need to be assessed thoroughly.

The notion of searching for a "reversible" dementia (implying that nothing can be done to help the person with an "irreversible" dementia) is only helpful in so far as it prompts a consideration of the myriad causes of intellectual decline. In a study of 107 demented older persons, 16 improved 6 months after their initial assessment.[61] Eleven were patients with "reversible" dementia, but they showed a deteriorating course typical of Alzheimer's disease on further follow-up. The five remaining patients with "irreversible" dementia who improved did so after concurrent conditions, such as congestive heart failure, depression, and anemia, were addressed. Classifying dementia as reversible (treatable) or irreversible (not treatable) may unnecessarily compromise patient management. Instead, all demented persons must be considered to be at increased risk for secondary treatable conditions,[61,62] not to mention that caregivers require attention in the care of dementia patients.

One helpful scheme (Exhibit 7–2) that organizes the differential diagnosis of dementia and aids the clinician's memory was suggested by Cummings and Benson.[63] By considering a hierarchy of clinical features, the dementias can be systematically reviewed in the clinician's mind.

---

**Exhibit 7–2** Classification of the Major Causes of Dementia Based on the Occurrence of Features of Cortical and Subcortical Dysfunction

Cortical dementias
- Alzheimer's disease
- Frontal lobe degeneration

Subcortical dementias
- Extrapyramidal syndromes
  - Parkinson's disease
  - Huntington's disease
  - Progressive supranuclear palsy
  - Wilson's disease
  - Spinocerebellar degeneration
  - Idiopathic basal ganglia calcification
- Hydrocephalus
- Dementia syndrome of depression
- White matter diseases
  - Multiple sclerosis
  - Human immunodeficiency virus encephalopathy
- Vascular dementias
  - Lacunar state
  - Binswanger's disease

Combined cortical and subcortical features
- Multi-infarct dementias
- Infectious dementias
  - Slow-virus dementias
  - General paresis
- Toxic and metabolic encephalopathies
  - Systemic illnesses
  - Endocrinopathies
  - Deficiency states
  - Drug intoxications
  - Heavy metal exposure
- Miscellaneous dementia syndromes
  - Post-traumatic
  - Post-anoxic
  - Neoplastic

*Source:* Adaped with permission from JL Cummings and DF Benson, *Dementia: A Clinical Approach*, Woburn, MA, Butterworth-Heinemann, © 1983.

First, are the features consistent with a cortical dementia such as Alzheimer's or Pick's disease? Alzheimer's disease is characterized by an insidious onset with a progressive deteriorating course. Typically, memory is affected early on. Clinical criteria for the clinical diagnosis of Alzheimer's disease reported by McKhann et al. aid in the evaluation of patients with dementia.[64] Of course, a definite diagnosis of Alzheimer's disease requires histopathologic evidence obtained at autopsy, but a diagnosis of probable and possible Alzheimer's disease can be made clinically using the criteria set forth by the National Institute of Neurological and Communicative Disorders and Stroke-Alzheimer's Disease and Associated Disorders Association Task Force on Alzheimer's Disease. Probable Alzheimer's disease may be diagnosed with the following criteria:[64]

1. Dementia established by clinical examination and by the MMSE or a similar examination
2. Deficits in two or more areas of cognition
3. Progressive worsening of memory and other cognitive functions
4. No disturbance of consciousness (to distinguish from delirium)
5. Onset most often after the age of 65 years
6. No systemic disorder or other brain disease that could account for the findings

The diagnosis of Alzheimer's disease is supported by progressive deterioration in specific functions such as language, impaired activities of daily living, and evidence of cerebral atrophy on computed tomography (CT) scan. *DSM-IV* criteria for dementia of the Alzheimer type include multiple cognitive deficits (e.g., memory impairment, aphasia, apraxia, agnosia, and disturbance of executive function) and interference with social and occupational roles (Exhibit 7–3).[50]

A scale developed as a tool to assist in the differential diagnosis of dementia, specifically for the diagnosis of Alzheimer's disease, is the Inventory of Diagnostic Clinical Features of Dementia of the Alzheimer Type.[65] A maximum score of 20 is possible, attained by persons with uncomplicated dementia of the Alzheimer type. The higher scores (14 or greater) reflect greater consistency with the diagnosis of Alzheimer's disease and lower scores with other diagnoses.

In retrospective and prospective studies, the inventory was highly accurate in differentiating persons with Alzheimer's disease from those who have dementia from another etiology. This inventory (Exhibit 7–4) gives greater weight to loss of intellectual functions than to

**Exhibit 7–3** Diagnostic Criteria for Dementia of the Alzheimer Type

A. The development of multiple cognitive deficits manifested by both:
  (1) memory impairment (impaired ability to learn new information or to re-call previously learned information)
  (2) one (or more) of the following cognitive disturbances:
    (a) aphasia (language disturbance)
    (b) apraxia (impaired ability to carry out motor activities despite intact motor function)
    (c) agnosia (failure to recognize or identify objects despite intact sensory function)
    (d) disturbance in executive functioning (i.e., planning, organizing, sequencing, and abstracting)
B. The cognitive deficits in criteria A1 and A2 each cause significant impairment in social or occupational functioning and represent a significant decline from a previous level of functioning.
C. The course is characterized by gradual onset and continuing cognitive decline.
D. The cognitive deficits in criteria A1 and A2 are not due to any of the following:
  (1) other central nervous system conditions that cause progressive deficits in memory and cognition (e.g., cerebrovascular disease, Parkinson's disease, Huntington's chorea, subdural hematoma, normal-pressure hydro-cephalus, or brain tumor)
  (2) systemic conditions that are known to cause dementia (e.g., hypothy-roidism, vitamin $B_{12}$ or folic acid deficiency, niacin deficiency, hypercal-cemia, neurosyphilis, or HIV infection)
  (3) substance-induced conditions
E. The deficits do not occur exclusively during the course of a delirium.
F. The disturbance is not better accounted for by another Axis I disorder (e.g., major depressive disorder or schizophrenia).

*Source:* Reprinted with permission from the *Diagnostic and Statistical Manual of Mental Disorders,* 4th ed. © 1994 American Psychiatric Association.

motor abnormalities. Atypical presentations of dementia of the Alzheimer type or mixed diagnoses may fail to be identified because of the absence of multiple areas of intellectual impairment assessed by the inventory.[65,66] The scoring scheme of the inventory reflects the generally normal results of motor examination of persons with Alzheimer's disease and the early impairment of language and memory. Demented persons who present with signs or symptoms of a movement disorder should suggest to the practitioner a diagnosis other than primary degenerative (cortical) dementia.

Patients with Pick's disease, the other primary cortical dementia, have personality changes with poor judgment and social graces, but

**Exhibit 7–4** Inventory of Diagnostic Clinical Features of Senile Dementia of the Alzheimer Type

| Mental Functions | 0 | 1 | 2 |
|---|---|---|---|
| Memory | Normal or forgetfulness that improves with cues | Recalls one or two of three words, spontaneous, incompletely aided by prompting | Disoriented, unable to learn three words in 3 min, recall not aided by prompting |
| Visuospatial | Normal or clumsy drawings, minimal distortions | Flattening, omissions, distortions | Disorganized, unrecognizable copies of models |
| Cognition | Normal or impairment of complex abstractions and calculations | Fails to abstract simple proverbs and has difficulty with mathematical problems | Fails to interpret even simple proverbs or idioms, acalculia |
| Personality | Disinhibition or depression | Appropriately concerned | Unaware or indifferent, irritability not uncommon |
| Language | Normal | Anomia, mild comprehension deficits | Fluent aphasia with anomia, decreased comprehension paraphasia |

| Motor Functions | 0 | 1 | 2 |
|---|---|---|---|
| Speech | Mute, severely | Slurred, amelodic, dysarthric | Normal hypophonic |
| Psychomotor speed | Slow, long latency to response | Hesitant responses | Normal, prompt responses |
| Posture | Abnormal, flexed, extended, or distorted | Stooped or mildly distorted | Normal, erect |
| Gait | Hemiparetic, ataxic, apractic, or hyperkinetic | Shuffling, dyskinetic | Normal |
| Movements | Tremor, akinesia, rigidity, or chorea | Imprecise, poorly coordinated | Normal |

*Source:* Adapted with permission from J Cummings and D Benson, Dementia of the Alzheimer Type: An Inventory of Diagnostic Clinical Features, *Journal of American Geriatric Society,* Vol. 34, pp. 12–19, © 1986, Lippincott Williams & Wilkins.

with strikingly preserved memory, language, and visuospatial skills early in the course of the dementia. Pathologic changes in Pick's disease occur primarily in the temporal and frontal lobes of the brain.

Is there evidence of a halting progression to the disorder with spotty mental status deficits associated with a history of hypertension or strokes? Vascular dementia, which is thought to be the result of strokes or cerebrovascular disease,[67] may be more common than previously appreciated.[68,69] Several lines of evidence now suggest that cognitive impairment in older adults is associated with vascular lesions in the central nervous system, even without dementia.[69–78] Some individuals exhibit changes of Alzheimer's disease occurring in the context of multiple infarcts (mixed dementia). Small infarcts, strategically located, may be associated with increased vulnerability to Alzheimer's disease.[79] Thus, the relationship between cardiovascular disease risk factors, such as lipid and apolipoprotein profiles, dementia, and stroke, is complex indeed.

Vascular factors have long been thought to influence mental health in late life. For example, describing changes in the brains of patients with dementing illness, one influential writer, Dr. Benjamin Ball, wrote in 1881, "Localised softening caused the more severe states of cognitive impairment."[80] Even as late as the 1960s, many of the mental disturbances of late life were ascribed to atherosclerosis.[80,81] The realization that most dementia appeared to be related to neuropathologic changes described by Alzheimer in 1906 largely discredited the notion of atherosclerotic dementia. Now recent evidence has rekindled interest in the role of vascular factors in dementia,[82] including Alzheimer's disease,[83–85] and even in depression arising in late life.[86] Medicine is in the early stages in the investigation of how cardiovascular disease risk factors, such as hypertension, diabetes, high cholesterol, smoking, and atrial fibrillation, contribute to cognitive impairment in late life.

In the clinical examination of the person with vascular dementia, the practitioner should look for spasticity in the limbs, hyperreflexia, plantar extensor reflexes, and an abnormal gait. The personality is relatively preserved. The CT scan reveals evidence of infarcts in only half of patients suspected of having vascular dementia.[87] Criteria of *DSM-IV* for vascular dementia are similar to the criteria for dementia of the Alzheimer type except that focal neurologic signs and symptoms are present or imaging studies reveal cerebrovascular disease.[50]

Senile dementia of the Binswanger's type, described over 100 years ago, is a type of vascular dementia more commonly recognized because of new imaging techniques, particularly magnetic resonance imaging.[88] Patients with this type of dementia have an insidious onset of dementia with gait disturbance, urinary incontinence, and neurologic signs early in the course of the illness. Diagnostic criteria include at least two of the following: hypertension or other known cardiovascular risk factors; evidence of cerebrovascular disease; evidence of subcortical features, such as abnormal gait or muscular rigidity; and subcortical attenuation of white matter on brain scan.[89] The pathologic condition relates to infarctions in the white matter just below the cortex, resulting in isolation of cortex from deeper structures. Risk factors (e.g., diabetes and hypertension) for small artery disease may predispose persons to senile dementia of the Binswanger's type.[90,91]

Recognition of vascular dementia assumes particular importance when considered with hypertension treatment or modification of other cardiovascular risk factors. Some investigators believe there is a "therapeutic window" within which blood pressure should be controlled. When blood pressure was lowered below this optimal range, the persons with vascular dementia exhibited further cognitive decline.[92] In contrast, persons who stop smoking benefit by showing less cognitive decline.[93] The Hachinski Ischemic Score (Exhibit 7–5) has been devised to help distinguish vascular dementia from other types of dementia. Persons with a score of 7 or more are said to be more

---

**Exhibit 7–5** Hachinski Ischemic Score

1. Abrupt onset (2)
2. Stepwise deterioration (1)
3. Fluctuating course (2)
4. Nocturnal confusion (1)
5. Relative preservation of personality (1)
6. Depression (1)
7. Somatic complaints (1)
8. Emotional incontinence (1)
9. History of hypertension (1)
10. History of strokes (2)
11. Evidence of associated atherosclerosis (1)
12. Focal neurologic symptoms (2)
13. Focal neurologic signs (2)

The score for each feature is noted in parentheses. A score of greater than 7 suggests a vascular component to the dementia.

*Source:* Adapted with permission from VC Hachinski et al., Cerebral Blood Flow in Dementia, *Archives of Neurology* Vol. 32, p. 634. Copyright © 1975, American Medical Association.

likely to have vascular dementia or at least a vascular component to their dementia.[94] An extensive review of the literature by Liston and LaRue led the authors to conclude that a low Hachinski Ischemic Score could help exclude vascular dementia because ischemic lesions severe enough to produce a dementia would be expected to be severe enough to cause the associated neurologic changes and elevate the score.[94]

Is there evidence of a movement disorder? Parkinson's disease is a subcortical process associated with a dementia. The person's intellectual processes seem to be "slowed" along with his or her movements. Frequently, there is a superimposed depression. Subcortical dementias classically are associated with abnormalities of the motor system, such as stooped posture, increased muscle tone, and abnormal movements and gait.[63] Other subcortical dementias are associated with Huntington's chorea, progressive supranuclear palsy, and Wilson's disease. The concept of cortical and subcortical types of dementia is not as clearcut as it would seem. Some of the features generally reported to be characteristic of one type may be found in the other, such as aphasia being present in persons with subcortical dementia.[95] Dementia with Lewy bodies is characterized by pathology in the cortical region[96] but results in features that include movement disorder. In people with Lewy body dementia, deficits in memory and visuospatial ability occur as in Alzheimer's disease, but so do fluctuating cognition, recurrent visual hallucinations, and motor features resembling Parkinson's disease.[97]

Is there an affective component to the dementia? Persons who vigorously complain of memory impairment often are depressed (or have early Alzheimer's disease or both). Those suffering from dementia syndrome of depression, on close continued observation, may be able to learn new facts and might give a detailed account of their memory loss. Depression as a precursor of intellectual impairment is discussed more fully later in this chapter.

Is the classic triad of normal pressure hydrocephalus present? Normal pressure hydrocephalus is characterized by the triad of gait disturbance, urinary incontinence, and dementia. Physical examination reveals spasticity in the legs with hyperreflexia and plantar extension reflexes. Of course, the classic triad need not be present. The CT examination shows dilated ventricles, but there may be considerable overlap with other dementias.[98]

Is there evidence of a toxic process? Prescription medications are among the greatest offenders, but hidden alcohol abuse must be considered as well.[99–104] Commonly used medicines (e.g., propranolol or digoxin) may cause an altered mental state as the only side effect.

Some medicines (e.g., the benzodiazepines) can precipitate a delirium or seizures when discontinued.

Is there evidence of a metabolic abnormality? Electrolyte imbalance, such as hyponatremia, can result in a confused mental state. Calcium abnormalities can cause lethargy. Hypoxia or hypercarbia, as could result from pulmonary or cardiac disease, may also cause confusion.

Is there evidence of an endocrine abnormality? Testing for apathetic hyperthyroidism or for occult hypothyroidism should be part of the complete workup for dementia. Are the electrolytes suggestive of an adrenal problem? Is there evidence of a nutritional deficiency, such as deficiency of thiamine, niacin, or vitamin B12? Thiamine deficiency, which is associated with alcohol abuse, may result in Wernicke's encephalopathy or organic amnestic syndrome. Niacin deficiency is associated with dementia. Vitamin B12 deficiency may result in psychologic changes without concomitant macrocytosis.

Is there evidence of an infection such as meningitis? Of course, reliable diagnosis would require lumbar puncture. Lumbar puncture probably is not very helpful applied indiscriminately to the diagnosis of dementia; it should be reserved for specific circumstances, such as acute deterioration with fever. Neurosyphilis is an unusual cause of dementia today but can be present even with a negative rapid plasma reagin test. Creutzfeldt-Jakob disease is a rapidly progressing dementia caused by a slow virus and characterized by myoclonus in its late stages and a burst–silence pattern on electroencephalography. Dementia secondary to human immunodeficiency virus is perhaps the newest addition to the list. The acquired immune deficiency syndrome could be important to keep in mind, particularly when risk factors, such as sexual exposure to high-risk persons or the use of blood products, are present.[105,106]

Are there focal neurologic signs suggestive of an intracranial process such as a neoplasm or a chronic subdural hematoma? Is there a history of trauma followed by changes in mental state? A complete mental status examination may reveal deficits that point to involvement of an otherwise "silent" area of the brain. Cranial CT rarely may find a mass lesion presenting as dementia when focal signs are absent.

Finally, is there more than one process occurring simultaneously? Are there concurrent medical illnesses that could be more optimally treated? In other words, is an overlying delirium resulting in deterioration of the mental status with pre-existing dementia? Over 30% of persons with dementia have more than one disorder contributing to the persistence of the dementia.[107] The need to consider alternative conditions rather than ascribing the changes to a deterioration of dementia cannot be overemphasized when persons who carry a diagnosis of dementia have acute changes in their ability to function.

## MENTAL STATUS ASSESSMENT INSTRUMENTS

Many short mental status screening instruments have been devised to assist clinicians. Some screening instruments for intellectual functioning were devised for the sole purpose of assessing mental status, and others form part of a total instrument that includes measures of functional status and/or psychiatric illness. Further information on instruments to assess mental state may be found in the *Geropsychology Assessment Resource Guide*[108] and in *Measuring Health: A Guide to Rating Scales and Questionnaires.*[109] Instruments that are commonly endorsed for clinical practice will be reviewed, bearing in mind that other strategies are being developed to achieve the goals of a brief and accurate scale to assess mental status (see Froehlich et al.,[110] Solomon and Pendlebury,[111] and Lorentz et al.[112]).

The sensitivity and specificity of a test are used to assess performance of the test at specific cut points. Sensitivity and specificity are characteristics of tests that do not change with the prevalence of the disease in a population. Simply stated, the sensitivity of a test is the proportion of those persons with a disease who are detected by the test. Specificity is the proportion of those who are free of disease who are identified as such by the test. A related concept is the predictive value of a test result. The predictive value of a positive test is the proportion of persons that has a positive test and truly has the disease. The rest of the group, those with a positive result but without disease, are considered to have false-positive results. The predictive value of a negative test is the proportion of persons who has a negative test and truly does not have the disease. The rest of the group, those with a negative result but with the disease, have false-negative results.

The predictive value of a test varies as the prevalence of the disease in the population varies. The more common the disease is in the population to be tested, the greater is the predictive value of a positive test, but as the predictive value of a negative test goes down, the number of false-negative results increases. This makes intuitive sense because it would seem that the more common the disease the more likely it is that a positive test result is true. Conversely, it will be less likely that a negative test represents a "true" negative. In a nursing home, for example, where the prevalence of dementia is presumably

higher than in the general population, the predictive value of a negative screening test is diminished compared with the value of a negative test in community-dwelling older adults.

In contrast is the case of a less common disease. The lower the
prevalence of the disease in the population to be tested the greater is
the predictive value of a negative test, but the predictive value of a
positive test goes down; the number of false-positive results increases.
Again, it would seem intuitive that the rarer a disease is, a positive test
is more likely to be wrong rather than truly indicating someone with
the rare illness.

In addition to simple detection of the demented state, the mental
status assessment instruments can stratify persons with regard to the
severity of dementia. Many of the instruments designed specifically
for this purpose also include some assessment of functional ability,
the dementia rating scales, discussed in Chapter 4. Because a score is
generated by some of the mental status assessment instruments discussed in this section, stratification is possible merely on that basis.
Mental status assessment instruments may exhibit threshold or ceiling effects. In other words, persons beyond a certain level of severity
of dementia score the same despite some differences in degree. In a
population with a predominance of severely demented persons, for
example, an instrument would not be useful for following change if
all severely affected individuals performed equally poorly. By the
same token, in a population of relatively well older persons, an easy
test will be insensitive to mildly demented persons, who may be able
to perform well on it, whereas on a more discriminating test, they
would have difficulties. This is vividly illustrated by the case of a patient who studied for the MMSE. She was being admitted to a retirement home and was disappointed when the physician did not ask her
"those questions" her friend had told her about. She had studied the
"answers" to the examination based on information from her friend,
who was a resident in the home.[113]

## Folstein MMSE

The MMSE[114] is one of the most widely employed tests of cognitive
function and is one of the best studied.[115,116] Five cognitive functions
underlie the items in the MMSE: concentration, language, orientation, memory, and attention.[117] Population-based norms are readily
available according to age and educational level.[28,116] The MMSE consists of two parts (Exhibit 7–6). The first part requires verbal responses

**Exhibit 7–6** The Folstein Mini-Mental State Examination (MMSE)

| *Maximum Score* | |
|---|---|
| | *Orientation* |
| 5 | What is the (year) (season) (date) (day) (month)? |
| 5 | Where are we (state) (county) (town) (hospital) (floor)? |
| | *Registration* |
| 3 | Name three objects: one second to say each. Then ask the patient all three after you have said them. Give one point for each correct answer. Repeat them until he or she learns all three. Count trials and record number. |
| | *Attention and calculation* |
| 5 | Begin with 100 and count backward by 7 (stop after five answers). Alternatively, spell "world" backward. |
| | *Recall* |
| 3 | Ask for the three objects repeated above. |
| | *Language* |
| 2 | Show a pencil and a watch and ask the patient to name them. |
| 1 | Repeat the following: "No ifs, ands, or buts." |
| 3 | A three-stage command: "Take a paper in your right hand, fold it in half, and put it on the floor." |
| 1 | Read and obey the following: (show written item) CLOSE YOUR EYES |
| 1 | Write a sentence. |
| 1 | Copy a design (complex polygon). |
| 30 | Total score possible |

*Source:* "Mini-mental state." a practical method for grading the cognitive state of patients for the clinician. *Journal of Psychiatric Research,* 12(3):189–198, © 1975, 1998 Mini Mental LLC. The copyright in the Mini Mental State Examination is wholly owned by the Mini Mental LLC, a Massachusetts limited liability company. For information about how to obtain permission to use or reproduce the Mini Mental State Examination, please contact John Gonsalves, Jr., Administrator of the Mini Mental LLC, at 31 St. James Avenue, Suite I, Boston, Massachusetts 02116—(617)587-4215.

only and assesses orientation, memory, and attention. The three words used to test memory are left up to the examiner, leaving the possibility that this question could vary in difficulty. The items "apple, table, penny" were used in the Epidemiologic Catchment Area Program.[116] In addition to serial 7s, the individual is asked to spell "world" backward, and the best score may be taken for calculating the total score. A "chess-move" strategy is used to score the "world" item (i.e., the number of transpositions required to spell "DLROW" yields the number of errors).[118] The second part evaluates the ability to write a sentence, name objects, follow verbal and written commands, and copy a complex polygon. The maximum score is 30. The test is not timed. A telephone version of the MMSE is available for special purposes.[119]

In the original work with the MMSE, normal older persons scored a mean of 27.6. Patients with dementia, depression with cognitive impairment, and affective disorders formed a continuum with the mean scores for these groups of 9.7, 19, and 25, respectively. Not only did the demented persons score the lowest and the depressed ones the highest, but after treatment for depression, the depressed persons with cognitive impairment showed improvement in their scores. The demented individuals had no change, as would be expected.[114]

The MMSE was administered to patients undergoing cranial CT scanning referred from neurologic and psychiatric services at the University of Iowa. Patients whose CT scan showed no cerebral atrophy had a mean score of 26.4. Those with focal brain lesions scored 25.3, which was not significantly different from the group without atrophy. Patients with atrophy alone had a mean score of 18.0. Thus, the MMSE correlates to some degree with structural changes in the brain.[120]

Although one report failed to show a difference in sensitivity between the MMSE and the Short Portable Mental Status Questionnaire (SPMSQ),[121] others have suggested that the sensitivity of the MMSE is better than that of the SPMSQ,[122,123] with an ability to pick up cognitive impairment closer to 90% rather than 50% (Table 7–2). The sensitivity of an instrument such as the MMSE, which, unlike the SPMSQ, tests recent memory, written and spoken language, and construction ability (drawing), in addition to orientation, would be expected to be better because a broader range of intellectual functions is sampled.

In any case, when the MMSE reveals that the individual is impaired, additional diagnostic testing and mental status examination are indicated to define the disorder further, as would be true for any brief screening instrument. This is an acceptable practice in general medical settings using the MMSE as part of a routine screen of older persons.[13]

The sensitivity of the MMSE was 76% when 126 patients on neurosurgical and neurologic wards were tested, and a cutoff score of 23 was used to differentiate impaired from normal patients.[124] The mean age of these patients was 49.9. Patients with bilateral hemispheric damage or with left hemispheric damage scored around 23, whereas control subjects and patients with right hemispheric damage scored around 28. Thus, the instrument detects left hemispheric dysfunction better than it does right hemispheric dysfunction. This

**Table 7–2** Sensitivity, Specificity, and Predictive Value of the Folstein Mini-Mental State Examination (MMSE)

|  | *Clinical Examination Consistent with Dementia* | *Clinical Examination Not Consistent with Dementia* |  |
|---|---|---|---|
| Score indicates impairment | Agrees | False positive | Predictive value of a positive test is 60%–93% |
| Score indicates no impairment | False negative | Agrees | Predictive value of a negative test is 77%–95% |
|  | Sensitivity is 50%–87% | Specificity is approximately 90% |  |

A cutoff score of 24 is used to indicate dementia.

*Sources:* Adapted from *Journal of Neurology, Neurosurgery, and Psychiatry,* © 1984, Vol. 47, pp. 496–499, with permission from the BMJ Publishing Group; *Psychological Medicine*, Vol. 12, No. 2, pp. 397–408, © 1982; *Journal of the American Geriatric Society*, Vol. 28, No. 38, pp. 381–384, © 1980, Lippincott Williams & Wilkins.

asymmetrical detection of dysfunction was also shown to be true for the Cognitive Capacity Screen, to be discussed later in this chapter.[125] In the study of Dick et al., there was excellent agreement between the results of the MMSE and those of the Wechsler Adult Intelligence Scale.[124] Dropping the cutoff score to 20 or 21 decreased the sensitivity of the instrument but allowed a greater number of normal persons to be classified correctly.

There is some question as to the adjustment of scores on mental status screening instruments based on the educational level of the subject. A low score may imply more severe intellectual impairment among persons with high educational attainment. As the education level increases, one expects the specificity of an instrument to rise; an abnormal test result probably really is abnormal because one would expect better performance from an educated person. Conversely, sensitivity goes down as educational level increases; a "normal" or "negative" test result occurs in an impaired person. For example, the sensitivity of the MMSE was 93% in a population with less than an eighth-grade education but fell to 71% for the individual with more than eight grades of schooling.[123,126] Psychometric studies of the MMSE have not revealed strong differential functioning of specific items according to educational status.[127,128]

Lower scores may occur among patients with less education who are not demented.[116,129] Normative data on the MMSE based on age and educational attainment were provided by Crum et al.[116] and in the report from AHCPR.[28] Among persons with 0 to 4 years of education, a cutoff point of 19 represents the 75th percentile (in other words, 75% of community-dwelling adults with 0 to 4 years of education would score below 19 on the MMSE). Corresponding cutoff points are for persons with 5 to 8 years of schooling, 23 and below; for 9 to 12 years of schooling, 27 and below; for schooling at the college level and beyond, 29 and below.[116] The person should be asked how much schooling he or she has had to assist in interpreting scores. It should be remembered that the MMSE and other mental status instruments serve as only one component in assessment of dementia, along with criteria in Exhibit 7–3.

## Short Portable Mental Status Questionnaire

One of the simpler tests widely used to assess mental status is the SPMSQ developed by Pfeiffer.[130] This test comprises 10 questions dealing with orientation, personal history, remote memory, and calculations (Exhibit 7–7). The Kahn-Goldfarb Mental Status Questionnaire[131]

---

**Exhibit 7–7** Short Portable Mental Status Questionnaire (SPMSQ)

1. What is the date today?
2. What day of the week is it?
3. What is the name of this place?
4. What is your telephone number? (If the patient does not have a phone: What is your street address?)
5. How old are you?
6. When were you born?
7. Who is the president of the United States now?
8. Who was the president just before that?
9. What was your mother's maiden name?
10. Subtract 3 from 20 and keep subtracting 3 from each new number you get, all the way down.

*Source:* Adapted with permission from E. Pfeiffer, A short portable mental status questionnaire for the assessment of organic brain deficit in elderly patients, *Journal of the American Geriatric Society*, Vol. 23, pp. 433–441, © 1975, Lippincott Williams & Wilkins.

is also a 10-item instrument; it is the prototype of short mental state examinations and is similar to the SPMSQ.

The final error score of the SPMSQ is modified by various factors. The number 1 is subtracted from the error score if the person has less than a high school education. More than three errors would identify the person as impaired. In the administration of this test, the examiner must keep in mind that the date must be exact, the birth date must be exact, the mother's maiden name does not require verification, and calculations must be done in their entirety and correctly.

A questionnaire such as this is compact, is easy to use, and requires no special materials. It would appear to meet the minimal criteria for face validity, being a mental status examination covering orientation, remote memory, and calculation. There is no task to assess short-term memory. How well the instrument performs for the assessment of cognitive functioning in clinical situations needs to be determined. Compared with a neuropsychiatric examination, how does the SPMSQ fare?

To evaluate the SPMSQ, it is necessary to return to the statistical concepts of sensitivity, specificity, and the predictive value of a positive or negative test discussed previously. When administered to community-dwelling older adults, the specificity is found to be better than 90%.[121,132] The sensitivity, the ability of the test to detect impairment, is not as great and may be as low as 50%.[121] This means that although 90% of normal older persons are identified correctly as not impaired, as few as half of the demented persons are detected. Thus, there are few false-positive results but many false-negative results. In another study, the sensitivity was found to be 82%, but the SPMSQ could not clearly differentiate mildly impaired from normal older persons.[133] Other studies have found good performance of the SPMSQ in clinical settings.[134,135] Fillenbaum et al. examined the performance of the SPMSQ in a large community sample of older adults, finding that SPMSQ scores were less affected by ethnicity and educational level when scoring adjusted for these factors.[136]

If one wished to be sure to detect as many cases of dementia as possible for further assessment, more stringent test requirements might be used. Fewer errors than the recommended four would then be acceptable as indicating a positive test. This was suggested in a Finnish study, which demonstrated that by using three errors as indicative of a positive test, sensitivity increased from 76% to 86%.[132]

Unlike the sensitivity and specificity, the predictive value of a positive and of a negative test result will vary depending on the prevalence of cognitive impairment in the study or practice population. In published data,[121,130] the predictive value of a positive test is around 90%; that of a negative test is 70% to 80%. Thus, in older populations, a positive test, indicating impairment, has a 90% probability of being correct, whereas a negative test has about an 80% chance of being correct (Table 7–3).

Put another way, of those who are determined to be impaired by their score on the SPMSQ, 90% are indeed found to be impaired by a "gold standard," namely, a complete mental status examination and psychiatric evaluation. The predictive value of a normal (i.e., negative) SPMSQ is about 80% in a community-dwelling population of older persons; 20% will have detectable cognitive impairment on more thorough testing. In a nursing home setting, where the prevalence of dementia is presumably higher, the predictive value of a negative test falls to around 70%; thus, 30% with a satisfactory score do not have normal cognitive functioning.

The SPMSQ is entirely verbal and easy to memorize. The clinician may consider supplementing the SPMSQ with the written parts of the mental status examination (e.g., signing name, writing a sentence, and drawing) discussed earlier in this chapter, particularly if the instrument is used as a periodic screening assessment of mental status. A more complete examination would be done if the SPMSQ detects in-

**Table 7–3** Sensitivity, Specificity, and Predictive Value of the Short Portable Mental Status Questionnaire (SPMSQ)

|  | Clinical Examination Consistent with Dementia | Clinical Examination Not Consistent with Dementia |  |
| --- | --- | --- | --- |
| Score indicates impairment | Agrees | False positive | Predictive value of a positive test is up to 90% |
| Score indicates no impairment | False negative | Agrees | Predictive value of a negative test is 70%–80% |
|  | Sensitivity is 50%–82% | Specificity is approximately 90% |  |

Four errors are used as a cutoff score to indicate dementia.

Sources: Data from the Journal of the American Geriatric Society, Vol. 23, pp. 433–441, © 1979; Vol. 27, pp. 263–269, © 1979; Vol, 28, pp. 381–384, © 1980, Lippincott Williams & Wilkins.

tellectual impairment or if the presenting complaint is related to confusion or personality change. In either case, knowledge of the prior performance of the individual is clearly of value.

### Orientation and Nonorientation Items

The SPMSQ and the MMSE rely heavily on questions of orientation. As indicated by the low sensitivity of both tests, the common practice of using orientation-type questions to screen for dementia may miss as many as half of such persons. A brief example illustrates this pitfall of using an interview heavily weighted toward orientation-type questions: A 66-year-old woman presented at the request of her family because of difficulty with memory. The patient's daughter stated that on several occasions the patient had forgotten the names of some family members and friends. The patient was still driving, keeping her checkbook, cooking, and performing the usual activities of daily living. Her SPMSQ score was 10 (no errors). Further mental status testing revealed she could not recall three items, copy a simple diagram, or write an organized sentence. Thus, orientation-type questions alone failed to identify a problem. Had just the SPMSQ been given, the intellectual deficits would have remained undetected.

Klein et al. reported on the sensitivity and specificity of various components of the MMSE.[137] The components of the examination were divided into two broad categories: orientation items (i.e., does the person know the day, month, year, city, and hospital?) and nonorientation items (i.e., can the person subtract 7 serially from 100, spell the word "world" backward, and recall three items after 5 minutes?).

Items of orientation had uniformly low sensitivity. Demented persons not uncommonly were oriented and therefore would have been missed by the unwary examiner using this type of question exclusively. Examiners need to recall that low sensitivity means that a low proportion of those with dementia is actually detected by the test. On the other hand, nonorientation items were highly sensitive in detecting dementia, but because many normal older persons also encountered difficulty with these items, the specificity was low. Recall that low specificity means that a low proportion of normal persons is identified as "normal" by the test. The clinical importance of this distinction between orientation and nonorientation items lies in interpreting the answers to the items (Table 7–4). The individual who knows where he or she is and the date may still be intellectually impaired.

**Table 7–4** Sensitivity and Specificity of Orientation and Nonorientation Items of the Mental Status Examination

| Item | Sensitivity (%) | Specificity (%) |
|---|---|---|
| *Orientation items* | | |
| Day | 52.8 | 91.7 |
| Month | 56.9 | 96.5 |
| Year | 51.4 | 98.6 |
| City | 15.3 | 100.0 |
| Hospital | 20.8 | 100.0 |
| *Nonorientation items* | | |
| Serial 7s (to 79) | 97.2 | 50.0 |
| "World" spelled backward | 94.4 | 61.8 |
| Recall of all three items | 97.2 | 43.1 |
| Recall of at least two items | 80.6 | 74.3 |
| Serial 7s (to 79) or "world" backward and recall of at least two items | 100.0 | 49.3 |

*Source:* Reprinted with permission from LE Klein et al., Univariate and multivariate analyses of the mental state examination, *Journal of the American Geriatric Society*, Vol. 33, pp. 483–488, © 1985, Lippincott Williams & Wilkins.

## Cognitive Capacity Screen

A 30-question Cognitive Capacity Screen[138] was used in the detection of "organic brain syndromes" in patients with medical illness (Exhibit 7–8). Those patients with scores of less than 20 (maximum score of 30) were more likely to meet clinical criteria for dementia. A low test score could reflect a condition other than dementia, of course, such as a low educational level. Conversely, a high test score would not exclude the possibility of a focal abnormality. Most psychiatric patients tested scored greater than 20 on the test. The scale is a bit more cumbersome than the SPMSQ or the MMSE but includes some areas not tested by others, such as abstraction ability (Questions 18 and 19 deal with similarities).

A high proportion of hospitalized patients given the Cognitive Capacity Screen were found to be impaired, as indicated by a score of less than 20. The same study found that 11 patients in the control group (18%) also scored less than 20; however, when these patients were examined carefully, only one met the criteria for dementia.[139] The investigators did not examine the patients with a normal score to see whether any demented patients were missed.

**Exhibit 7–8** Cognitive Capacity Screen

1. What day of the week is this?
2. What month?
3. What day of the month?
4. What year?
5. What place is this?
6. Repeat these numbers: 8 7 2.
7. Say them backward.
8. Repeat these numbers: 6 3 7 1.
9. Listen to these numbers: 6 9 4. Count 1 through 10 out loud, then repeat 6 9 4. (Help if needed. Then use numbers 5 7 3.)
10. Listen to these numbers: 8 1 4 3. Count 1 through 10 out loud, then repeat 8 1 4 3.
11. Beginning with Sunday, say the days of the week backward.
12. 9 plus 3 is?
13. Add 6 (to the previous answer or "to 12").
14. Take away 5 ("from 18").

Repeat these words after me and remember them; I will ask for them later: HAT, CAR, TREE, TWENTY-SIX.

15. The opposite of fast is slow. The opposite of up is _____ .
16. The opposite of large is _____ .
17. The opposite of hard is _____ .
18. An orange and a banana are both fruits. Red and blue are both _____ .
19. A penny and a dime are both _____ .
20. What were those words I asked you to remember? (HAT)
21. (CAR)
22. (TREE)
23. (TWENTY-SIX)
24. Take away 7 from 100, then take away 7 from what is left and keep going: 100 minus 7 is ____ .
25. Minus 7 ____ .
26. Minus 7 ____ . (Write down answers; check correct subtraction of 7)
27. Minus 7 ____ .
28. Minus 7 ____ .
29. Minus 7 ____ .
30. Minus 7 ____ .

Total correct (maximum score: 30) ____ .

*Source:* Reproduced, with permission from: J Jacobs et al., Screening for organic mental syndromes in the medically ill, *Annals of Internal Medicine*, © 1977; 86: pp. 40–46, American College of Physicians.

On a neuropsychologic service, the Cognitive Capacity Screen had a sensitivity of 49% and a specificity of 90%.[125] The sensitivity was increased when the examination was combined with a Memory for Designs test, which identified the patients with right hemispheric lesions missed by the Cognitive Capacity Screen. It was suggested that the Cognitive Capacity Screen misses right hemispheric lesions (only two of the seven patients with such lesions were detected by the test). Patients with diffuse brain injury may be easier to detect with screening instruments because patients with focal lesions may have deficits that the test does not elicit.[125]

The propensity to miss structural lesions was emphasized in a study comparing results on the Cognitive Capacity Screen with those found on neurologic examination. The sensitivity in consecutive admissions to a neurologic service was 73%; the specificity was 90%.[138] The predictive value of a positive test was 93%; that of a negative test was 67%. Of nine patients with a false-negative test, five were found to have a moderate degree of dementia, and all nine had focal (or multifocal) cerebral disease such as brain tumor or abscess. Seven of these patients had obvious neurologic deficits, such as hemiparesis.

## Kokmen Short Test of Mental Status

The Kokmen Short Test of Mental Status attempts to sample a wide range of intellectual tasks, including some not tested by the SPMSQ and the MMSE, such as abstraction.[35] This assessment instrument (Exhibit 7–9) was given to 93 "nondemented" patients on a general neurologic consult service and to 87 demented persons living at home. The latter group included 67 individuals with Alzheimer's disease. When a score of 29 points or less was used to classify a patient as demented (total maximum score is 38), the sensitivity to detect dementia was 95.5%, and the specificity was 91.4%. The Kokmen Short Test of Mental Status as well as the next instrument to be discussed was included with others as recommended tools in the AHCPR guidelines on Alzheimer's disease.[28]

## Orientation-Memory-Concentration Test

A six-item Orientation-Memory-Concentration (OMC) Test (Exhibit 7–10) with weighted items has shown that 90% of older persons without mental impairment have a weighted error score of 6 or less.[140]

**Exhibit 7–9** The Kokmen Short Test of Mental Status

*Orientation*
  Full name, address, building, city, state, day of the week or month, month, year.
Score one point for each correct response.
  Maximum: 8

*Attention*
  Digit repetition (start with five, go to six and then seven if correct). Record the
best performance and score the number of digits repeated forward correctly.
  Maximum: 7

*Learning*
  Remember the following: apple, Mr. Johnson, charity, tunnel. Give a maximum
of four trials to learn all words and record the number of words learned and the
number of trials to learn them. Score one point per word learned but subtract one
less than the number of trials to do so from the number of words learned.
  Maximum: 4

*Arithmetic calculation*
  Do the following: 5 times 13, 65 minus 7, 58 divided by 2, and 11 plus 29. Score
one point for each correct answer.
  Maximum: 4

*Abstraction*
  How are the following alike? An orange and a banana, a horse and a dog, a table
and a bookcase. Score one point for each definitely abstract answer.
  Maximum: 3

*Information*
Who is the President now?
Who was the first President?
How many weeks are there in a year?
Define "island."
Score one point for each correct answer.
  Maximum: 4

*Construction*
  Draw the face of a clock showing 11:15 and copy a picture of a three-dimensional
cube (which the patient may view while copying). Score, for each drawing, two
points for an adequate conceptual drawing, one for a less than complete drawing,
and zero if the patient is unable to perform the task.
  Maximum: 4

*Recall*
  Recall the four items from the learning task. Score one point for each word recalled.
  Maximum: 4

*Source:* Adapted with permission from E Kokmen et al, *Mayo Clinics Proceedings*, Vol. 62, pp. 282–283, © 1987, Mayo Foundation.

**Exhibit 7–10** Orientation-Memory-Concentration Test

| Items | Maximum Error | Score | Weight | Total |
|---|---|---|---|---|
| 1. What year is it now? | 1 | _____ | × 4 | _____ |
| 2. What month is it now? | 1 | _____ | × 3 | _____ |
| Memory phrase. Repeat this phrase after me: John Brown, 42 Market Street, Chicago | | | | |
| 3. About what time is it? (within one hour) | 1 | _____ | × 3 | _____ |
| 4. Count backward from 20 to 1. | 2 | _____ | × 2 | _____ |
| 5. Say the months in reverse order. | 2 | _____ | × 2 | _____ |
| 6. Repeat the memory phrase. | 5 | _____ | × 2 | _____ |
| | | | Total score: | _____ |

   Score one point for each incorrect response; maximum weighted error score equals 28. Over 90% of normal elders have a weighted score of 6 or less. Scores greater than 10 are suggestive of mental impairment.

   *Source: American Journal of Psychiatry*, Vol. 140, p. 739, 1983. Copyright © 1983, the American Psychiatric Association. Reprinted by permission.

Weighted error scores of 10 or more were consistent with the presence of dementia in most patients. The memory phrase and the months backward questions are among the first items to be answered wrong as dementia develops. The OMC Test certainly is an example of a test that is short and convenient for use by the primary care practitioner. In a comparison with the SPMSQ, the OMC Test performed favorably but identified more older persons as cognitively impaired.[136] Test scores from this short instrument were highly correlated to scores from the longer MMSE and may be highly suitable for use in primary care settings.[141–143]

## Category Fluency

   The test of category fluency, or the set test, is a simple test in which one asks the person to name as many items as he or she can in each of four sets or categories.[144] The four sets are fruits, animals, colors, and towns. A maximum of 10 is allowed in each set for a maximum score of 40. The test is not timed. A score of less than 15 is abnormal, and 80% of demented older persons scored in this range. Conversely, no one with an affective disorder scored less than 15, and only 2 of 146 ostensibly normal older persons did so (1%). This certainly compares favorably with the tests outlined earlier.

The value of the set test was demonstrated in a University of Iowa study.[145] Simply stated, eight psychologic tests were given to a group of normal older persons and to a group with the diagnosis of dementia. The investigators then proceeded to determine which tests best differentiated the two groups. Two items stood out in discrimination ability. One was the ability to remember designs, and the other task was a variation of the set test (i.e., the production of a list of words beginning with a given target letter). Presented as a "school-type" test in the examination of the nervous system, the set test would seem to be less likely to offend most older patients. Category fluency is sometimes considered a measure of executive functioning, that is, indicative of frontal lobe functioning.

## Clock-Drawing Task

In the clock-drawing task, the individual is presented with a pen and a piece of paper on which a 4- to 6-inch circle is drawn and asked to write the numbers and draw the hands of the clock to show "10 past 11." Although there are several versions of the clock-drawing task (e.g., differing in whether the circle outline is provided or must be drawn by the person and the time to be represented), the clock-drawing task may be useful in eliciting some signs of cognitive impairment and assessing persons with dementia.[53–59,146–148] The clock-drawing task no doubt taps into multiple cognitive and motor functions rather than attempting to assess specific domains, such as memory, and serves as a practical method of screening and assessment that is acceptable to most people. Patients with left-sided hemispheric damage may tend to get the "gestalt" of the clock correct (e.g., there are lines at the 12, 3, 6, and 9 o'clock positions, but no numbers) because of language deficits. Right-sided lesions may result in clocks with readable numbers that are grouped all to one side. Clocks drawn by persons with Alzheimer's disease may exhibit all of these and other features, such as perseveration (repetition of the same number all around the clock).

A qualitative evaluation of changes noted by reviewing the dated drawings in the medical record will be sufficient in most clinical applications. However, investigators have provided scales to rank the drawing for completeness and correctness[54] or to rate specific components of the clock drawn and combine the ratings into a score. The clock-drawing interpretation scale recommended by Mendez et al.[55] falls into this latter category (Exhibit 7–11). Other scoring methods are found in other sources.[56,57,148,149] Simplified and more objective methods than the Mendez scoring criteria have been suggested,[57,148] but none is standard.

Persons with Alzheimer's disease and other dementias score significantly worse than older adults without dementia,[53-55] and when a scoring threshold is used, the clock-drawing task shows good sensitivity and specificity in comparison with a diagnosis of dementia.[57] The clock-drawing task was found to be highly sensitive and specific for moderate to severe cognitive impairment in a large representative

---

**Exhibit 7–11** Clock-Drawing Interpretation Scale

Ask the patient to draw a clock and indicate the time as "ten after eleven." Score one point for each item.
1. There is an attempt to indicate a time in some way.
2. All marks or items can be classified as part of a closure figure, a hand, or a symbol for clock numbers.
3. There is a totally closed figure without gaps (closure figure).

Score only if symbols for clock numbers are present.
4. A "2" is present and is pointed out in some way for the time.
5. Most symbols are distributed as a circle without major gaps.
6. Three or more clock quadrants have one or more appropriate numbers: 12–3, 3–6, 6–9, and 9–12 per respective clockwise quadrant.
7. Most symbols are ordered in a clockwise or rightward direction.
8. All symbols are totally within a closure figure.
9. An "11" is present and is pointed out in some way for the time.
10. All numbers 1–12 are indicated.
11. There are no repeated or duplicated number symbols.
12. There are no substitutions for Arabic or Roman numerals.
13. The numbers do not go beyond the number 12.
14. All symbols lie about equally adjacent to a closure figure edge.
15. Seven or more of the same symbol type are ordered sequentially.

Score only if one or more hands are present.
16. All hands radiate from the direction of a closure figure center.
17. One hand is visibly longer than another hand.
18. There are exactly two distinct and separable hands.
19. All hands are totally within a closure figure.
20. There is an attempt to indicate a time with one or more hands.

*Source:* Adapted with permission from MF Mendez et al., Development of scoring criteria for the clock-drawing task in Alzheimer's disease, *Journal of the American Geriatric Society,* Vol. 40, pp. 1095–1099, © 1992, Lippincott Williams & Wilkins.

sample of adults aged 75 years and older.[150] Poor scores were associated with increased rates of death after 5 years of follow-up. Unfortunately, the clock-drawing task may not be immune to an effect of the level of educational attainment of the patient. Mean scores of patients with more education were higher than scores of persons with less than 9 years of schooling.[146] There is a need for more standardization of the administration and scoring of the clock-drawing task. This task may be thought of as a supplement to other mental status assessment instruments such as the MMSE.[148]

## SUMMARY OF MENTAL STATUS ASSESSMENT

Assessing the mental status of patients is important, especially on initial workup for an older adult admitted to a hospital or nursing home and whenever behavior, mental status, or level of functioning is a cause for concern. Changes in mental state can be more confidently assessed when a baseline has been established. Assessment of mental status must be considered within the context of the individual's functional status, the physical examination (especially vision and hearing), the history from an informant, and the total clinical picture. Mental status questionnaires can be used in combination with the written parts of the mental status examination to provide a record of performance for the medical chart; the record can then be used for following the progression of cognitive impairment or as a baseline assessment. Some persons will need more careful delineation of mental status and would benefit from formal neuropsychologic testing, particularly when presentation or course does not follow expected patterns.

### REFERENCES

1. Shepherd M, Cooper B, Brown AC, Kalton GW. *Psychiatric Illness in General Practice*. London: Oxford University Press; 1966.

2. Regier DA, Narrow WE, Rae DS, Manderscheid RW, Locke BZ, Goodwin FK. The de facto US mental and addictive disorders system: Epidemiologic Catchment Area prospective 1-year prevalence rates of disorders and services. *Arch Gen Psychiatry*. 1993;50:85–94.

3. Gallo JJ, Marino S, Ford D, Anthony JC. Filters on the pathway to mental health care: II: Sociodemographic factors. *Psychol Med*. 1995;25:1149–1160.

4. Cooper-Patrick L, Gallo JJ, Powe NR, Steinwachs DM, Eaton WW, Ford DE. Mental health service utilization by African-Americans and whites: The Baltimore Epidemiologic Catchment Area Follow-Up. *Medical Care*. 1999;37:1034–1045.

5. Wang PS, Berglund P, Kessler RC. Recent care of common mental disorders in the United States. *J Gen Intern Med*. 2000;15:284–292.

6. Gallo JJ, Marino S, Ford D, Anthony JC. Filters on the pathway to mental health care: II: Sociodemographic factors. *Pyschol Med*. 1995;25:1149–1160.

7. Snowden LR, Pingitore D. Frequency and scope of mental health service delivery to African Americans in primary care. *Ment Health Serv Res*. 2002;4:123–130.

8. Sager MA, Dunham NC, Schwantes A, Mecum L, Halverson K, Harlowe D. Measurement of activities of daily living in hospitalized elderly: A comparison of self-report and performance-based methods. *J Am Geriatr Soc*. 1992;40:457–462.

9. Jacobs J, Bernhard MR, Delgado A, et al. Screening for organic mental syndromes in the medically ill. *Ann Intern Med*. 1977;86:40–46.

10. McCartney JR, Palmatee LM. Assessment of cognitive deficit in geriatric patients: A study of physician behavior. *J Am Geriatr Soc*. 1985;33:467–471.

11. Callahan CM, Hendrie HC, Tierney WM. Documentation and evaluation of cognitive impairment in elderly primary care patients. *Ann Intern Med*. 1995;122: 422–429.

12. Larson EB. Recognition of dementia: Discovering the silent epidemic. *J Am Geriatr Soc*. 1998;46:1576–1577.

13. Iliffe S, Booroff A, Gallivan S, Goldenberg E, Morgan P, Haines A. Screening for cognitive impairment in the elderly using the mini-mental state examination. *Br J Gen Pract*. 1990;40:277–279.

14. Cooper B, Eastwood R. *Primary Health Care and Psychiatric Epidemiology*. New York: Tavistock/Routledge; 1992.

15. Cooper B, Bickel H. Population screening and the early detection of dementing disorders in old age: A review. *Psychol Med*. 1984;14:81–95.

16. Ross GW, Abbott RD, Petrovitch H. Frequency and characteristics of silent dementia among elderly Japanese-American men. *JAMA*. 1997;277:800–805.

17. Valcour VG, Masaki KH, Curb JD, Blanchette PL. The detection of dementia in the primary care setting. *Arch Intern Med*. 2000;160:2964–2968.

18. Schneider LS, Reynolds CF, Lebowitz BD, Friedhoff AJ. *Diagnosis and Treatment of Depression in Late Life: Results of the NIH Consensus Development Conference*. Washington, DC: American Psychiatric Association; 1994.

19. Francis J, Kapoor WN. Prognosis after hospital discharge of older medical patients with delirium. *J Am Geriatr Soc*. 1992;40:601–606.

20. Marcantonio ER, Goldman L, Mangione CM, et al. A clinical prediction rule for delirium after elective noncardiac surgery. *JAMA*. 1994;271:134–139.

21. Fields SD, MacKenzie R, Charlson ME, et al. Cognitive impairment: Can it predict the course of hospitalized patients? *J Am Geriatr Soc*. 1986;34:579–585.

22. Murray AM, Levkoff SE, Wetle TT, et al. Acute delirium and functional decline in the hospitalized elderly patient. *J Gerontol*. 1993;48:M181–M186.

23. O'Keeffe ST, Lavan JN. Predicting delirium in elderly patients: Development and validation of a risk-stratification model. *Age Ageing*. 1996;25:317–321.

24. Inouye SK, Charpentier PA. Precipitating factors for delirium in hospitalized elderly persons: Predictive model and interrelationship with baseline vulnerability. *JAMA*. 1996;275:852–857.

25. Cooper JK, Mungas D, Weiler PG. Relation of cognitive status and abnormal behaviors in Alzheimer's disease. *J Am Geriatr Soc*. 1990;38:867–870.

26. Henderson AS, Huppert FA. The problem of mild dementia. *Psychol Med*. 1984;14:5–11.

27. Warshaw G. Are mental status questionnaires of clinical value in everyday office practice? An affirmative view. *J Fam Pract*. 1990;30:194–197.

28. Costa PT, Williams TF, Somerfield M, et al. *Early Identification of Alzheimer's Disease and Related Dementias, Clinical Practice Guidelines, No 19*. Rockville, MD: US Department of Health and Human Services, Public Health Service, Agency for Health Care Policy and Research; 1996. AHCPR Publication Number 97-0703.

29. Kapp MB, Bigot A. *Geriatrics and the Law*. New York: Springer Publishing; 1985.

30. Auerbach SH, Cicerone KD, Levin HS, Tranel D. What you can learn from neuropsychologic testing. *Patient Care*. 1994;28:97–116.

31. Strub RL, Black FW. *The Mental Status Examination in Neurology*, 2nd ed. Philadelphia: FA Davis; 1985.

32. Jones TV, Williams ME. Rethinking the approach to evaluating mental functioning of older persons: The value of careful observations. *J Am Geriatr Soc*. 1988;36: 1128–1134.

33. Fry PS. *Depression, Stress, and Adaptations in the Elderly: Psychological Assessment and Intervention*. Rockville, MD: Aspen Publishers, 1986.

34. Feher EP, Doody R, Pirozzolo FJ, Appel SH. Mental status assessment of insight and judgment. *Clin Geriatr Med*. 1989;5:477–498.

35. Kokmen E, Naessens JM, Offord KP. A short test of mental status: Description and preliminary results. *Mayo Clin Proc*. 1987;62:281–288.

36. Mattis S. Mental status examination for organic mental syndrome in the elderly patient. In Bellak L, Karasu TB, eds. *Geriatric Psychiatry*. New York: Grune & Stratton; 1976:77–121.

37. LaRue A. Memory loss and aging: Distinguishing dementia from benign senescent forgetfulness and depressive pseudodementia. *Psychiatr Clin N Am*. 1982;5:89–103.

38. Blum JE, Jarvik LF, Clark ET. Rate of change on selective tests of intelligence: A twenty-year longitudinal study of aging. *J Gerontol*. 1970;25:171–176.

39. Gallo JJ, Stanley L, Zack N, Reichel W. Multi-dimensional assessment of the older patient. In: Reichel W, ed. *Clinical Aspects of Aging*, 4th ed. Baltimore: Williams & Wilkins; 1995:15–30.

40. Erilsen CW, Hamlin RM, Daye C. Aging adults and rate of memory scan. *Bull Psychon Soc*. 1973;1:259–260.

41. Smith ME. Delayed recall of previously memorized material after fifty years. *J Gen Psychol*. 1963;102:3–4.

42. Grut M, Jorm AF, Fratiglioni L, Forsell Y, Viitanen M, Winblad B. Memory complaints of elderly people in a population survey: Variation according to dementia stage and depression. *J Am Geriatr Soc*. 1993;41:1295–1300.

43. Crook T, Bartus RT, Ferris SH, et al. Age-associated memory impairment: Proposed diagnostic criteria and measures of clinical change: Report of a National Institute of Mental Health work group. *Dev Neuropsychol*. 1986;2:261–276.

44. Kral VA. Senescent forgetfulness: Benign and malignant. *J Can Med Assoc*. 1962; 86:257–260.

45. Rediess S, Caine ED. Aging-associated cognitive changes: How do they relate to the diagnosis of dementia? *Curr Opin Psychiatry*. 1993;6:531–536.

46. Working Party of the International Psychogeriatric Association in collaboration with the World Health Organization. Aging-associated cognitive decline. *Int Psychogeriatr*. 1994;6:63–68.

47. Blackford RC, La Rue A. Criteria for diagnosing age-associated memory impairment: Proposed improvements from the field. *Dev Neuropsychol.* 1989;5:295–306.

48. Small GW, Okonek A, Mandelkern MA, et al. Age-associated memory loss: Initial neuropsychological and cerebral metabolic findings of a longitudinal study. *Int Psychogeriatr.* 1994;6:23–44.

49. Huppert FA, Brayne C, O'Connor DW. *Dementia and Normal Aging.* Cambridge, Cambridge University Press; 1994.

50. American Psychiatric Association. *Diagnostic and Statistical Manual of Mental Disorders,* 4th ed. Washington, DC: American Psychiatric Association; 1994.

51. Blazer DG. *Depression in Late Life,* 2nd ed. St. Louis: CV Mosby; 1993.

52. Damasio AR. Aphasia. *N Engl J Med.* 1992;326:531–539.

53. Wolf-Klein GP, Silverstone FA, Levy AP, Brod MS. Screening for Alzheimer's disease by clock drawing. *J Am Geriatr Soc.* 1989;37:730–737.

54. Sunderland T, Hill JL, Mellow AM, et al. Clock drawing in Alzheimer's disease: A novel measure of dementia severity. *J Am Geriatr Soc.* 1989;37:725–729.

55. Mendez MF, Ala T, Underwood KL. Development of scoring criteria for the clock drawing task in Alzheimer's disease. *J Am Geriatr Soc.* 1992;40:1095–1099.

56. Tuokko H, Hadjistavropoulos T, Miller JA, Beattie BL. The clock test: A sensitive measure to differentiate normal elderly from those with Alzheimer's disease. *J Am Geriatr Soc.* 1992;40:579–584.

57. Watson YI, Arfken CL, Birge SJ. Clock completion: An objective screening test for dementia. *J Am Geriatr Soc.* 1993;41:1235–1240.

58. Shuttleworth EC. Memory function and the clinical differentiation of dementing disorders. *J Am Geriatr Soc.* 1982;30:363–366.

59. Lipowski ZJ. Delirium (acute confusional states). *JAMA.* 1987;258:1789–1792.

60. Inouye SK, van Dyck CH, Alessi CA, Balkin S, Siegal AP, Horwitz RJ. Clarifying confusion: The confusion assessment method: A new method for detection of delirium. *Ann Intern Med.* 1990;113:941–948.

61. Larson EB, Reifler BV, Featherstone HJ, et al. Dementia in elderly outpatients: A prospective study. *Ann Intern Med.* 1984;100:417–423.

62. Maletta GJ. The concept of "reversible" dementia: How nonreliable terminology may impair effective treatment. *J Am Geriatr Soc.* 1990;38:136–140.

63. Cummings JL, Benson DF. *Dementia: A Clinical Approach,* 2nd ed. Stoneham, MA: Butterworth-Heinemann; 1992.

64. McKhann G, Drachman D, Folstein M, et al. Clinical diagnosis of Alzheimer's disease: Report of the NINCDS-ADRDA work group under the auspices of Department of Health and Human Services Task Force on Alzheimer's Disease. *Neurology.* 1984;34:939–944.

65. Cummings JL, Benson DF. Dementia of the Alzheimer type: An inventory of diagnostic clinical features. *J Am Geriatr Soc.* 1986;34:12–19.

66. Coen RF, O'Mahoney D, Bruce I, Lawlor BA, Walsh JB, Coakley D. Differential diagnosis of dementia: A prospective evaluation of the DAT inventory. *J Am Geriatr Soc.* 1994;42:16–20.

67. Emery VOB, Gillie EX, Smith JA. Reclassification of the vascular dementias: Comparisons of infarct and noninfarct vascular dementias. *Int Psychogeriatr.* 1996; 8:33–61.

68. Larson EB. Illness causing dementia in the very elderly. *N Engl J Med.* 1993;328: 203–205.

69. Skoog I. Risk factors for vascular dementia: A review. *Dementia.* 1994;5:137–144.

70. Yao H, Sadoshima S, Ibayashi S. Leukoariosis and dementia in hypertensive patients. *Stroke.* 1992;23:1673–1677.

71. Breteler MM, van Swieten JC, Bots ML. Cerebral white matter lesions, vascular risk factors, and cognitive function in a population-based study: The Rotterdam Study. *Neurology.* 1994;44:1246–1252.

72. Breteler MM, van Amerongen NM, van Swieten JC. Cognitive correlates of ventricular enlargement and cerebral white matter lesions on magnetic resonance imaging: The Rotterdam Study. *Stroke.* 1994;25:1109–1115.

73. Manolio TA, Kronmal RA, Burke GL. Magnetic resonance abnormalities and cardiovascular disease in older adults. *Stroke.* 1994;25:318–327.

74. De Reuck J, Crevitz L, De Coster W. Pathogenesis of Biswanger chronic progressive subcortical encephalopathy. *Neurology.* 1980;30:920–928.

75. Awad IA, Johnson PC, Spetzler RF, Hodak JA. Incidental subcortical lesions identified on magnetic resonance imaging in the elderly: II: Postmortem pathological correlations. *Stroke.* 1986;17:1090–1097.

76. Chimowitz MI, Estes ML, Furlan AJ, Awad IA. Further observations on the pathology of subcortical lesions identified on magnetic resonance imaging. *Arch Neurol.* 1992;49:747–752.

77. Price TR, Manolio TA, Kronmal RA, et al. Silent brain infarction on magnetic resonance imaging and neurological abnormalities in community-dwelling older adults: The Cardiovascular Health Study, CHS Collaborative Group. *Stroke.* 1997;28:1158–1164.

78. Ferrucci L, Guralnik JM, Salive ME, et al. Cognitive impairment and risk of stroke in the older population. *J Am Geriatr Soc.* 1996;44:237–241.

79. Snowdon DA. Aging and Alzheimer's disease: Lessons from the Nun Study. *Gerontologist.* 1997;37:150–156.

80. Berrios GE. Dementia. In: Berrios GE, Porter R, eds. *A History of Clinical Psychiatry: The Origin and History of Psychiatric Disorders.* Washington Square, NY: New York University Press; 1995:34–51.

81. Dening TR. Stroke and other vascular disorders. In: Berrios GE, Porter R, eds. *A History of Clinical Psychiatry: The Origin and History of Psychiatric Disorders.* Washington Square, NY: New York University Press; 1995:72–85.

82. Devasenapathy A, Hachinski V. Vascular cognitive impairment: A new approach. In: Holmes C, Howard R, eds. *Advances in Old Age Psychiatry: Chromosomes to Community Care.* Bristol, PA: Wrightson Biomedical Publishing; 1997:79–95.

83. Steingart A, Hachinski VC, Lau C, et al. Cognitive and neurologic findings in demented patients with diffuse white matter lucencies on computed tomographic scan (leuko-ariosis). *Arch Neurol.* 1987;44:36–39.

84. Hofman A, Ott A, Breteler MMB, et al. Atherosclerosis, apolipoprotein E, and prevalence of dementia and Alzheimer's disease in the Rotterdam Study. *Lancet.* 1997; 349:151–154.

85. Snowdon DA, Greiner LH, Mortimer JA, Riley KP, Greiner PA, Markesbery WR. Brain infarction and the clinical expression of Alzheimer's disease: The Nun Study. *JAMA.* 1997;277:813–817.

86. Alexopoulos GS, Meyers BS, Young RC, Campbell S, Silbersweig D, Charlson M. "Vascular depression" hypothesis. *Arch Gen Psychiatry.* 1997;54:915–922.

87. Emery VOB, Gillie EX, Smith JA. Reclassification of the vascular dementias: Comparisons of infarct and noninfarct vascular dementias. *Int Psychogeriatr.* 1996;8:33–61.

88. Olsen CG, Clasen ME. Senile dementia of the Binswanger's type. *Am Fam Physician.* 1998;58:2068–2074.

89. Bennett DA, Wilson RS, Gilley DW, Fox JH. Clinical diagnosis of Binswanger's disease. *J Neurol Neurosurg Psychiatry.* 1990;53:1–5.

90. Roman GC. Senile dementia of the Binswanger type: A vascular form of dementia in the elderly. *JAMA.* 1987;258:1782–1788.

91. Mahler ME, Cummings JL, Tomiyasu U. Atypical dementia syndrome in an elderly man. *J Am Geriatr Soc.* 1987;35:1116–1126.

92. Meyer JS, Judd BW, Tawakina T, et al. Improved cognition after control of risk factors for multi-infarct dementia. *JAMA.* 1986;256:2203–2209.

93. Hachinski VC, Iliff LD, Zilhka E, et al. Cerebral blood flow in dementia. *Ann Neurol.* 1975;32:632–637.

94. Liston EH, LaRue A. Clinical differentiation of primary degenerative and multi-infarct dementia: A critical review of the evidence: II: Pathological studies. *Biol Psychiatry.* 1983;18:1467–1484.

95. Whitehouse PJ. The concept of subcortical and cortical dementia: Another look. *Ann Neurol.* 1986;19:1–6.

96. McKeith IG. Dementia with Lewy bodies. In: Holmes C, Howard R, eds. *Advances in Old Age Psychiatry: Chromosomes to Community Care.* Bristol, PA: Wrightson Biomedical Publishing; 1997:52–63.

97. McKeith LG, Galasko D, Kosaka K. Consensus guidelines for the clinical and pathologic diagnosis of dementia with Lewy bodies (DLB): Report of the Consortium on DLB International Workshop. *Neurology.* 1996;47:1113–1124.

98. Clarfield AM, Larson EB. Should a major imaging procedure (CT or MRI) be required in the workup of dementia? An opposing view. *J Fam Pract.* 1990;31:405–410.

99. Beresford TP. Alcoholism in the elderly. *Int Rev Psychiatry.* 1993;5:477–483.

100. Brody JA. Aging and alcohol abuse. *J Am Geriatr Soc.* 1982;30:123–126.

101. Gottheil E, Druley KA, Skoloda TE. *The Combined Problems of Alcoholism, Drug Addiction, and Aging.* Springfield, IL: Charles C. Thomas; 1985.

102. Wattis JP. Alcohol problems in the elderly. *J Am Geriatr Soc.* 1981;29:131–134.

103. Zimberg S. Alcohol abuse among the elderly. In: Carstensen LL, Edelstein BA, eds. *Handbook of Clinical Gerontology.* New York: Pergamon Press; 1987:57–65.

104. Widner S, Zeichner A. Alcohol abuse in the elderly: Review of epidemiology research and treatment. *Clin Gerontol.* 1991;11:3–18.

105. Moss RJ, Miles SH. AIDS and the geriatrician. *J Am Geriatr Soc.* 1987;35:460–464.

106. Sabin TD. AIDS: The new "great imitator" [editorial]. *J Am Geriatr Soc.* 1987;35: 467–468.

107. Larson EB, Reifler BV, Sumi SM, et al. Diagnostic evaluation of 200 elderly outpatients with suspected dementia. *J Gerontol.* 1985;40:536–543.

108. National Center for Cost Containment. *Geropsychology Assessment Resource Guide.* Milwaukee, WI: US Department of Commerce, National Technical Information Service; 1993.

109. McDowell I, Newell C. *Measuring Health: A Guide to Rating Scales and Questionnaires,* 2nd ed. New York: Oxford University Press; 1996.

110. Froehlich TE, Robison JT, Inouye SK. Screening for dementia in the outpatient setting: The time and change test. *J Am Geriatr Soc.* 1998;46:1506–1511.

111. Solomon PR, Pendlebury WW. Recognition of Alzheimer's disease: The 7-minute screen. *Fam Med.* 1998;30:265–271.

112. Lorentz WJ, Scanlan JM, Borson S. Brief screening tests for dementia. *Can J Psychiatry.* 2002;47:723–733.

113. Keating HJ. "Studying" for the Mini-Mental Status Exam [letter]. *J Am Geriatr Soc.* 1987;35:594–595.

114. Folstein MF, Folstein SE, McHugh PR. "Mini-Mental State": A practical method for grading the cognitive state of patients for the clinician. *J Psychiatr Res.* 1975;12:189–198.

115. Tombaugh TN, McIntyre NJ. The Mini-Mental State Examination: A comprehensive review. *J Am Geriatr Soc.* 1992;40:922–935.

116. Crum RM, Anthony JC, Bassett SS, Folstein MF. Population-based norms for the Mini-Mental State Examination by age and educational level. *JAMA.* 1993;269:2386–2391.

117. Jones RN, Gallo JJ. Dimensions of the Mini-Mental State Examination among community dwelling older adults. *Psychol Med.* 2000;30:605–618.

118. Gallo JJ, Anthony JC. Misperception in the scoring of the MMSE [letter]. *Can J Psychiatry.* 1994;39:382.

119. Brandt J, Spencer M, Folstein M. The telephone interview for cognitive status. *Neuropsychiatry Neuropsychol Behav Neurol.* 1988;1:11–17.

120. Tsai L, Tsuang MT. The Mini-Mental State test and computerized tomography. *Am J Psychiatry.* 1979;136:436–439.

121. Fillenbaum G. Comparison of two brief tests of organic brain impairment, the MSQ and the short portable MSQ. *J Am Geriatr Soc.* 1980;28:381–384.

122. Roth M, Tym E, Mountjoy CQ, et al. CAMDEX: A standardised instrument for the diagnosis of mental disorder in the elderly with special reference to the early detection of dementia. *Br J Psychiatry.* 1986;149:698–709.

123. Anthony JC, LeResche L, Niaz U, von Korff M, Folstein MF. Limits of the "Mini-Mental State" as a screening test for dementia and delirium among hospital patients. *Psychol Med.* 1982;12:397–408.

124. Dick JPR, Guiloff RJ, Stewart A, et al. Mini-Mental State Examination in neurological patients. *J Neurol Neurosurg Psychiatry.* 1984;47:496–499.

125. Webster JS, Scott RR, Nunn B, et al. A brief neuropsychological screening procedure that assesses left and right hemispheric function. *J Clin Psychol.* 1984;40:237–240.

126. Kittner SJ, White LR, Farmer ME, et al. Methodological issues in screening for dementia: The problem of education adjustment. *J Chronic Dis.* 1986;39:163–170.

127. Jones RN, Gallo JJ. Education and sex differences in the Mini-Mental State Examination: Effects of differential item functioning. *J Gerontol Psychol Sci.* 2002;57:548–558.

128. Jones RN, Gallo JJ. Education bias in the Mini-Mental State Examination. *Int Psychogeriatr.* 2001;13:299–310.

129. Uhlmann RF, Larson EB. Effect of education on the Mini-Mental State Examination as a screening test for dementia. *J Am Geriatr Soc.* 1991;39:876–880.

130. Pfeiffer E. A short portable mental status questionnaire for the assessment of organic brain deficit in elderly patients. *J Am Geriatr Soc.* 1975;23:433–441.

131. Kahn RL, Goldfarb AI, Pollack M. Brief objective measures for the determination of mental status in the aged. *Am J Psychiatry.* 1960;117:326–328.

132. Erkinjuntt T, Sulkava R, Wikstrom J, et al. Short Portable Mental Status Questionnaire as a screening test for dementia and delirium among the elderly. *J Am Geriatr Soc.* 1987;35:412–416.

133. Smyer MA, Hofland BF, Jonas EA. Validity study of the Short Portable Mental Status Questionnaire for the elderly. *J Am Geriatr Soc.* 1979;27:263–269.

134. Dalton JE, Pederson SL, Blom BE, et al. Diagnostic errors using the Short Portable Mental Status Questionnaire with a mixed clinical population. *J Gerontol.* 1987;42:512–514.

135. Wolber G, Romaniuk M, Eastman E, et al. Validity of the Short Portable Mental Status Questionnaire with elderly psychiatric patients. *J Consult Clin Psychol.* 1984;52:712–713.

136. Fillenbaum GG, Landerman LR, Simonsick EM. Equivalence of two screens of cognitive functioning: The Short Portable Mental Status Questionnaire and the Orientation-Memory-Concentration Test. *J Am Geriatr Soc.* 1998;46:1512–1518.

137. Klein LE, Roca RP, McArthur J, et al. Univariate and multivariate analyses of the mental state examination. *J Am Geriatr Soc.* 1985;33:483–488.

138. Kaufman DM, Weinberger M, Strain JJ, et al. Detection of cognitive deficits by a brief mental status examination: The Cognitive Capacity Screening Examination. *Gen Hosp Psychiatry.* 1979;1:247–254.

139. Omer H, Foldes J, Toby M, et al. Screening for cognitive deficits in a sample of hospitalized geriatric patients: A re-evaluation of a brief mental status questionnaire. *J Am Geriatr Soc.* 1983;31:266–268.

140. Katzman R, Brown T, Fuld P, Peck A, Schechter R, Schimmel H. Validation of a short orientation-memory-concentration test of cognitive impairment. *Am J Psychiatry.* 1983;140:734–739.

141. Lorentz WJ, Scanlan JM, Borson S. Brief screening tests for dementia. *Can J Psychiatry.* 2002;47:723–733.

142. Brooke P, Bullock R. Validation of a 6-item cognitive impairment test with a view to primary care usage. *Int J Geriatr Pyschiatry.* 1999;14:936–940.

143. Stuss DT, Meiran N, Guzman A, Lafeche G, Wilmer J. Do long tests yield a more accurate diagnosis of dementia than short tests? A comparison of 5 neuropsychological tests. *Arch Neurol.* 1996;53:1033–1039.

144. Issacs B, Kennie AT. The set test as an aid to the detection of dementia in old people. *Br J Psychiatry.* 1973;123:467–470.

145. Eslinger PJ, Damasio AR, Benson AL, et al. Neuropsychologic detection of abnormal mental decline in older persons. *JAMA.* 1985;253:670–674.

146. Ainslie NK, Murden RA. Effect of education on the clock-drawing dementia screen in nondemented elderly persons. *J Am Geriatr Soc.* 1993;41:249–252.

147. Rook KS, Catano R, Dooley D. The timing of major life events: Effects of departing from the social clock. *Am J Community Psychol.* 1989;17:233–258.

148. Stahelin HB, Monsch AU, Spiegel R. Early diagnosis of dementia via a two-step screening and diagnostic procedure. *Int Psychogeriatr.* 1997;9(Suppl 1):123–130.

149. van der Burg M, Bouwen A, Stessens J, Ylieff M, Fontaine O, de Lepeleire J, Buntix F. Scoring clock tests for dementia screening: a comparison of two scoring methods. *International J Geriatr Psychiatry.* 2004;19:685–689.

150. Nishiwaki Y, Breeze E, Smeeth L, Bulpitt CJ, Peters R, Fletcher AE. Validity of the clock-drawing test as a screening tool for cognitive impairment in the elderly. *Am J Epidemiol.* 2004;160:797–807.

# 8

# *Depression Assessment*

Joseph J. Gallo and Marsha N. Wittink

**M**ood is to affect as climate is to weather.[1] The mood disorders include major depression, dysthymia, and bipolar (manic-depressive) disorder. Publication of Diagnosis and Treatment of Depression in Late Life: Results of the NIH Consensus Development Conference called attention to depression in late life in primary care by including a chapter highlighting the primary care setting.[2] The Consensus Panel update on depression in late life continued to emphasize the importance of the primary care sector for older adults who are depressed.[3] *Clinical Practice Guideline for the Detection, Diagnosis, and Treatment of Depression in Primary Care*, published by the Agency for Health Care Policy and Research, pointed out that the course of major depression, as well as other poorly characterized mood disturbances, among older persons is not well understood.[4] The Institute of Medicine's report, *The Second Fifty Years: Promoting Health and Preventing Disability*, observed that a better definition of depression in older adults would facilitate effective studies of depression in late life in the community.[5] Finally, *Healthy People 2000*, a report from the Department of Health and Human Services, acknowledged the role that the primary care sector plays in maintaining good health of older persons.[6] Clearly, if intervening in depression and suicide in late life is possible, primary care physicians and other health professionals in primary care are in a position to do so.[7–9]

Clinical and epidemiologic studies using symptoms scales, similar to the ones discussed in the following sections, show that the prevalence of depression increases with age, whereas epidemiologic studies using the standard criteria show a decrease in prevalence of depression with age.[10] At the same time, suicide rates increase with age.[11] Thus, depression in older persons presents a paradox; depression prevalence in epidemiologic studies decreases with age, whereas suicides increase with age. Although many factors contribute to suicide in the aged, it seems that (1) the criteria for major depression are not age specific, (2) medical problems and functional impairment contribute to preoccupation with death and suicide, and (3) hopelessness, not sadness, may be more pertinent in predicting suicide risk.

Older persons may not feel comfortable raising concerns of a psychologic nature to their physicians. An older person may believe that it is an imposition on the physician's time that should be occupied with "real" problems. The primary care provider, who has an intimate knowledge of the older person and family, should assess the person for the possibility of depression. Asking about feelings indicates that feelings are appropriate subjects for discussion and are not a waste of time. Older adults may view a psychologic problem as a sign of weakness, as something to be ashamed of or as meaning that they are "crazy."[12] For all of these reasons, the presentation of depression may be quite different in older adults than in younger persons, discussed at length elsewhere.[13,14]

Some studies indicate that screening for depression may be useful because recognition by the physician leads to attention to the problem and treatment or referral.[15–17] German et al.,[18] working in a general medical outpatient setting, screened patients of all ages using the General Health Questionnaire (GHQ). Feedback on a randomized group of patients was given to the physicians in training consisting of the GHQ score and its interpretation. Patients were examined 6 months later. The screening procedure resulted in a significantly increased rate of detection when compared with major depression only for the patients aged 65 years and older (63% recognition among the patients for whom the doctor received feedback of GHQ score vs. 41% for the patients for whom no feedback was given). There was a trend toward greater efforts to manage depression among the group for whom the doctor received feedback.[18] The use of a screening diagnostic questionnaire may increase recognition, but recognition may be less clearly tied to treatment in older persons than in younger persons.[19] These studies add evidence to the argument that screening for depression may be worthwhile among older persons in general medical outpatient settings, and the notion of screening deserves further investigation. However, it seems likely that to improve treatment will require more intensive intervention than the use of assessment instruments in screening mode.

The diagnostic features of a major depressive episode are delineated in the fourth edition of the *DSM-IV* of the American Psychiatric Association and are reproduced in Exhibit 8–1.[1] These symptoms of depression should be sought in the complete evaluation, but especially when mental impairment is a consideration or in the setting of significant life events in which loss is a theme (e.g., bereavement or recent diagnosis of cancer). Has the individual felt "blue" or "down in the dumps?" The question "How are your spirits with everything that is going on with you?" may open a discussion related to depression. Has he or she lost interest in activities that were enjoyed previously? How is his or her "energy level?" How well is the person sleeping? Is he or she eating? Does he or she feel useless or like life is not worth living? Does the family give the history that its loved one has withdrawn from usual activities? Is he or she using alcohol, sedatives, or tranquilizers to excess?

Anxious, somatic, or hypochondriacal complaints without sadness in older adults felt to be clinically depressed have been observed by experienced clinicians.[20,21] Feelings of helplessness[22] and hopelessness[23] may play a more central role in depression among older persons than younger persons. Other aspects of depression that may be characteristic for older adults are not included in the standard criteria (e.g., perceived cognitive deficit[24] or irritability[25]). Anxiety symptoms may accompany depression, persisting even after depression has improved.[26] Fogel and Fretwell[20] observed that because many depressed older adults do not complain of depression, a diagnosis of depression emphasizes a symptom that does not speak to the illness experience of the older person.

An older adult with numerous somatic complaints may be depressed but may deny feeling blue. It may then be hard to convince him or her and the family that depression is the diagnosis because mood disturbance is denied by the individual. The family may misinterpret depressive symptoms as grouchiness, hostility, laziness, or merely complaining.[12,27] Hypochondriasis may serve as a plea for help, to displace anxiety, as a manifestation of unresolved guilt, and as a way to manipulate the environment.[28] In community samples,

**Exhibit 8–1** Diagnostic Criteria for a Major Depressive Episode

A. Five (or more) of the following symptoms have been present during the same 2-week period and represent a change from previous functioning; at least one of the symptoms is either (1) depressed mood or (2) loss of interest or pleasure.
   Note: Do not include symptoms that are clearly due to a general medical condition, or mood-incongruent delusions or hallucinations.
   (1)  depressed mood most of the day, nearly every day, as indicated by either subjective report (e.g., feels sad or empty) or observation made by others (e.g., appears tearful). Note: In children and adolescents, can be irritable mood.
   (2)  markedly diminished interest or pleasure in all, or almost all, activities most of the day, nearly every day (as indicated by either subjective account or observation made by others).
   (3)  significant weight loss when not dieting or weight gain (e.g., a change of more than 5% of body weight in a month), or decrease or increase in appetite nearly every day. Note: In children, consider failure to make expected weight gains.
   (4)  insomnia or hypersomnia nearly every day.
   (5)  psychomotor agitation or retardation nearly every day (observable by others, not merely subjective feelings of restlessness or being slowed down).
   (6)  fatigue or loss of energy nearly every day.
   (7)  feelings of worthlessness or excessive or inappropriate guilt (which may be delusional) nearly every day (not merely self-reproach or guilt about being sick).
   (8)  diminished ability to think or concentrate, or indecisiveness, nearly every day (either by subjective account or as observed by others).
   (9)  recurrent thoughts of death (not just fear of dying), recurrent suicidal ideation without a specific plan, or a suicide attempt or a specific plan for committing suicide.
B. The symptoms do not meet criteria for a Mixed Episode.
C. The symptoms cause clinically significant distress or impairment in social, occupational, or other important areas of functioning.
D. The symptoms are not due to the direct physiological effects of a substance (e.g., a drug of abuse, a medication) or a general medical condition (e.g., hypothyroidism).
E. The symptoms are not better accounted for by Bereavement, i.e., after the loss of a loved one, the symptoms persist for longer than 2 months or are characterized by marked functional impairment, morbid preoccupation with worthlessness, suicidal ideation, psychotic symptoms, or psychomotor retardation.

*Source:* Reprinted with permission from the *Diagnostic and Statistical Manual of Mental Disorders,* Fourth Edition. © 1994, American Psychiatric Association.

the dysphoria/anhedonia criterion for major depression was less likely to be endorsed by persons 65 years of age and older for the 1 month before interview, even adjusting for differences caused by the level of the symptoms of depression and for characteristics thought to influence the reporting of symptoms, such as gender and level of educational attainment.[29] This raises the possibility that the criteria in use for major depression may not be uniformly valid across all age groups.[30] The person who denies sadness may yet have significant depression.[14-31]

Although depression seems to decrease with age in some studies, hopelessness seems to increase with age. This is important because hopelessness, rather than dysphoria, seems to be an important concomitant of suicidal ideation and suicide.[32,33] Community surveys that permit direct age comparisons of the level of hopelessness are uncommon, but employing the Beck Hopelessness Scale, Greene found a clear and statistically significant trend to increasing levels of hopelessness with advancing age in Dublin among 396 community residents.[34] This dovetails with the work showing that dysphoria is less likely to be endorsed by persons aged 65 years and older[29] because it means that to identify older persons at risk for depression and suicide, the physician must consider cognitions related to hopelessness and subsyndromal distress. In other words, the older person must be asked about feelings of helplessness and hopelessness in the context of physical illness, paying close attention to depression and thoughts of death in these circumstances. Suicide risk may be increased among older persons who live alone or who are male, are recently bereaved, or have a history of psychiatric disorders, including drug or alcohol abuse.

Depression can affect performance on mental status tests. When cognitive impairment is suspected, depression should be considered. The person with the appearance of cognitive impairment secondary to depression remains oriented and with coaxing can perform cognitive tests. Clues that dementia may be secondary to depression include recent onset and rapid progression, a family history of depressive disorders, a personal history of affective disorders, and onset of the disorder after the age of 60 years.[34] A more valuable concept regards depression as frequently coexisting with dementia: patients can be diagnosed with both Alzheimer's dementia and depression.[35] An observer-rated scale specifically for depression in dementia, the National Institute of Mental Health (NIMH) Dementia Mood Assessment Scale, is available.[36] Persons found to have some cognitive impairment with accompanying depression may be at risk for developing dementia.[37,38] A plausible estimate is that 20% of individuals with Alzheimer's disease suffer from a major depressive syndrome.[39,40] Treatment with antidepressants may be the only way to prove that a concomitant depression exists.[2,41,42] Treatment of depression could improve cognitive deficits that are mistakenly ascribed to a primary degenerative dementia and improve overall functioning.[43]

The relationship of physical illness and medication effects to depression is particularly important for older adults because physical illness and medication use are more common with advancing age. Depression may be a direct manifestation of a physical disorder or medication, may be a reaction to the diagnosis of a chronic illness, or may coexist in a person with physical illness. For example, stroke is especially likely to result in depression if certain brain regions are injured.[44] Depression in persons with cardiovascular disease, on the other hand, may arise as a reaction to functional limitations or to anxiety over sexual issues. The classic lesion associated with depression is carcinoma of the pancreas. Other conditions are pernicious anemia (even without megaloblastic changes or anemia); hypothyroidism; hyperthyroidism; parathyroid and adrenal disease; chronic subdural hematoma; untreated congestive heart failure; systemic vasculitis; infections such as hepatitis, influenza, and encephalitis; drug toxicity from drugs such as propranolol and diazepam; and alcoholism.[45–48]

An argument can be made that some standardized instrument be used to screen older persons for affective disorder (especially in relationship to stressful life events such as institutionalization) in the same way that tests can be used to assess cognitive impairment.[49] The instrument might be used to assess the mood of caregivers who themselves are older.[50] When older adults express hopelessness, anxiety, or unexplained somatic complaints or the score on a brief measure indicates possible depression, the criteria of the depression syndrome should be sought (see Exhibit 8–1). At the same time, significant depression may occur in persons who do not fulfill these criteria.[14,31] The following sections discuss several brief instruments that can be used to uncover depression or psychologic distress.

## DEPRESSION SCALES

Symptom scales can be useful to screen for depression or general psychologic distress. Consideration must be given to two dimensions when trying to define depression: symptom patterns and severity. Symptom pattern refers to the type of symptoms that form the items of the scale (e.g., somatic complaints, hopelessness, or irritability). When items in a scale are summed to obtain a score, the implicit assumption is that the symptoms are given equal weight. Persons with higher scores are assumed to be more depressed, but this does not necessarily account for the severity of symptoms being experienced. Although clinical judgment remains paramount, the scales can assist in determining whether the person is making satisfactory progress or needs further assessment or referral. Finally, when scales are used, the time frame for the assessment, such as "in the past 2 weeks," should be specified.

## Geriatric Depression Scale

The Geriatric Depression Scale (GDS) has been recommended for clinical use by the Institute of Medicine[5] and is included as a routine part of comprehensive geriatric assessment in *A Core Curriculum in Geriatric Medicine.*[51] Introduced almost 2 decades ago,[52] the GDS is finding increasing use in research on depression in older adults.

The GDS is a questionnaire consisting of 30 items to be answered "yes" or "no," a considerable simplification over scales that use a five-category response set (Exhibit 8–2). The questionnaire is scored by assigning one point for each answer that matches the "yes" or "no" in the parentheses after the written question. A score of 10 or 11 is usually used as the threshold to separate patients into depressed and non-depressed groups.

The GDS was devised by choosing from 100 statements felt by the investigators to relate to seven common characteristics of depression in later life.[52,53] In particular, the 100 items could be grouped a priori into several domains: (1) somatic concern, (2) lowered affect, (3) cognitive impairment, (4) feelings of discrimination, (5) impaired motivation, (6) lack of future orientation, and (7) lack of self-esteem.[52] Based on administration of the items to 46 depressed and normal older adults, the best 30 items were selected by noting their correlation to the total score (the total number of the 100 items present). Somatic symptoms such as anorexia and insomnia did not correlate highly with the total score and were dropped from the final instrument. The GDS was then administered to 20 normal older persons and 51 older persons who were in treatment for depression to evaluate the performance of the new 30-item instrument. Using a cutoff score of 11 or above to designate depressed individuals, the test was 84% sensitive and 95% specific for the diagnosis of depression.[52] Subsequent studies have demonstrated the value of the GDS.[54–60]

Persons with dementia were excluded from formative studies of the GDS, but Brink was the first to suggest that the GDS may have uncertain validity in the presence of dementia.[61] Insensitivity of the GDS to dementia was suggested by a study of older adults from a compre-

**Exhibit 8–2** Geriatric Depression Scale

---

1. Are you basically satisfied with your life? (no)
2. Have you dropped many of your activities and interests? (yes)
3. Do you feel that your life is empty? (yes)
4. Do you often get bored? (yes)
5. Are you hopeful about the future? (no)
6. Are you bothered by thoughts that you just cannot get out of your head? (yes)
7. Are you in good spirits most of the time? (no)
8. Are you afraid that something bad is going to happen to you? (yes)
9. Do you feel happy most of the time? (no)
10. Do you often feel helpless? (yes)
11. Do you often get restless and fidgety? (yes)
12. Do you prefer to stay home at night, rather than go out and do new things? (yes)
13. Do you frequently worry about the future? (yes)
14. Do you feel that you have more problems with memory than most? (yes)
15. Do you think it is wonderful to be alive now? (no)
16. Do you often feel downhearted and blue? (yes)
17. Do you feel pretty worthless the way you are now? (yes)
18. Do you worry a lot about the past? (yes)
19. Do you find life very exciting? (no)
20. Is it hard for you to get started on new projects? (yes)
21. Do you feel full of energy? (no)
22. Do you feel that your situation is hopeless? (yes)
23. Do you think that most persons are better off than you are? (yes)
24. Do you frequently get upset over little things? (yes)
25. Do you frequently feel like crying? (yes)
26. Do you have trouble concentrating? (yes)
27. Do you enjoy getting up in the morning? (no)
28. Do you prefer to avoid social gatherings? (yes)
29. Is it easy for you to make decisions? (no)
30. Is your mind as clear as it used to be? (no)

   Score one point for each response that matches the yes or no answer after the question.

   *Source:* Adapted from *Journal of Psychiatric Research*, Vol. 17, JA Yesavage and TL Brink, Development and Validation of a Geriatric Depression Screening Scale: A Preliminary Report. © 1983, with permission from Elsevier Science.

---

hensive evaluation clinic.[62] A total of 72 persons with Alzheimer's disease were compared with 70 cognitively intact persons. Overall, the GDS was found to be useful in the detection of depression, but for a demented group, the GDS performance was no better than chance. For those with dementia, there was no cutoff that yielded a sensitivity and specificity greater than 65%. Another study by Burke et al.[63] did not show any difference in performance with cognitive impairment. In this study, the diagnoses were obtained prospectively (i.e., after the GDS was administered). The authors explain the discrepancy between the studies as caused by differences in the case ascertainment. Despite memory impairment, demented persons in this particular study were often consistent in their responses to questions about depression; however, persons with dementia may deny symptoms of depression in the same way that they deny memory difficulties.[64]

Kafonek et al.[65] studied the GDS at an academic nursing home. Of 169 eligible admissions, 134 gave consent for the study, and 70 completed the examination. Residents were classified with regard to depression by a psychiatrist using the criteria of the third edition of the *Diagnostic and Statistical Manual (DSM-III)* and were blinded to the results of the GDS. By clinical examination, 59% of the residents were demented, 19% were delirious, and 21% were depressed. Using a cutoff of 13/14, the GDS was 47% sensitive and 75% specific for the diagnosis of depression for the residents as a group. Importantly, the investigators found that GDS sensitivity was markedly diminished in the subset that scored less than 24 on the Mini-Mental State Examination (MMSE). In the current study, sensitivity dropped from 75% in the resident subset scoring normally on the MMSE to 25% in the subset scoring in the abnormal range. In other words, the GDS may not be suitable for detecting depression in the presence of dementia, which is a common type of impairment in nursing homes.

Finally, Parmelee et al.[66] examined 708 persons with a mean age of 84 years and found that 43% had symptoms of depression, 12% meeting criteria for major depression, even in the face of cognitive impairment. The article sets forth very clearly the thorough attempts made at verifying diagnostic accuracy and reasons for nonparticipation. The GDS showed good agreement with observer ratings of depression whether or not there was dementia. The investigators felt that the GDS gave reliable data as long as cognitive deficits were not so severe as to preclude comprehension of the questions.

A short version of the GDS has been published.[67] The 15 questions of the shorter version are 1–4, 7–9, 10, 12, 14, 15, 17, and 21–23. Scores of 5 or more may indicate depression, according to the authors. Eighty-one volunteers from a continuing-care community and a foster grandparent program were randomized to receive either the long GDS form or the short GDS form and 2 weeks later the alternative instrument.[68] The correlation coefficient for the scores on the two instruments was 0.66, indicating very high agreement. Using the GDS short form, Cwikel and Ritchie[69] interviewed 285 community respondents aged 65 years and older, and a subset of 71 was examined by a clinician. A preliminary study of 20 cases and 20 controls showed that the threshold of 6/7 had the best sensitivity and specificity. Using a threshold of 6/7, the sensitivity was 72%, and specificity was 57% for a *DSM-III* diagnosis of major depression. Persons without formal education were more likely to score in the depressed range on the GDS short form. It remains to be seen how specific the GDS is to geriatric depression and how specific to depression as opposed to general psychologic distress; however, the GDS can be usefully applied in general medical settings. In using the GDS, it must be remembered that potentially important signals of depression in older people are not included in the GDS, such as sleep disturbance, somatic symptoms, and appetite disturbance with weight loss.

## Zung Self-Rating Depression Scale

The Zung Self-Rating Depression Scale comprises 10 positive and 10 negative statements (Exhibit 8–3).[70] The statements are answered with the following phrases: "a little of the time," "some of the time," "a good part of the time," or "most of the time." The responses are scored from 1 to 4 in such a way that a higher score indicates greater depression. The score may be expressed as a percentage of 80, which is the maximum score attainable.

The Zung Self-Rating Depression Scale has been validated for a university outpatient psychiatric population.[71,72] Older persons apparently score higher than other groups.[73] In one study, community-dwelling older adults without psychiatric impairment had a score similar to that which would be considered borderline for the population as a whole.[74] Eighty-eight percent of patients with the diagnosis of depression by psychiatric examination had a score of 50 or greater, and 88% of patients who were not depressed had a score less than 50.[73,75]

In a study that compared the Zung Self-Rating Depression Scale with psychiatric examination, the sensitivity was 77%, and the specificity was 82%. The predictive value of a positive test (for this study, a cutoff of 60 was used) was 65%; for a negative test, it was 89%.[76] The Zung scale contains more physical symptoms than other scales, and older adults, even when not depressed, tend to score higher than younger adults.[73]

**Exhibit 8–3** The Zung Self-Rating Depression Scale

1. (−) I feel downhearted and blue.
2. (+) Morning is when I feel the best.
3. (−) I have crying spells or feel like it.
4. (−) I have trouble sleeping at night.
5. (+) I eat as much as I used to.
6. (+) I still enjoy sex.
7. (−) I notice that I am losing weight.
8. (−) I have trouble with constipation.
9. (−) My heart beats faster than usual.
10. (−) I get tired for no reason.
11. (+) My mind is as clear as it used to be.
12. (+) I find it easy to do the things I used to.
13. (−) I am restless and can't keep still.
14. (+) I feel hopeful about the future.
15. (−) I am more irritable than usual.
16. (+) I find it easy to make decisions.
17. (+) I feel that I am useful and needed.
18. (+) My life is pretty full.
19. (−) I feel that others would be better off if I were dead.
20. (+) I still enjoy the things I used to do.

Statements are answered "a little of the time," "some of the time," "a good part of the time," or "most of the time." The responses are given a score of 1 to 4, arranged so that the higher the score, the greater the depression: the statements designated with (+) are given "1" for response "most of the time," while those with (−) are given a "4" for "most of the time"

*Source:* Reprinted with permission from WWK Zung, A Self-Rating Scale, *Archives of General Psychiatry*, Vol. 12, p. 65. © 1965, American Medical Association.

## The GHQ

The GHQ is a 60-item self-administered instrument whose purpose is to detect the presence of a psychiatric disorder.[77] A scaled version has been devised consisting of 28 items testing four general categories (seven questions each) that include somatic symptoms, anxiety and insomnia, social dysfunction, and depression (Exhibit 8–4). The GHQ is unusual among assessment questionnaires in that it was developed specifically for use in the primary care setting and has been used throughout the world.

Using the GHQ, respondents rate the presence of anxious and depressive symptoms over the past few weeks into one of four categories: "not at all" (coded 1), "no more than usual" (coded 2), "more

**Exhibit 8–4** Items from the Scaled US Version of the General Health Questionnaire (GHQ)

A. *Somatic symptoms*
   A1. Been feeling in need of some medicine to pick you up?
   A2. Been feeling in need of a good tonic?
   A3. Been feeling run down and out of sorts?
   A4. Felt that you are ill?
   A5. Been getting any pains in your head?
   A6. Been getting a feeling of tightness or pressure in your head?
   A7. Been having hot or cold spells?

B. *Anxiety and insomnia*
   B1. Lost much sleep over worry?
   B2. Had difficulty staying asleep?
   B3. Felt constantly under strain?
   B4. Been getting edgy and bad-tempered?
   B5. Been getting scared or panicky for no reason?
   B6. Found everything getting on top of you?
   B7. Been feeling nervous and uptight all the time?

C. *Social dysfunction*
   C1. Been managing to keep yourself busy and occupied?
   C2. Been taking longer over the things you do?
   C3. Felt on the whole you were doing things well?
   C4. Been satisfied with the way you have carried out your tasks?
   C5. Felt that you are playing a useful part in things?
   C6. Felt capable of making decisions about things?
   C7. Been able to enjoy your normal day-to-day activities?

D. *Depression*
   D1. Been thinking of yourself as a worthless person?
   D2. Felt that life is entirely hopeless?
   D3. Felt that life isn't worth living?
   D4. Thought of the possibility that you might do away with yourself?
   D5. Found at times you couldn't do anything because your nerves were too bad?
   D6. Found yourself wishing you were dead and away from it all?
   D7. Found that the idea of taking your own life kept coming into your mind?

There are four responses for each question: score 1 for either of the two answers consistent with depression and 0 for the other two.

*Source:* Adapted with permission from DP Goldberg and VF Hiller, A Scaled Version of the General Health Questionnaire. *Psychological Medicine*, Vol. 9, No. 1, pp. 139–145. © 1979, Cambridge University Press.

than usual" (coded 3), or "much more than usual" (coded 4). Good-child and Duncan-Jones[78] recommended a modified scoring method in which certain symptoms rated "no more than usual" are considered positive responses, reasoning that the GHQ may otherwise fail to detect chronic distress in persons screened for psychologic distress in general medical settings.

In a British general practice, using a score of 4 or 5 as a cutoff, with higher scores indicating psychiatric illness, the scale has an 88% sensitivity (i.e., 88% of respondents with a psychiatric disorder are correctly classified) and an 84% specificity (i.e., 84% of the normal respondents are correctly classified).[79] Similar results were obtained in an American practice; when compared with the examination of a psychiatrist who did not know the result of the GHQ, the sensitivity was 86% with a specificity of 77%.[80]

As mentioned previously, the use of a screening instrument to detect depression in primary medicine can be valuable to increase awareness of depression in primary care practices.[81] In contrast to expectations, older persons as a group did not have any more somatic symptoms on the scale than did the younger subjects. Despite the use of idioms such as "strung up" and "keyed up," the GHQ appears to be sensitive to both anxiety and depression in outpatients, has been used all over the world, and is very well-studied.[15,82–91]

## Beck Depression Inventory

The Beck Depression Inventory (BDI) is an instrument that addresses 21 characteristics of depression: mood, pessimism, sense of failure, satisfaction, guilt, sense of punishment, disappointment in oneself, self-accusations, self-punitive wishes, crying spells, irritability, social withdrawal, indecisiveness, body image, function at work, sleep disturbance, fatigue, appetite disturbance, weight loss, preoccupation with health, and loss of libido.[92,93] Graber and Toth[94] and Gallo et al.[95] illustrated versions of the instrument. The BDI is administered by an interviewer, although it has been adapted for use as a self-administered instrument. Individual items are scored as 0, 1, 2, or 3. As reported in a study by Beck et al.,[96] a score of greater than 21 was indicative of severe depression, with about 75% sensitivity and 92% specificity; the value of a positive test in that sample (only 5% of subjects were over 55 years of age) was 75%, and that of a negative test was 92%. Compared with the *DSM-III* criteria for depression, the instrument was 100% sensitive (no missed cases) and 90% specific when a cutoff score of 10 was used to indicate depression in an adult sample with a mean age of about 40 years.[97]

Older adults participating in a psychiatric inpatient program were administered the BDI with good results. Using a score of 11 or greater as indicative of depression, the instrument had 93% sensitivity and

81% specificity. The predictive value of a positive test was 93%.[98] Medically ill older adults over the age of 60 years were administered the BDI on referral to a geriatric clinic. At a cutoff point of 10, the BDI was 89% sensitive and 82% specific when compared with a standardized diagnostic interview.[56]

In a study involving 526 patients in a primary care medical setting, a threshold score of 13 was used as indicative of depression; with this cutoff score, the sensitivity was 79%, and the specificity was 77% for all age groups.[99] The authors suggested using a cutoff score of 10 despite the greater number of false-positive results in order to avoid missing any cases of depression. In another study, a cutoff score of 10 was used for a group of 31 older medical outpatients; the BDI proved to be 89% sensitive and 82% specific as regarded in the detection of depression.[57] In a study sample with a prevalence of depression estimated at about 12%, using 10 as a cutoff score was found to miss few depressed patients.[49]

A short version of the BDI (i.e., the 21 items are reduced to 13) was shown to identify cases of depression as well as the longer instrument. The self-administered 13-item BDI takes 5 minutes to complete. The questions are identical to those in the larger instrument except that the order of the responses is reversed—the patient reads the most negative statements first. Scores of 5 to 7 are consistent with mild depression; scores of 8 to 15 indicate a moderate depression, and scores of 16 or greater show severe depression.[93]

The number of responses for each item in the Beck instruments is a source of potential confusion to the older patient, especially when some degree of mental impairment is present. As is the case with other instruments, older persons with numerous somatic complaints and difficulties may answer the items in such a way as to reflect these multiple physical complaints, rather than depression. The value of a positive test could be considerably lower in a primary care population where the prevalence of major depression would presumably be lower than in a psychiatric practice.[49] This is not necessarily a disadvantage as long as the examiner is prepared to confirm results by clinical interview. A short version of the BDI was recommended for use in primary care by the Depression Guidelines Panel.[4]

## Center for Epidemiologic Studies Depression Scale

The Center for Epidemiologic Studies Depression Scale (CES-D) (Exhibit 8–5) was developed by the Center for Epidemiologic Studies at

**Exhibit 8–5** Center for Epidemiologic Studies Depression Scale

---

**Instructions for questions:** Below is a list of the ways you might have felt or behaved. Please tell me how often you have felt this way during the past week.

> Rarely or none of the time (less than 1 d)
> Some or a little of the time (1–2 d)
> Occasionally or a moderate amount of the time (3–4 d)
> Most or all of the time (5–7 d)

---

*During the past week:*
1. I was bothered by things that usually don't bother me.
2. I did not feel like eating; my appetite was poor.
3. I felt that I could not shake off the blues even with help from my family or friends.
4. I felt that I was just as good as other people.
5. I had trouble keeping my mind on what I was doing.
6. I felt depressed.
7. I felt that everything I did was an effort.
8. I felt hopeful about the future.
9. I thought my life had been a failure.
10. I felt fearful.
11. My sleep was restless.
12. I was happy.
13. I talked less than usual.
14. I felt lonely.
15. People were unfriendly.
16. I enjoyed life.
17. I had crying spells.
18. I felt sad.
19. I felt that people dislike me.
20. I could not get "going."

*Source:* Reprinted from the Center for Epidemiologic Studies, National Institute of Mental Health.

---

the NIMH for use in studies of depression in community samples.[100–102] The CES-D contains 20 items. Respondents are asked to report the amount of time they have experienced symptoms during the past week by choosing one of the following phrases: "rarely or none of the time"—less than 1 day—score 0; "some or a little of the time"—1 to 2 days—score 1; "occasionally or a moderate amount of time"—3 to 4 days—score 2; "most or all of the time"—5 to 7 days—score 3. Typically, a threshold of 17 and above is taken as defining "caseness,"[103] although higher cutoff points (e.g., 24 and above) have been suggested.[104] Among patients in a medical setting, an inordinate number of false positives were generated with higher thresholds on the CES-D, but a higher threshold of 27 was associated with greater specificity.[105] The CES-D did not seem to be biased by somatic complaints in a large community survey of persons aged 55 years and older.[106] Zimmerman and Coryell called attention to the lack of correlation to *DSM-IV* criteria and proposed a revision that would include criteria such as suicidal ideation and psychomotor agitation or retardation,[107] and modifications of the CES-D are in development.[14]

## REFERENCES

1. American Psychiatric Association. *Diagnostic and Statistical Manual of Mental Disorders,* 4th ed. Washington, DC: American Psychiatric Association; 1994.

2. NIH Consensus Development Panel on Depression in Late Life. Diagnosis and treatment of depression in late life. *JAMA.* 1992;268:1018–1024.

3. Lebowitz BD, Pearson JL, Schneider LS, et al. Diagnosis and treatment of depression in late life: Consensus statement update. *JAMA.* 1997;278:1186–1190.

4. Depression Guideline Panel. *Depression in Primary Care: Volume 1. Detection and Diagnosis: Clinical Practice Guideline,* No. 5. Rockville, MD: US Department of Health and Human Services, Public Health Service, Agency for Health Care Policy and Research; 1993. AHCPR Publication Number 93-0550.

5. Institute of Medicine. *The Second Fifty Years: Promoting Health and Preventing Disability.* Washington, DC: National Academy Press; 1992.

6. Department of Health and Human Services. *Healthy People 2000: National Health Promotion and Disease Prevention Objectives.* Washington, DC: US Government Printing Office; 1991. DHHS Publication No. PHS 91-50213.

7. Rabins PV. Prevention of mental disorders in the elderly: Current perspectives and future prospects. *J Am Geriatr Soc.* 1992;40:727–733.

8. Conwell Y. Suicide in elderly patients. In: Schneider LS, Reynolds CF, Lebowitz BD, Friedhoff AJ, eds. *Diagnosis and Treatment of Depression in Late Life: Results of the NIH Consensus Development Conference.* Washington, DC: American Psychiatric Association; 1994:397–418.

9. Gallo JJ, Rabins PV, Iliffe S. The "research magnificent" in late life: Psychiatric epidemiology and the primary health care of older adults. *Int J Psychiatry Med.* 1997;27:185–204.

10. Newmann JP. Aging and depression. *Psychol Aging.* 1989;4:150–165.

11. National Center for Health Statistics. *Vital Statistics of the United States.* 1988, Vol. II: Mortality, Part A. Washington, DC: US Public Health Service; 1991.

12. Chaisson-Stewart GM. The diagnostic dilemma. In: Chaisson-Stewart GM, ed. *Depression in the Elderly: An Interdisciplinary Approach.* New York: John Wiley & Sons; 1985:18–43.

13. Gallo JJ, Rabins PV. Depression without sadness: Alternative presentations of depression in late life. *Am Fam Physician.* 1999;60(3):820–826.

14. Gallo JJ, Gonzales J. Depression and other mood disorders. In: Adelman A, Daly M, eds. *Twenty Common Problems in Geriatrics.* New York: McGraw-Hill; 2001;14:205–235.

15. Higgins ES. A review of unrecognized mental illness in primary care. Prevention, natural history, and efforts to change the course. *Arch Fam Med.* 1994;3:908–917.

16. Ormel J, Van den Brink W, Koeter MWJ, et al. Recognition, management and outcome of psychological disorders in primary care: A naturalistic follow-up study. *Psychol Med.* 1990;20:909–923.

17. Gonzales JJ, Norquist G. Mental health consultation-liaison interventions in primary care. In: Miranda J, Hohmann AA, Attkisson CC, Larson DB, eds. *Mental Disorders in Primary Care.* San Francisco: Jossey-Bass Publishers; 1994:347–373.

18. German PS, Shapiro S, Skinner EA, et al. Detection and management of mental health problems of older patients by primary care providers. *JAMA.* 1987;257:489–493.

19. Valenstein M, Kales H, Mellow A, et al. Psychiatric diagnosis and intervention in older and younger patients in a primary care clinic: Effect of a screening and diagnostic instrument. *J Am Geriatr Soc.* 1998;46:1499–1505.

20. Fogel BS, Fretwell M. Reclassification of depression in the medically ill elderly. *J Am Geriatr Soc.* 1985;33:446–448.

21. Salzman C, Shader RI. Depression in the elderly: I: Relationship between depression, psychologic defense mechanisms and physical illness. *J Am Geriatr Soc.* 1978;26:253–260.

22. Depure RA, Monroe SM. Learned helplessness in the perspective of the depressive disorders: Concepts and definitional issues. *Abnorm Psychol.* 1978;87:3–20.

23. Abramson LY, Metalsky GI, Alloy LB. Hopelessness depression: A theory based subtype of depression. *Psychol Rev.* 1989;96:358–372.

24. Weiss IK, Nagel CL, Aronson MK. Applicability of depression scales to the old person. *J Am Geriatr Soc.* 1986;34:215–218.

25. Rohrbaugh RM, Siegal AP, Giller EL. Irritability as a symptom of depression in the elderly. *J Am Geriatr Soc.* 1988;36:736–738.

26. Blazer D, Hughes DC, Fowler N. Anxiety as an outcome symptom of depression in the elderly and middle-aged adults. *Int J Geriatr Psychiatry.* 1989;4:273–278.

27. Roth M. Differential diagnosis of psychiatric disorders in old age. *Hosp Pract.* 1986;21(7):111–138.

28. Blazer D, Siegler IC. *A Family Approach to Health Care of the Elderly.* Menlo Park, CA: Addison-Wesley Publishing; 1984.

29. Gallo JJ, Anthony JC, Muthen BO. Age differences in the symptoms of depression: A latent trait analysis. *J Gerontol Psychol Sci.* 1994;49:P251–P264.

30. Henderson AS. Does ageing protect against depression? *Soc Psychiatry Psychiatr Epidemiol.* 1994;29:107–109.

31. Gallo JJ, Rabins PV, Lyketsos CG, Tien AY, Anthony JC. Depression without sadness: Functional outcomes of nondysphoric depression in later life. *J Am Geriatr Soc.* 1997;45:570–578.

32. Beck AT, Steer RA, Beck JS, Newman CF. Hopelessness, depression, suicidal ideation, and clinical diagnosis of depression. *Suicide Life Threat Behav.* 1993;23:139–145.

33. Beck AT, Steer RA, Kovacs M. Hopelessness and eventual suicide: A 10-year prospective study of patients hospitalized with suicidal ideation. *Am J Psychiatry.* 1985;142:559–563.

34. Greene SM. Levels of measured hopelessness in the general population. *Br J Clin Psychol.* 1981;20:11–14.

35. Whitehouse PJ. The concept of subcortical and cortical dementia: Another look. *Ann Neurol.* 1986;19:1–6.

36. Sunderland T, Alterman IS, Yount D, et al. A new scale for the assessment of depressed mood in demented patients. *Am J Psychiatry.* 1988;145:955–959.

37. Rabins PV, Merchant A, Nestadt G. Criteria for diagnosing reversible dementia caused by depression: Validation by 2-year follow-up. *Br J Psychiatry.* 1984;144:488–492.

38. Devanand DP, Sano M, Tang MX, et al. Depressed mood and the incidence of Alzheimer's disease in the elderly living in the community. *Arch Gen Psychiatry.* 1996; 53:175–182.

39. Rovner B, Broadhead J, Spencer M. Depression in Alzheimer's disease. *Am J Psychiatry.* 1989;146:350–353.

40. Wragg RE, Jeste DV. Overview of depression and psychosis in Alzheimer's disease. *Am J Psychiatry.* 1989;146:577–589.

41. Reynolds CF, Kupfer DJ, Hoch CC, et al. Two-year follow-up of elderly patients with mixed depression and dementia: Clinical and electroencephalographic sleep findings. *J Am Geriatr Soc.* 1986;34:793–799.

42. Caine ED. Pseudodementia. *Arch Gen Psychiatry.* 1981;38:1359–1364.

43. Reifler BV, Larson E, Hanley R. Coexistence of cognitive impairment and depression in geriatric outpatients. *Am J Psychiatry.* 1982;139:623–626.

44. Morris PLP, Robinson RG, Raphael B. Prevalence and course of post-stroke depression in hospitalized patients. *Int J Psychiatry Med.* 1990;20:327–342.

45. Murray AM, Levkoff SE, Wetle TT, et al. Acute delirium and functional decline in the hospitalized elderly patient. *J Gerontol.* 1993;48:M181–M186.

46. Lipowski ZJ. Delirium (acute confusional states). *JAMA.* 1987;258:1789–1792.

47. Beresford TP. Alcoholism in the elderly. *Int Rev Psychiatry.* 1993;5:477–483.

48. Lehmann HE. Affective disorders in the aged. *Psychiatr Clin North Am.* 1982;5:27–48.

49. Kamerow DB, Campbell TL. Is screening for mental health problems worthwhile in family practice? *J Fam Pract.* 1987;25:181–187.

50. Gallo JJ. The effect of social support on depression in caregivers of the elderly. *J Fam Pract.* 1990;30:430–436.

51. Cobbs EL, Duthie EH, Murphy JB, eds. *Geriatric Review Syllabus: A Core Curriculum in Geriatric Medicine,* 4th ed. New York: American Geriatrics Society; 1999.

52. Brink TL, Yesavage JA, Lum O, et al. Screening tests for geriatric depression. *Clin Gerontol.* 1982;1:37–43.

53. Yesavage JA, Brink TL. Development and validation of a geriatric depression screening scale: A preliminary report. *J Psychiatr Res.* 1983;17:37–49.

54. O'Riordan TG, Hayes JP, O'Neill D. The effect of mild to moderate dementia on the Geriatric Depression Scale and on the General Health Questionnaire. *Age Ageing.* 1990;19:57–61.

55. Hyer L, Blount J. Concurrent and discriminant validities of the Geriatric Depression Scale with older psychiatric patients. *Psychol Rep.* 1984;54:611–616.

56. Magni G, Shifano F, de Leo D. Assessment of depression in an elderly medical population. *J Affective Disord.* 1986;11:121–124.

57. Norris JT, Gallagher D, Wilson A, Winograd CH. Assessment of depression in geriatric medical outpatients: The validity of two screening measures. *J Am Geriatr Soc.* 1987;35:989–995.

58. Koenig HG, Meador KG, Cohen HJ. Self-rated depression scales and screening for major depression in the older hospitalized patient with medical illness. *J Am Geriatr Soc.* 1988;36:699–706.

59. Rapp SR, Parial SA, Walsh DA. Detecting depression in elderly medical inpatients. *J Consult Clin Psychol.* 1988;56:509–513.

60. Harper RG, Kotik-Harper D, Kirby H. Psychometric assessment of depression in an elderly general medical population: Over- or underassessment? *J Nerv Ment Dis.* 1990;178:113–119.

61. Brink TL. Limitations of the GDS in cases of pseudodementia. *Clin Gerontol.* 1984;2:60–61.

62. Burke WJ, Houston MJ, Boust SJ. Use of the Geriatric Depression Scale in dementia of the Alzheimer type. *J Am Geriatr Soc.* 1989;37:856–860.

63. Burke WJ, Nitcher RL, Roccaforte WH, Wengel SP. A prospective evaluation of the Geriatric Depression Scale in an outpatient geriatric assessment center. *J Am Geriatr Soc.* 1992;40:1227–1230.

64. Feher EP, Larrabee GJ, Crook TH. Factors attenuating the validity of the Geriatric Depression Scale in a dementia population. *J Am Geriatr Soc.* 1992;40:906–909.

65. Kafonek S, Ettinger WH, Roca R. Instruments for screening for depression and dementia in a long-term care facility. *J Am Geriatr Soc.* 1989;37:29–34.

66. Parmelee PA, Katz IR, Lawton MP. Depression among institutionalized aged: Assessment and prevalence estimation. *J Gerontol.* 1989;44:M22–M29.

67. Yesavage JA. The use of self-rating depression scales in the elderly. In: Poon LW, ed. *Clinical Memory Assessment of Older Adults.* Washington, DC: American Psychological Association; 1986.

68. Alden D, Austin C, Sturgeon R. A correlation between the Geriatric Depression Scale long and short forms. *J Gerontol.* 1989;4:P124–P125.

69. Cwikel J, Ritchie K. Screening for depression among the elderly in Israel: An assessment of the Short Geriatric Depression Scale (S-GDS). *Isr J Med Sci.* 1989;25:131–137.

70. Zung WWK. A self-rating depression scale. *Arch Gen Psychiatry.* 1965;12:63–70.

71. Zung WWK, Richards DB, Short MF. Self-rating depression scale in an outpatient clinic: Further validation of the SDS. *Arch Gen Psychiatry.* 1965;13:508–515.

72. Zung WWK. Factors influencing the self-rating depression scale. *Arch Gen Psychiatry.* 1967;16:543–547.

73. Zung WWK. Depression in the normal aged. *Psychosomatics.* 1967;8:287–292.

74. Freedman N, Bucci W, Elkowitz E. Depression in a family practice elderly population. *J Am Geriatr Soc.* 1982;30:372–377.

75. Moore JT, Silimperi DR, Bobula JA. Recognition of depression by family medicine residents: The impact of screening. *J Fam Pract.* 1978;7:509–513.

76. Okimoto JT, Barnes RF, Veith RC, et al. Screening for depression in geriatric medical patients. *Am J Psychiatry.* 1982;139:799–802.

77. Goldberg DP. *The Detection of Psychiatric Illness by Questionnaire.* London: Oxford University Press; 1972.

78. Goodchild ME, Duncan-Jones P. Chronicity and the General Health Questionnaire. *Br J Psychiatry.* 1985;146:55–61.

79. Goldberg DP, Hillier VF. A scaled version of the General Health Questionnaire. *Psychol Med.* 1979;9:139–145.

80. Goldberg DP, Rickels K, Downing R, Hesbacher P. A comparison of two psychiatric screening tests. *Br J Psychiatry.* 1976;129:61–67.

81. German PS, Shapiro S, Skinner EA. Mental health of the elderly: Use of health and mental health services. *J Am Geriatr Soc.* 1985;33:246–252.

82. Clarke DM, Smith GC, Herrman HE. A comparative study of screening instruments for mental disorders in general hospital patients. *Int J Psychiatry Med.* 1993;23:323–337.

83. Cleary PD, Goldberg ID, Kessler LG, Nycz GR. Screening for mental disorders among primary care patients. *Arch Gen Psychiatry.* 1982;39:837–840.

84. Ford DE, Anthony JC, Nestadt GR, Romanoski AJ. The General Health Questionnaire by interview: Performance in relation to recent use of health services. *Med Care.* 1989;27:367–375.

85. Lindsay J. Validity of the General Health Questionnaire (GHQ) in detecting psychiatric disturbance in amputees with phantom pain. *J Psychosom Res.* 1986;30:277–281.

86. Lobo A, Perez-Echeverria M, Jimenez-Aznarez A, et al. Emotional disturbances in endocrine patients: Validity of the scaled version of the General Health Questionnaire (GHQ-28). *Br J Psychiatry.* 1990;152:807–812.

87. Marino S, Bellantuono C, Tansella M. Psychiatric morbidity in general practice in Italy: A point-prevalence survey in a defined geographical area. *Soc Psychiatry Psychiatr Epidemiol.* 1990;25:67–72.

88. Rand EH, Badger LW, Coggins DR. Toward a resolution of contradictions: Utility of feedback from the GHQ. *Gen Hosp Psychiatry.* 1988;10:189–196.

89. Samuels JF, Nestadt G, Anthony JC, Romanoski AJ. The detection of mental disorders in the community setting using a 20-item interview version of the General Health Questionnaire. *Acta Psychiatr Scand.* 1994;89:14–20.

90. Simon GE, VonKorff M, Durham ML. Predictors of outpatient mental health utilization by primary care patients in a Health Maintenance Organization. *Am J Psychiatry.* 1994;151:908–913.

91. Von Korff M, Shapiro S, Burke JD, et al. Anxiety and depression in a primary care clinic: Comparison of Diagnostic Interview Schedule, General Health Questionnaire, and practitioner assessments. *Arch Gen Psychiatry.* 1987;44:152–156.

92. Gallagher D. The Beck Depression Inventory and older adults: Review of its development and utility. In: Brink TL, ed. *Clinical Gerontology: A Guide to Assessment and Intervention.* New York: Haworth Press; 1986:149–163.

93. Beck AT, Beck RW. Screening depressed patients in family practice: A rapid technique. *Postgrad Med.* 1972;52:81–85.

94. Graber MA, Toth PP. *The University of Iowa Family Practice Handbook.* St. Louis: Mosby; 1997.

95. Gallo JJ, Reichel W, Andersen LM. *Handbook of Geriatric Assessment.* Gaithersburg, MD: Aspen Publishers; 1988.

96. Beck AT, Ward CH, Mendelson M, et al. An inventory for measuring depression. *Arch Gen Psychiatry.* 1961;4:53–63.

97. Oliver JM, Simmons ME. Depression as measured by the *DSM-III* and the Beck Depression Inventory in an unselected adult population. *J Consult Clin Psychol.* 1984;52:892–898.

98. Gallagher D, Breckenridge J, Steinmetz J, et al. The Beck Depression Inventory and Research Diagnostic Criteria: Congruence in an older population. *J Consult Clin Psychol.* 1983;51:945–946.

99. Nielsen AC, Williams TA. Depression in ambulatory medical patients: Prevalence by self-report questionnaire and recognition by nonpsychiatric physicians. *Arch Gen Psychiatry.* 1980;37:999–1004.

100. Radloff LS. The CES-D Scale: A self-report depression scale for research in the general population. *Appl Psychol Meas.* 1977;1:385–401.

101. Comstock GW, Helsing KJ. Symptoms of depression in two communities. *Psychol Med.* 1976;6:551–563.

102. Eaton WW, Kessler LG. Rates of symptoms of depression in a national sample. *Am J Epidemiol.* 1981;114:528–538.

103. Katon W, Schulberg HC. Epidemiology of depression in primary care. *Gen Hosp Psychiatry.* 1992;14:237–247.

104. Husaini BA, Neff JA, Harrington JB, et al. Depression in rural communities: Validating the CES-D Scale. *J Community Psychol.* 1980;8:20–27.

105. Schulberg HC, Saul M, McClelland M, Ganguli M, Christy W, Frank R. Assessing depression in primary medical and psychiatric practices. *Arch Gen Psychiatry.* 1985;42:1164–1170.

106. Foelker GA, Shewchuk RM. Somatic complaints and the CES-D. *J Am Geriatr Soc.* 1992;40:259–262.

107. Zimmerman M, Coryell W. Screening for major depressive disorder in the community: A comparison of measures. *Psychol Assess.* 1994;6:71–74.

# 9

# Substance Use
# and Abuse Assessment

Faika Zanjani and David Oslin

S ubstance use examination in clinical settings aids in the detection of substance abuse/dependence (i.e., alcohol use, drug misuse, and nicotine use) and provides screening for risky substance use patterns (current or past) for the prevention of possible abuse/dependency problems and/or identification of potential interactions with other mental and physical health conditions. The gold standard for assessing substance misuse is a comprehensive diagnostic interview and/or the Addiction Severity Index,[1] but both are lengthy in duration. As an alternative, brief screening tools can be used. The AUDIT-C, MAST-G/ SMAST-G, and CAGE appear to be the most sensitive tools for assessing and differentiating types of substance use in the older population. However, new developments need to provide a more efficient and comprehensive process for detecting substance problems for the growing older adult population.

Substance use is a reversible risky health behavior. Assessing substance use in the geriatric population is extremely salient considering the unique characteristics of this population. It is well known that the geriatric population is a group with heightened physical and mental disability;[2] consequently, it is matched with exposure to multiple treatments in various forms (i.e., therapy, prescription medication, herbal, and radiation). In addition, it has also been well documented that improper substance use (i.e., alcohol, drugs, and tobacco) can increase the incidence of co-morbidities[3] and interfere in the treatment process,[4] therefore increasing medical complexity and costs. Regardless, there is a significant prevalence of substance misuse in the older population. Various studies have indicated that within the older population 19.1% are at-risk drinkers, and 8.9% are heavy drinkers,[5] 54.2% are moderate drinkers,[4] 10.2% reported cocaine use, 8.3% reported heroin use, 3.1% reported sedative use, 2.3% reported marijuana use,[3] 21.2% were using prescription drugs not advised for geriatric patients,[6] and on average, 16% smoked tobacco.[7]

Considering that several ubiquitous goals for older adults are the compression of morbidity (delaying onset of disease), physical and mental independence, and prevention of premature mortality, it is relevant to identify and formulate screening and assessments that can indicate substance misuse to prevent further morbidity in this segment of the population. The focus on this chapter is to introduce substance use screening and assessment tools for alcohol, drug, and tobacco misuse that have been used and documented in the current literature. It will be apparent in this review that some areas, such as alcohol assessments, have been much more established and empirically tested, whereas others, such as drug and tobacco assessments, still require further scientific inquiry to benefit the geriatric population accurately. It will also be apparent that there are not many devices for specific use in the geriatric population.

Before introducing substance abuse criteria and screening/assessment tools, it is salient to discuss briefly the benefit and purpose of substance use screening and assessment in clinical settings. An obvious reason is the detection of substance abuse/dependence (i.e., alcohol use, drug misuse, and nicotine use), a disease in itself that can have extremely negative physical and mental health consequences, especially if left untreated. However, a less obvious reason for screening is to identify risky substance use patterns (current or past) for the prevention of abuse/dependency problems and/or identification of potential interactions with other mental and physical health conditions. Given that any use of nicotine or an illicit substance should lead to an intervention, the distinctions between at-risk use, dependence, and nonproblematic use are of concern exclusively with alcohol consumption. Heavy drinking, even in the absence of abuse and dependence, can be detrimental to the care of older adults; however, moderate drinking may be associated with certain health benefits. For instance, alcohol can have negative interactions with many medications commonly used by older persons and can have detrimental impacts on health and psychologic distress.[8] At-risk drinking is described in more detail later in the chapter.

It is also important to recognize past problems with alcohol or other substances as relevant to the current care of an older adult. Although it is not clear whether all patients should be screened for past problems, patients should be asked about past problems with substances at some point in routine care. Past problems can have a negative impact on the incidence and/or treatment for physical and mental illnesses or even be a risk factor for abuse/dependence.[9] Some evidence suggests that past substance problems can affect an individual's ability to adapt to new environments,[10] depression levels,[9] and brain atrophy.[11] Screening will provide a better indication of the patient's history and identify past substance use for understanding individual risks for certain health complications.

## CLASSIFICATION

According to *Diagnostic and Statitical Manual (DSM-IV)* criteria, substance abuse is categorized by 12 months of one or more of the following symptoms: recurrent substance use resulting in (1) a failure to fulfill major obligations at work, school, or home; (2) situations in which it is physically hazardous; (3) legal problems; and (4) persistent or recurrent social or interpersonal problems caused or exacerbated by the effects of the substance. Substance dependence requires specific classifications for alcohol, amphetamines, cannabis, cocaine, hallucinogens, inhalants, nicotine, opioids, phencyclidine, sedatives/hypnotics/anxiolytics, and polysubstance use. These classifications are universal and hence applicable to the entire population regardless of age, sex, and race. Although these criteria were validated in younger individuals, some criteria may be less applicable to older adults (i.e., school, driving, or work). This does not exclude older adults from having dependency; however, the criterion may simply make it harder for older adults to reach abuse/dependence status. It is also important to understand that within the *DSM* criteria there are no specific quantity limits incorporated with the diagnosis of substance use; the criteria merely focus on the presence of specific scenarios/outcomes.

Experts in the field of geriatric addiction have defined substance use disorders, emphasizing a broader public health view of identification to include at-risk drinking as well as substance abuse/dependence. Most investigators and clinicians with expertise in the field define at-risk use by measuring the quantity and frequency of the substance consumed over a defined period. Instruments such as a 5- to 7-day diet record or a quantity and frequency index are easily administered and provide discrete information about substance use. In addition, using the same methods, researchers have gone ahead and determined risky and/or hazardous criteria levels to identify individuals who are at-risk of developing more severe abuse/dependency problems for alcohol consumption (i.e., averaging two drinks a day). The quantity and frequency of use may be inadequate in identifying how substances affect a patient psychodynamically, socially, physiologically, or functionally, especially across age groups.

## ALCOHOL CONSUMPTION

The US Preventive Task Force has recently recommended alcohol screening and behavioral counseling for all adults in primary care settings.[12] The criteria they have recommended for defining the limits of moderate drinking for young and middle-aged adults is two standard drinks or less per day for men and one drink or less per day for women and persons older than 65 years of age.[13] Therefore, developmentally, male adults need to cut down on their drinking as they age in order not to be considered a risky drinker. The two universal assessment tools mentioned as the most popular were Alcohol Use Disorders Identification Test (AUDIT)[14] for screening and CAGE (feeling the need to Cut down, Annoyed by criticism, Guilty about drinking, and need for an Eye-opener in the morning)[15] for differentiating types of drinkers (i.e., at-risk, dependent). The CAGE is particularly useful in identifying alcohol dependence but is less sensitive to identification of at-risk drinking. The methods used for screening should be directly related to the goals and availability for follow-up of positives. In other words, if the clinical staff has the capacity to complete brief interventions and prevention services, then the goal of screening should be to identify at-risk and alcohol dependent patients. In this instance, the CAGE may not be appropriate. Additionally, the US Preventive Task Force specified screening tools for pregnant women and adolescents; however, there was no mention for a precise tool to assess alcohol problems in the geriatric population.

Alternative assessment tools that have been used in the field are the AUDIT Consumption (AUDIT-C)[16] for screening, Michigan Alcoholism Screening Test (MAST),[17] Shortened Michigan Alcoholism Screening Test (SMAST),[18] Brief Michigan Alcoholism Screening Test (BMAST),[19] Michigan Alcoholism Screening Test Geriatric Version (MAST-G),[20] Shortened Michigan Alcoholism Screening Test Geriatric Version (SMAST-G),[21] and two questions from the Cyr and Wartman[22] for identifying problem drinking. The MAST-G and SMAST-G are the only assessment tools mentioned that have been specifically designed to concentrate on the geriatric population. In addition to these standardized tools, the Alcohol-Related Problems Survey (ARPS) was recently developed to assess alcohol use in connection with individual lifestyle factors. Evidence shows that ARPS is able to differentiate harmful, hazardous, and nonhazardous drinking in a geriatric sample[23] in the context of health status.

## AUDIT and AUDIT Consumption

AUDIT is comprised of 10 questions: 3 regarding alcohol frequency, 3 regarding alcohol dependence, and 4 regarding the consequences of alcohol use. Summation of the unevenly weighted (i.e., 0–4) responses equaling 8 or more is indicative of alcohol abuse problems.

AUDIT-C is comprised of three questions regarding alcohol frequency and patterns of alcohol consumption. Summation of the unevenly weighted (i.e., 0–5) responses equaling four or more for men/ three or more for women is indicative of alcohol use problems.

## CAGE

CAGE stands for Cut down, Annoyed, Guilty, and Eye-opener. There are four detailed yes/no questions. They are as follows: (1) Have you ever felt you should cut down on your drinking? (2) Have people annoyed you by criticizing your drinking? (3) Have you ever felt bad or guilty about your drinking? (4) Have you ever had a drink first thing in the morning to steady your nerves or to get rid of a hangover? Affirmations of two of these questions are indicative of an alcohol abuse problem.

## MAST, SMAST, BMAST, MAST-G, and SMAST-G

MAST is comprised of 24 yes/no questions; it was developed to measure alcohol abuse and dependence. Summation of the unevenly weighted (i.e., 1–5) responses equaling 5 or more is indicative of alcohol abuse problems. Therefore, affirmation of one heavily weighted score (i.e., 5) or a fewer lightly weighted scores could be indicative of alcohol problems. As a screening instrument, the MAST is considerably long and may not be adequate in certain populations. Therefore, a number of different versions of the MAST have been created, including two short versions (SMAST and BMAST) and a specific version for geriatric populations (MAST-G and SMAST-G). The SMAST-G (Appendix) is one of the two single tests validated within a geriatric population. This test is comprised of 10 yes/no questions and was developed to measure alcohol abuse and dependence in an older population. Summation of the evenly weighted responses (i.e., 1) equaling 2 or more may be indicative of alcohol problems.

### Cyr and Wartman (2 Questions)

These two questions are as follows: (1) Have you ever had a drinking problem? (2) When was your last drink? An individual is defined as having an alcohol abuse problem if they self-report as ever having a drinking problem and respond that their last drink was within 24 hours.

### ARPS

This self-report test is comprised of 60 items. There are 14 items that assess medical and psychiatric conditions, 12 items that assess symptoms of disease, 1 item on smoking behavior, 17 items on medication use, 6 items on physical functioning and health status, 2 items on frequency and quantity of alcohol use, 2 items on episodic drinking, 4 items on symptoms of alcohol abuse and dependence, 1 item on drinking and driving, and 1 item on gender. Harmful, hazardous, and nonhazardous classifications were based on a collaborative assessment of drinking pattern and health conditions.

All of these tests have their own sensitivities and specificities, with none serving as a gold standard specified for the geriatric population.[1] There have been some indications that the SMAST-G and CAGE individually and in combination are best suited for the geriatric population when compared with MAST and AUDIT[24,25] for identifying abuse/dependence. Another study has indicated that CAGE in combination with MCV-$\gamma$GT (biological marker test) may be the best indicator of alcohol misuse in the geriatric population.[5] Because of incongruence in diagnosis between quantity–frequency questions, binge drinking questions, AUDIT, CAGE, and questions of lifetime consumption, it was suggested that a collaboration of measures may be most effective for evaluating alcohol misuse in the geriatric population, at least until an optimal assessment is established.[26] However, the practicality and efficiency of this recommendation may be highly questionable considering the short amount of time available in clinical visits. Ideally, screening is conducted in a staged process, with positive screens leading to a formal assessment, which then determines the intervention approach.

Because there is not always sufficient time during a single clinical visit to assess all of the health needs of an older adult, computerized technology has been shown possibly to improve efficiency in the medical care system. The Computer Alcohol-Related Problems Survey (CARPS) is a computerized program that is used to evaluate self-reported alcohol behaviors and simultaneously provide patients with health education. This computerized assessment tool was found to distinguish effectively between hazardous, harmful, and binge drinkers in a geriatric population.[27] Most geriatric patients were able to complete CARPS while sitting in the waiting room for their appointments, thus possibly stimulating discussion about their substance use in their upcoming appointment. Ironically, most patients indicated that they have never spoken about alcohol with their physician (78%), which makes this not only a resourceful tool but one that incorporates a neglected area and could possibly stimulate discussion during office visits. In support of the clinical providers, there has been some indication that new problem drinkers may not accurately recall physician conversations in reference to alcohol behaviors.[28] Therefore, geriatric patients showing new symptoms of problem drinking should be provided with clear and concise recommendations to treat or prevent alcohol problems.

It is salient to assess alcohol behaviors of geriatric patients, whether using a short self-report or a multidimensional assessment. Unrecognized alcohol problems could lead to physical and mental withdrawal syndromes, liver/digestive system complications, pancreatitis, thiamine deficiency, neuropathy, dementia, and cardiomyopathy, in addition to negative social consequences.[29] Because this population has a higher likelihood of suffering from additional health conditions, assessing and then treating alcohol misuse can reduce the incidence of further co-morbidity and premature death and possibly improve the quality of life for geriatric individuals.

## DRUG USE

In the geriatric population, there are two types of drug misuse: illicit drug use[30] and medication misuse.[31] Illicit drug use is categorized in a similar manner to the way it is categorized in other age groups, being defined as an improper use of illegal chemical substances such as cannabis, cocaine, hallucinogens, inhalants, opioids, and phencyclidine. Medication misuse can be defined as (1) not following the dosage recommendations by overmedicating or undermedicating oneself, (2) taking medication without the intention to treat a health condition, and/or (3) taking medications as prescribed but without well-defined goals, leading to use without defined efficacy.

The gold standard for assessing illicit drug misuse is a comprehensive diagnostic interview.[1] An alterative to the diagnostic interview could be the Addiction Severity Index,[32] but both are lengthy. Because of the time constraints during clinical visits, the CAGE and MAST have been altered for the purposes of assessing illicit drug use.[1] However, there is no specified instrument for use in the geriatric population only. Nevertheless, a modified version of the CAGE, to assess for drug abuse for medications and drugs, was found to differentiate successfully older individuals with alcohol misuse and drug misuse and those without any substance abuse problems.[33]

### Modified CAGE

As in the original CAGE assessment, CAGE stands for Cut down, Annoyed, Guilty, and Eye-opener; however, it is modified to include aspects of drug use. There are four detailed yes/no questions. They are as follows: (1) Have you ever felt you should cut down on your drinking/drug use? (2) Have people annoyed you by criticizing your drinking/drug use? (3) Have you ever felt bad or guilty about your drinking/drug use? (4) Have you ever had a drink first thing in the morning to steady your nerves or to get rid of a hangover/drug use? Affirmations of two of questions are indicative of an abuse problem.

### MAST

This test is comprised of 24 yes/no questions and was developed to measure alcohol abuse and dependence. Summation of the unevenly weighted responses (i.e., 1–5) equaling 5 or more was indicative of alcohol abuse problems. Therefore, affirmation of one heavily weighted score (i.e., 5) could be indicative of abuse problems. However, to assess drug use, drinking language is substituted with language describing illicit drug use.

Objective assessments of illicit drug use employ toxicologic tests (i.e., radioimmunoassay, enzymatic immunoassay, fluorescence polarization immunoassay, thin-layer chromatography) of urine or blood specimens.[34] The sensitivity of these methods is dependent on the time lapse between illicit drug use and testing. It is ideal for the time lapse to be as short as possible for the most accuracy in identifying drug use. In addition, medications such as prescribed opiates may make interpretation of results difficult due to toxicology sensitivity to medication interactions. Therefore, considering that geriatric individuals are the greatest consumers of medication, objective toxicology tests may be less beneficial and accurate.

There seems to be no quick and easy assessment tool for identifying medication misuse. The tools that are currently available require comprehensive medication reporting as well as manual or computerized contrast/comparison to expert recommendations. One source for assessing medication misuse is drug utilization reviews (DURs).[35] DURs provide standards and criteria for proper drug use; however, these lists are designed for specific purposes and contexts. Therefore, DURs can vary from one institution to the next and are not necessarily always applicable to geriatric patients. A more common and universal tool for assessing improper prescription drug use in older persons is the Beers' List.[36,37] This listing categorizes drugs that are improper for use specifically in the older population. The Medication Appropriateness Index is another assessment tool that has also been used as another catalog for prescription drug accuracy for the older population.[38]

## DURs

DURs are expert consensus opinions for defining medication standards and/or explicit criteria for a single drug, class of drugs, or groups of drugs. These can be unique to context (i.e., health maintenance organizations, pharmacies, governmental agencies). For example, the Medicaid program uses DURs that have been developed for the Health Care Financing Administration.[39]

## Beers' List

Beers' List is a national guideline for physicians and pharmacists that serves the geriatric population. The list consists of criteria defining medications that generally should be avoided in geriatric patients, regardless of setting.

### Medication Appropriateness Index

The Medication Appropriateness Index uses implicit criteria to judge the appropriateness of medication prescribing, using the criteria to evaluate each medication individually. It measures the magnitude of inappropriate prescribing for most dimensions of drug use that are clinically relevant.

An alternative to these classification lists is a computerized system known as pharmaceutical benefit manager. This program can identify poor prescription patterns in an efficient automated approach. However, the geriatric population has limited access to such resources because of its exclusion in Medicare drug programs.[40]

Regardless of which tool is used to assess medication misuse, the first step to assessing prescription drug misuse is to have an accurate assessment of prescription drugs currently in use by a single geriatric individual. One obvious method would be computer records of all drugs recommended/prescribed, provided samples of, filled and purchased at pharmacies, and submitted to insurance plans. However, the problem is that individuals can have multiple clinicians prescribing medications, sometimes providing prescription samples to their patients, with several participating pharmacies and insurance coverages that most likely do not work in partnership.

Therefore, an alternative method to collecting accurate medication data may be simply to ask the individual for a list of medications that he or she is currently taking. However, errors may result from changes in memory associated with aging; therefore, a geriatric individual's recollection of his or her medications may be vulnerable to respondent accuracy.[41] The Brown Bag method could be an alternative approach to assessing proper medication use.[42,43] This method requires the individual to place all of his or her medications in current use into a bag to bring them to a certain location where the medications are recorded. At that time, details concerning their dose and adherence can be reviewed. The Brown Bag method can resolve individual recall inaccuracy for medications and overcome the lack of collaboration in the medication bureaucracies. However, this method may be exceedingly inappropriate in clinical visits but may be a method to pursue outside of clinical visits, yet in the realm of primary care.

It is salient to assess the drug misuse, both illicit drug use and medication misuse, behaviors of geriatric patients. With the exception of the modified versions of MAST-G and CAGE, the currently available tools are comprehensive but time consuming and could require multiple resources.

## TOBACCO USE

Tobacco assessments are imperative considering that the US Preventive Task Force recommends tobacco cessation counseling for all persons who use tobacco products.[1] There is a significant portion of geriatric smokers who believe that geriatric populations are too old to quit tobacco use, that they no longer suffer from the negative consequences of tobacco use, or that they cannot benefit from the cessation of tobacco use.[44] Therefore, tobacco assessments in the geriatric population are still salient.

Because of the lack of a scientific tobacco assessment tool produced or used for the geriatric population, an obvious method would be a simple counsel during clinical visits to assess for tobacco-related behaviors. When a geriatric patient indicates smoking, clinicians should recommend cessation treatment immediately.[45]

It is salient to assess the tobacco behaviors of geriatric patients even if the only probable tool is a brief question asking whether they smoke. Tobacco use is the leading cause of premature death compared with other health behaviors, such as inadequate diets and activity patterns, alcohol use, microbial agents, toxic agents, firearms, sexual behaviors, motor vehicle accidents, and illicit use of drugs.[46] Smoking has also been linked to the cause of lung cancer by stimulating abnormal cellular growth in the lungs[47] and cardiovascular diseases by certain cardiovascular risk factors, for example, a lack of physical exercise and obesity.[48] Because this population has a higher likelihood of suffering from additional conditions, assessing and then treating tobacco misuse can reduce the incidence of further co-morbidity and premature mortality and possibly improve the quality of life for geriatric individuals.

## BARRIERS TO THE USE OF SUBSTANCE USE ASSESSMENTS

The diagnostic assessments described for substance use disorders rely greatly on self-reported behavioral symptoms. Given that denial, as well as individual opinions regarding professional help, plays such a prominent role in the pathology of substance use disorders for the patient, information obtained by self-report probably underestimates any problems associated with substance use as well as the quantity and frequency of use. Mentioned previously, people's ability to remember past events or report past average consumption may deteriorate with advancing age. Outside of having more assessments tools tailored for the geriatric population, there is a need for more assessment tools that overcome patient memory inaccuracy, sensitivity, and denial concerns.

Geriatric individuals may not be assessed for substance use issues because clinicians may think it is a nonexistent problem. Substance abuse is a noteworthy problem for geriatric populations. There is substantial evidence alluding to a considerable number of geriatric patients with indications of alcohol misuse, illicit drug use, medication drug misuse, and tobacco use. Additionally, it is expected that with the increase in the geriatric population, caused by baby boomers reaching old age, there will be an estimated 2.5-times greater prevalence of older adults in need of substance use treatment.[49]

Clinicians may also fail to assess their geriatric patients for substance use issues because they may think their patient would not be willing to change. This is not true considering the evidence showing that substance use treatment programs are effective in older adults.[50] Because the geriatric population is a specialized group with unique cohort and individual effects, treatments need to be implemented accordingly. There has been some indication that there is a greater likelihood of change in substance use behaviors when age-specific interventions are facilitated.[51] Along the same lines, another barrier could be the idea that it is too late for geriatric patients to avoid negative health consequences by changing substance misuse behaviors. However, there is no scientific indication that geriatric populations are too old to achieve some health benefits from treatment of their substance use.

Finally, based on the review of substance use assessments, clinicians may have some difficulty finding proper assessment tools for their geriatric population. It is obvious that a need exists to have more assessments that are tailored to assess substance use in the geriatric population. In addition, there has been some evidence that not enough treatment facilities have been designed to serve specifically the geriatric population.[52] Having less than ideal assessment tools and a need for more treatment facilities could inadvertently cause hesitation for clinical substance use assessments in geriatric populations. This is also a major problem considering that the older population in the United States is growing rapidly. The US Census Bureau estimates by the year 2020, 18% compared with a current 12% of the population will be over the age of 65 years.[53] As the percentage of older persons nearly doubles over the next 25 years, the need for prevention, assessments, and treatment of substance use disorders and associated conditions will also grow. Considering that there is currently a weakness in this area, as the geriatric population grows, so will the severity of not having the appropriate treatment facilities and assessment tools.

## CONCLUSIONS/RECOMMENDATIONS

In every substance use assessment, it is first necessary to start by asking whether the patient drinks/uses illicit drugs or medications/uses any form of tobacco. In the case of substance use, further assessment is necessary to determine the level of severity for this behavior. In the case of no use, the patient should be asked about any past problems with substances. This will provide a better indication of the patient's history and his or her level of risk.

Despite the need for better screening/assessment tools to identify substance issues in older persons, it is still tremendously relevant to screen geriatric patients for substance use with the tools and knowledge currently available. The MAST-G or SMAST-G (Appendix) and CAGE appear to be most sensitive tools for assessing and differentiating types of substance use in older adults. However, new developments may provide a more efficient process to detecting substance problems in the older population. The ARPS and the CARPS are both multidimensional tools that incorporate substance use within the context of other health conditions and health behaviors. The strength of CARPS, however, is the fact that it not only assesses substance use in an efficient manner, but it also offers an educational health component. Indirectly, CARPS has also been shown to stimulate substance use conversation positively within primary care clinical visits.

It is recommended that not only do more assessments need to be developed and validated for use in the geriatric population, but these tools should incorporate the ideas of multidimensionality (i.e., incorporate alcohol, illicit drug use, medication misuse, and smoking). In addition, there is a need for temporal efficiency for ease of use in clinical visits and waiting rooms, maybe even in nonmedical locations. Incorporation of an educational component could provide a final progression, which may lead to self-initiation of substance use treatment. In order for this scientific development to be completely fruitful, clinicians need to ensure screening of their geriatric patients.

**REFERENCES**

1. US Preventive Task Force. *Guide to Clinical Preventive Services*. Baltimore: Williams & Wilkins; 1996.

2. Waern U. Health and disease at the age of sixty: Findings in a health survey of 60-year-old men in Uppsala and a comparison with men 10 years younger. *Uppsala J Med Sci.* 1978;83:153–156.

3. Weintraub E, Weintraub D, Dixon L, et al. Geriatric patients on a substance abuse consultation service. *Am J Geriatr Psychiatry.* 2002;10:337–342.

4. Onder G, Landi F, Vedova CD et al. Moderate alcohol consumption and adverse drug reactions among older adults. *Pharmaepidemiol Drug Safety.* 2002;11:385–392.

5. Di Bari M, Silvestrini G, Chiarlone M, et al. Features of excessive alcohol drinking in older adults distinctively captured by behavioral and biological screening instruments: An epidemiological study. *J Clin Epidemiol.* 2002;55:41–47.

6. Curtis LH, Ostbye T, Sendersky V, et al. Inappropriate prescribing for elderly Americans in a large outpatient population. *Am Med Assoc.* 2004;164:1621–1625.

7. Sulander T, Helakorpi S, Rahkkonen O, Nissinen A, Uutela A. Smoking and alcohol consumption among the elderly: Trends and associations 1985–2001. *Prev Med.* 2004;39(2):413–418.

8. Blow FC, Walton MA, Chermack ST, et al. Older adult treatment outcome following elder-specific inpatient alcoholism treatment. *J Subst Abuse Treat.* 2000;19:67–75.

9. McMahin RC, Malow R, Loewinger L. Substance abuse history predicts depression and relapse status among cocaine abusers. *Am J Addict.* 1999;8:1–8.

10. Lane SD, Cherek DR, Dougherty DM, et al. Laboratory measurement of adaptive behavior change in humans with a history of substance dependence. *Drug Alcohol Depend.* 1998;51:239–252.

11. Bjork JM, Grant SJ, Hommer DW. Cross-sectional volumetric analysis of brain atrophy in alcohol dependence: Effects of drinking history and comorbid substance use disorder. *Am J Psychiatry.* 2003;160:2038–2045.

12. US Preventive Task Force. Screening and behavioral counseling interventions in primary care to reduce alcohol misuse: Recommendation statement. *Ann Intern Med.* 2004;140: 554–556.

13. National Institute of Health. *The Physician's Guide to Helping with Alcohol Problems.* Bethesda, MD: National Institute on Alcohol Abuse and Alcoholism (NIAAA); 1995. NIH Publication No. 95-3769.

14. Saunders JB, Aasland OG, Babor TF, et al. Development of the Alcohol Use Disorders Identification Test (AUDIT): WHO collaborative project on early detection of person with harmful alcohol consumption—II. *Addiction.* 1993;88:791–804.

15. Ewing JA. Detecting alcoholism: The CAGE questionnaire. *JAMA.* 1984;252: 1905–1907.

16. Bush K, Kivlahan DR, McDonell MB, Fihn SD, Bradley KA. The AUDIT Alcohol Consumption Questions (AUDIT-C). *Arch Intern Med.* 1998;158:1789–1795.

17. Selzer ML. The Michigan Alcoholism Screening Test: The quest for a new diagnostic instrument. *Am J Psychiatry.* 1971;127:1653–1658.

18. Barry K, Fleming M. The Alcohol Use Disorders Identification Test (AUDIT) and the SMAST-13: Predictive validity in a rural primary care sample. *Alcohol.* 1993;17: 1188–1192.

19. Pokorny MD, Miller BA, Kaplan HB. The brief MAST: A shortened version of the Michigan Alcohol Screening Test. *Am J Psychiatry.* 1972;129:342–345.

20. Blow FC, Brower KG, Schulenberg JE, et al. The Michigan Alcoholism Screening Test-Geriatric Version (MAST-G): A new elderly-specific screening instrument. *Alcoholism Clin Exp Res.* 1992;19:372.

21. Blow FC, Gillespie BW, Barry KL, et al. Brief screening for alcohol problems in elderly populations using the Short Michigan Alcoholism Screening Test-Geriatric Version (SMAST-G). *Alcoholism Clin Exp Res.* 1998;22(Suppl):131A.

22. Cyr MG, Wartman SA. The effectiveness of routine screening questions in the detection of alcoholism. *JAMA.* 1988;259:51–54.

23. Fink A, Morton SC, Beck JC, et al. The alcohol-related problems survey: Identifying hazardous and harmful drinking in older primary care patients. *J Am Geriatr Soc.* 2002;50:1717–1722.

24. Beullens J, Aertgeeerts B. Screening for alcohol abuse and dependence in older people using *DSM* criteria: A review. *Aging Mental Health* 2004;8(1):76–82.

25. Moore AA, Seeman T, Morgenstern H, Beck JC, Reuben DB. Are there differences between older persons who screen positive on the CAGE Questionnaire and the Short Michigan Alcoholism Screening Test-Geriatric Version? *J Am Geriatr Soc.* 2002;50:858–862.

26. Reid MC, Tinetti ME, O-Connor PG, Kosten TR, Concato J. Measuring alcohol consumption among older adults: A comparison of available methods. *Am J Addictions* 2003;12:211–219.

27. Nguyen K, Fink A, Beck JC, Higa J. Feasibility of using an alcohol-screening and health education system with older primary care patients. *J Am Board Fam Pract.* 2001;14:7–15.

28. Conigliareo J, Lofgren RP, Hanusa BH. Screening for problem drinking: Impact on physician behavior and patient drinking habits. *J Gen Intern Med.* 1998;13:251–256.

29. National Institute on Alcohol Abuse and Alcoholism. *Alcohol and Health: Eighth Special Report to the Health and Human Services.* Rockville, MD: US Department of Health and Human Services, National Institutes of Health; 1993. (NIH Publication No. 94-3699.)

30. Anderson TL, Levy JA. Marginality among older injectors in today's illicit drug culture: Assessing the impact of ageing. *Addiction.* 2003;98:761–770.

31. Hanlon JT, Schmader KE, Boult C, et al. Use of inappropriate prescription drugs by older people. *J Am Geriatr Soc.* 2002;50:26–34.

32. McLellan AT, Lubrosky L, Woody GE, et al. An improved diagnostic evaluation instrument for substance abuse patients: The Addiction Severity Index. *J Nervous Mental Disord.* 1980;168:26–33.

33. Hinkin CH, Castellon SA, Dickson-Fuhrman E, et al. Screening for drug and alcohol abuse among older adults using a modified version of the CAGE. *Am J Addict.* 2001;10:319–326.

34. Catlin D, Cowan D, Donike M, et al. Testing urine for drugs. *Clin Chim Acta.* 1992;207:S13–S26.

35. Knapp DA. Development of criteria for drug utilization review. *Clin Pharmacol Theory.* 1991;5:600–602.

36. Beers MH. Explicit criteria for determining potentially inappropriate medication use by the elderly: An update. *Arch Intern Med.* 1997;157:1531–1536.

37. Fick DM, Cooper JW, Wade WE, Waller JL, Maclean JR, Beers MH. Updating the Beers criteria for potentially inappropriate medication use in older adults: Results of a US consensus panel of experts. *Arch Intern Med.* 2003;163:2716–2724.

38. Hanlon JT, Schmader JE, Samsa GP. A method for assessing drug therapy appropriateness. *J Clin Epidemiol.* 1992;45:1045–1051.

39. Knapp D, Erwin G. Screening criteria for outpatient drug use review: Final report to HCFA. Baltimore, MD: University of Maryland School of Pharmacy; 1992.

40. McLeod PJ, Huang AR, Tamblyn RM, et al. Defining inappropriate practices in prescribing for the elderly: A national consensus panel. *Canadian Med Assoc J.* 1997;156: 385–391.

41. Taylor DSA, Smiciklas-Wright H. The quality of survey data obtained from elderly adults. *J Nutr Elderly.* 1993;13:11–21.

42. Williams ME, Pulliam CC, Hunter R, et al. The short-term effect of interdisciplinary medication review on function and cost in ambulatory elderly people. *J Am Geriatr Soc.* 2004;52:93–98.

43. Spiers MV, Kutzik DM. Self-reported memory of medication use by the elderly. *Am J Health-System Pharm.* 1995;52:985–990.

44. Burns DM. Cigarette smoking among the elderly: Disease consequences and the benefits of cessation. *Am J Health Promot.* 2000;14:357–361.

45. Appel DW, Aldrich TK. Smoking cessation in the elderly. *Clin Geriatr Med.* 2003;19:1–21.

46. McGinnus JM, Foege WH. Actual causes of death in the United States. *JAMA.* 1993;270:2207–2212.

47. Center for Chronic Disease Prevention and Health Promotion: Centers for Disease Control. Smoking-attributable mortality and years of potential life lost—United States, 1990. *Morbid Mortal Weekly Rep.* 1993;42:645–648.

48. Centers for Disease Control. *Reducing the Health Consequences of Smoking: 25 Years of Progress: A Report of the Surgeon General.* Rockville, MD: US Department of Health and Human Services, Public Health Service, CDC, Center for Chronic Disease Prevention and Health Promotion; DHHS publication no (CDC) 1989;89–8411.

49. Gfroerer J, Penne M, Pemberton M, Folsom R. Substance abuse treatment need among older adults in 2020: The impact of the aging baby-boom cohort. *Drug Alcohol Depend.* 2003;69:127–135.

50. Bratzler DW, Oehlert WH, Austelle A. Smoking in the elderly: It's never too late to quit. *J Oklahoma State Med Assoc.* 2002;95:185–191.

51. Schonfeld L, Dupree LW. Treatment approaches for older problem drinkers. *Int J Addict.* 1995;30:1819–1842.

52. Schultz SK, Arndt S, Liesveld J. Locations of facilities with special programs for older substance abuse clients in the US. *Int J Geriatr Psychiatry.* 2003;18:839–843.

53. Spencer G. *Projections of the Population of the United States, by Age, Sex, and Race: 1988 to 2080,* vol. Series P-25. Washington, DC: USGPO. US Department of Commerce, 1989.

# Appendix
## MAST-G

1. After drinking, have you ever noticed an increase in your heart rate or beating in your chest?
2. When talking with others, do you ever underestimate how much you actually drank?
3. Does alcohol make you sleepy so that you often fall asleep in your chair?
4. After a few drinks, have you sometimes not eaten or been able to skip a meal because you didn't feel hungry?
5. Does having a few drinks help you decrease your shakiness or tremors?
6. Does alcohol sometimes make it hard for you to remember parts of the day or night?
7. Do you have certain rules for yourself that you won't drink before a certain time of the day?
8. Have you lost interest in hobbies or activities you used to enjoy?
9. When you wake up in the morning, do you ever have trouble remembering part of the night before?
10. Does having a drink help you sleep?
11. Do you hide your alcohol bottles from family members?
12. After a social gathering, have you ever felt embarrassed because you drank too much?
13. Have you ever been concerned that drinking might be harmful to your health?
14. Do you like to end the evening with a nightcap?
15. Did you find your drinking increased after someone close to you died?
16. In general, would you prefer to have a few drinks at home rather than go out to social events?
17. Are you drinking more now than in the past?
18. Do you usually take a drink to relax or calm your nerves?
19. Do you drink to take your mind off your problems?
20. Have you ever increased your drinking after experiencing a loss in your life?
21. Do you sometimes drive when you have had too much to drink?
22. Has a doctor or nurse ever said he or she was worried or concerned about your drinking?
23. Have you ever made rules to manage your drinking?
24. When you feel lonely, does having a drink help?

Scoring: If the person answered "yes" to five or more questions, responses are indicative of an alcohol problem.

# Appendix
## SMAST-G

1. When talking with others, do you ever underestimate how much you actually drink?
2. After a few drinks, have you sometimes not eaten or been able to skip a meal because you didn't feel hungry?
3. Does having a few drinks help decrease your shakiness or tremors?
4. Does alcohol sometimes make it hard for you to remember parts of the day or night?
5. Do you usually take a drink to relax or calm your nerves?
6. Do you drink to take your mind off problems?
7. Have you ever increased your drinking after experiencing a loss in your life?
8. Has a doctor or nurse ever said that he or she was worried or concerned about your drinking?
9. Have you ever made rules to manage your drinking?
10. When you feel lonely, does having a drink help?

Scoring: If the person answered "yes" to two or more questions, encourage a talk with the doctor.

# 10

## *Activities of Daily Living and Instrumental Activities of Daily Living Assessment*

Joseph J. Gallo

The preservation of function has become a prominent theme in geriatrics.[1,2] The emphasis has appropriately changed from an exclusive concern with delaying mortality to a focus on avoiding morbidity, that is, to preserving function[3,4] and extending active life expectancy.[5] Functional status captures the concept of quality of life in ways that an emphasis on medical diagnoses does not.[6,7] Functional assessment is the key to understanding the impact of medical illness on the older person and family and is the cornerstone of geriatric rehabilitation.[8,9] The typical catalog of medical problems is not sufficient to answer questions about functional capability, such as the ability to dress or use the toilet. Brief methods are emphasized in this chapter to encourage ongoing functional assessment in the office and in other settings.

### FOCUS ON FUNCTION

Functioning in daily life may be examined on several levels. Performance in social and occupational roles comprises one level.[10,11] The tasks demanded every day, such as driving or using public transportation, comprise another. Activities necessary for persons in a modern society such as using the telephone or automatic teller machine are commonplace. On another plane are the personal care tasks, such as dressing, bathing, and toileting. Older adults and others who have difficulty with these tasks must compensate for the disability.

The capacity to function independently is poorly described by the constellation of medical diseases alone. Performance on mental status testing does not necessarily predict functional status.[12,13] Similarly, the severity of disease as measured by standard laboratory tests does not necessarily imply disability. Functional status should be assessed directly and independently of medical and laboratory abnormalities or cognitive impairment.

A 70-year-old woman with diabetes mellitus, hypertension, and congestive heart failure was hospitalized for urinary incontinence. Urologic studies were normal, and the patient was discharged home in her husband's care. Two weeks later, she was again admitted for "mental status changes" because she was noted to be increasingly disoriented and incontinent. Her daughter related slow intellectual impairment over the course of at least a year. Mental status testing revealed global intellectual deficits in orientation, memory, calculations, and visuospatial skills. Review of the chart from the previous hospitalization showed no documented mental status examination with which to compare findings. It was believed the patient had Alzheimer's disease with superimposed delirium secondary to medication.

Specific functional loss in older adults is not determined by the locus of disease—urinary incontinence may not indicate disease confined to the urinary tract. Because of the family's difficulty in caring for this patient, she required nursing home care. In a situation with better functional ability or social support, she may have been able to stay at home. Thus, the problem list alone did not give all of the information needed to make recommendations.

Cognitive impairment does not necessarily imply an inability to perform enough activities to maintain independent living. Scores on the Short Portable Mental Status Questionnaire (SPMSQ) were only weakly correlated to the ability of older adults to care for themselves. Of 32 persons with moderate to severe impairment on the SPMSQ, 9 were living completely independently, and another 10 needed assistance with only dressing.[14] This observation is borne out by experience. Severely impaired persons may perform quite well in a familiar home setting.

Functional assessment can help the practitioner focus on the person's capabilities, and when there is a change, appropriate resources can be rallied and a search for medical illness initiated. The sometimes delicate state of homeostasis makes the older adult vulnerable to disability from a variety of sources. Going beyond the medical model is critical because medical or psychiatric illness may present as a nonspecific deterioration in functional status. It is not enough to enumerate the medical problems and treat them in isolation. When a medical illness is diagnosed, how it affects the older person's functional capacity must always be considered. Conversely, the person's functional status must be considered in formulating the treatment plan.

Consider an 83-year-old man who lives alone and has a history of paraplegia since an early age with confinement to a wheelchair, osteoarthritis, scoliosis, atrial fibrillation with controlled ventricular response on digoxin, a suprapubic catheter for a neurogenic bladder, cataracts, and poor dental hygiene with full dentures. This patient's mental status is normal. Despite his physical limitations and medical problems, he lives in his home alone with the periodic visits from his niece and visiting nurses. Suppose one knew that this person was not able to transfer from his wheelchair to the toilet or to the bed or that he was incapable of taking his medication properly. One can see how difficulty in one of these areas might change the situation and temper one's judgment about a person's ability to reside at home. Except for walking, this person's functional status is good.

The multitude of medical, social, and psychologic challenges presented by the older adult can overwhelm health care professionals. They should attack small problems with major consequences first. Ameliorating problems that interfere with safe driving and ambulation would be an important focus for intervention. Among the illnesses or complaints presented by the older person, which one or two are presenting the most difficulty in terms of functional capacity? For example, cataracts might present more difficulty with eating, shopping, and meal preparation than osteoarthritis. The physician should look closely at the less serious although treatable conditions that contribute to disability. Correction of minor problems could enhance the person's quality of life. Something as simple as modifying the diuretic drug dosing schedule to obviate the need for evening and nightly trips to the bathroom may enhance the sleep of the older person and his or her caregiver.

Asking about driving habits and accidents is an important inquiry but also signals that more basic tasks, such as shopping, dressing, and bathing, are probably adequately performed. Driving is given special attention in a separate chapter. Difficulties with the telephone or improper use of medications may signal cognitive impairment[15] or depression.[16]

The information from functional assessment has an important, practical role in advising and counseling clients and their families and in following clients after significant medical events.[10] A functional scale has been used to predict the need for institutionalization (at least on a temporary basis) after hip fracture.[17] This scale consists of components assessing physical health (e.g., vision, hearing, and mental status), ambulatory ability, daily activities, social situation (e.g., lives alone, with spouse, or in nursing home), and disabilities (e.g., incontinence, paralysis, amputation, decubitus, and contracture). The Functional Rating Scale for the Symptoms of Dementia, discussed later, is also an example of a functional assessment questionnaire that evaluates the need for nursing home placement in the patient with dementia.[18] The Determination of Need Functional Assessment is an example of a rating scale that has been specifically developed to evaluate the risk for nursing home placement and to assist with care planning for community-based services.[19,20]

Functional ability is prognostic of mortality. For example, a retrospective study compared persons who died within 1 year of placement in a nursing home with those who survived. The latter group was found to be more independent, especially in bathing and dressing.[21] Mortality was also associated with poor functioning after hospitalization.[22] The inability to perform tasks such as traveling, shopping, meal preparation, housework, and handling money predicts mortality as well.[23,24] An inability to perform simple tasks such as carrying a bag of groceries predicts further functional decline[25] and institutionalization.[26]

A person's home can speak volumes about the performance of activities of daily living (ADLs). How well arranged is the home for bathing and toileting? Are there obvious safety hazards (e.g., frayed wires, ashtrays near the bed, slippery floors or rugs, and firearms stored in the home of a person with dementia)? How well does the older person maneuver about the home (i.e., transfer and ambulation)? How well are nutritional needs met (i.e., food in the refrigerator, shopping, and cooking)? How well is the home maintained (i.e., shelter, cleanliness, and clutter)? In addition to the other benefits of home visits, such as the assessment of social support available to the patient, there is also less need for secondhand information about the functional ability of the older adult.[27,28]

Functional impairment can be listed independently of the problem list in the problem-oriented medical record. For example, two persons with rheumatoid arthritis may differ in their abilities to eat. The physician would then list "difficulty with feeding" independently of the medical diagnosis of rheumatoid arthritis. This helps quantify functional impairment and alerts other clinicians to the implications of the functional impairment (in this case, a problem with nutrition).

A complete problem-oriented medical record, listing functional as well as undefined problems, organizes them and helps establish priorities for solution. Seen as "building blocks," efforts to assist the patient are cumulative because some problems are selected for immediate attention, whereas others are worked on gradually. Medical diagnosis remains important, but functional assessment keeps the problems in perspective and provides a complementary viewpoint. Functional impairment should prompt a timely and thorough search for cognitive impairment, depression, substance abuse, adverse medication effects, and sensory impairment.[7]

Functional assessment can be a positive force in caring for older adults. Because so much professional training focuses on the negative aspects of age and its losses, taking care to determine functional capacity compels health professionals to see evaluation in a positive light. Despite multiple diseases, the patient functions well. How well does he or she function in his or her own environment? What adaptations and concessions have been made to make up for deficiencies? Finally, how can professionals and other caregivers promote and initiate adaptations to allow the most independent, fulfilling life possible? This is a taste of the kinds of issues facing clinicians who may use some of the instruments discussed later in this chapter to facilitate thinking along these lines.

## THE COMPONENTS OF FUNCTIONAL STATUS

A systematic approach to each domain of geriatric assessment, including functional assessment, is desirable. The items generally agreed on as composing functional assessment are the ADLs and the instrumental ADLs (IADLs), although other categorizations are possible.[29] The ADLs are the functions that are fundamental to independent living, such as dressing and bathing. The IADLs include more complex daily activities, such as using the telephone, housekeeping, and managing money. Statistical methods applied to self-report data on difficulty with activities resulted in similar groupings consisting of (1) activities related to mobility and exercise such as walking, (2) complex tasks such as paying bills and shopping, (3) self-care activities such as toileting, and (4) upper-extremity tasks such as grasping and reaching.[30] Driving and sexual functioning are other important arenas to consider in functional assessment and are discussed in other chapters.

Evaluation of functional status is not limited to the assessment of specific activities and tasks, although that is the emphasis here. Assessment may also include significant happenings in a person's life or family that have a bearing on the health status or situation (events of daily living), demands placed on the person from within or from the family and society (demands of daily living), the nature of the physical environment (environment of daily living), and the person's values and beliefs that determine decisions and responses regarding health care (values and beliefs in daily living).[31,32]

## ADLs

Just as is true for mental status testing instruments, ADL scales may have ceiling or threshold effects.[33] In other words, if the activities chosen for assessment are too easy, many persons will do well on the scale; thus, a prominent ceiling effect occurs. Such an ADL scale may be useful for assessing or defining frail older persons, but most community-dwelling older adults would be able to perform the activities on the list without much trouble.[34] Asking about driving and IADLs is apt to be more fruitful in functional assessment of ambulatory older persons.

The term "frailty" has been used to describe older adults whose management of day-to-day tasks is tenuous. The definition of frail has been couched in functional terms to describe those persons who need help performing ADLs,[35,36] with effects on behavior and quality of life.[37] A dynamic model assumes that it is the balance between assets and deficits that determines frailty; the assets and deficits are components of geriatric assessment, such as caregiver burden, resources, attitudes, and health status.[38] A change in status on one domain may tip the balance into frailty. Frail older adults may rely heavily on neighbors or family to perform routine jobs that fully independent persons do for themselves. Frailty implies health conditions that require frequent hospitalizations, medication, and visits to physicians' offices.

Ideally, practitioners need a set of questions that is quick and easy to administer periodically to detect older adults who are beginning to experience difficulty in the activities usually associated with independent living. Something similar to the Apgar score used to evaluate newborns might be desirable for this purpose. Details regarding the use of indexes of function and measurement theory can be found else-where.[1,33,39–43] Further theoretical considerations can be found in the Institute of Medicine Report *Disability in America*.[44] In the next section, specific instruments used to assess ADLs and IADLs are discussed.

## Katz Index of Activities of Daily Living

A basic schedule to assess ADLs, published in 1963, is the Katz Index of ADL, which includes bathing, dressing, toileting, transfer, conti-nence, and feeding (Exhibit 10–1).[45] It provides a framework for as-sessing the ability to live independently, or if deficiencies are found, it is the focal point for remediation. A person dependent in a single ac-tivity might need assistance at isolated times of the day, such as for bathing, but more help might be needed by persons dependent on as-sistance in many activities.

A three-tiered scale for the ADL is found to be more reliable and is reproducible even when scored by personnel with minimal training. The three-point scale might consist of the ratings "independent," "semi-independent" (needs a part-time assistant), and "dependent," rather than a checklist with four or five gradations defining how much assistance is required.[46]

Considering the basic ADL items in evaluation of an older person has several important advantages. For one, focusing on functional abilities allows matching of services to needs. For example, someone requiring assistance in only bathing may be maintained indepen-dently with an aide to perform the task once a week. In addition, key-ing in on specific tasks allows interventions to be more focused. In dealing with difficulty in dressing, a caregiver might try putting pic-ture labels on drawers, grouping items that belong together, and tak-ing the individual by the hand and starting the desired action as a cue. In other cases, multiple areas of dependence would make it clear that it is not possible to provide the necessary help to continue the multiple ADLs that keep the person at home.[45,47,48]

Subjective estimates of disease severity or mere use of a diagnostic label may not be as helpful as an emphasis on functional assessment. An individual with rheumatoid arthritis may have major functional deficits that could be improved with physical therapy, appliances, or the provision of help with key ADLs such as bathing. In the care of a patient after a stroke, following his or her progress on ADLs is useful.[49] In addition to matching services to needs, persons unable to perform

**Exhibit 10–1** Katz Index of Activities of Daily Living

1. *Bathing* (sponge, shower, or tub)
   I: receives no assistance (gets in and out of tub if tub is the usual means of bathing)
   A: receives assistance in bathing only one part of the body (such as the back or a leg)
   D: receives assistance in bathing more than one part of the body (or not bathed)

2. *Dressing*
   I: gets clothes and gets completely dressed without assistance
   A: gets clothes and gets dressed without assistance except in tying shoes
   D: receives assistance in getting clothes or in getting dressed or stays partly or completely undressed

3. *Toileting*
   I: goes to "toilet room," cleans self, and arranges clothes without assistance (may use object for support such as cane, walker, or wheelchair and may manage night bedpan or commode, emptying it in the morning)
   A: receives assistance in going to "toilet room" or in cleansing self or in arranging clothes after elimination or in use of night bedpan or commode
   D: doesn't go to room termed "toilet" for the elimination process

4. *Transfer*
   I: moves in and out of bed as well as in and out of chair without assistance (may be using object for support such as cane or walker)
   A: moves in and out of bed or chair with assistance
   D: doesn't get out of bed

5. *Continence*
   I: controls urination and bowel movement completely by self
   A: has occasional "accidents"
   D: supervision helps keep urine or bowel control; catheter is used, or is incontinent

6. *Feeding*
   I: feeds self without assistance
   A: feeds self except for getting assistance in cutting meat or buttering bread
   D: receives assistance in feeding or is fed partly or completely by using tubes or intravenous fluids

Abbreviations:  I, independent; A, assistance; D, dependent

*Source:* From Katz S, et al. Studies of illness in the aged: The index of ADL, activities of daily living scale, *JAMA*, Vol. 185, p. 915. © 1963, American Medical Association.

one or more of these ADLs may be at risk for hospitalization or nursing home placement.

## Barthel Index

The Barthel Index has also been used to assess ability for self-care, but the items are weighted to account for the amount of physical assistance that would be required if the individual is unable to carry out the function. In one study in a rehabilitative setting for patients with neuromuscular disorders, the Barthel Index was used to document improvement. Patients who did not improve their score during rehabilitation were believed to have poor potential for recovery.[50]

A modified Barthel Index has been devised and, when used to assess the need for home health services, correlated to the number of activities the person was able to do independently.[42,51] Persons scoring less than 60 on the modified Barthel Index (Table 10–1) were able to perform no more than 10 of the defined ADL and IADL tasks. A score of less than 60 was especially associated with the need for help in feed-

**Table 10–1** Modified Barthel Index

|  | Independent | | Dependent | |
|---|---|---|---|---|
|  | Intact | Limited | Helper | Null |
| Drink from cup/feed from dish | 10 | 5 | 0 | 0 |
| Dress upper body | 5 | 5 | 3 | 0 |
| Dress lower body | 5 | 5 | 2 | 0 |
| Don brace or prosthesis | 0 | 0 | −2 | 0 |
| Grooming | 5 | 5 | 0 | 0 |
| Wash or bathe | 4 | 4 | 0 | 0 |
| Bladder incontinence | 10 | 10 | 5 | 0 |
| Bowel incontinence | 10 | 10 | 5 | 0 |
| Care of perineum/clothing at toilet | 4 | 4 | 2 | 0 |
| Transfer, chair | 15 | 15 | 7 | 0 |
| Transfer, toilet | 6 | 5 | 3 | 0 |
| Transfer, tub or shower | 1 | 1 | 0 | 0 |
| Walk on level 50 yd or more | 15 | 15 | 10 | 0 |
| Up and down stairs for one flight or more | 10 | 10 | 5 | 0 |
| Wheelchair 50 yd (only if not walking) | 15 | 5 | 0 | 0 |

*Source:* Adapted with permission from Fortinsky RH et al. The use of functional assessment in understanding home care needs. *Med Care.* Vol. 19, No. 5, p. 491. © 1981, JB Lippincott Company.

ing, bathing, grooming, dressing, toileting, transferring, doing housework, and preparing meals.[51] The modified Barthel Index may be a
good indicator of the need for support in ADLs.

## IADLs

In addition to the ADLs, another set of activities required for independent living is the IADLs.[52,53] These activities are the more complex
and demanding skills of using the telephone, traveling, shopping,
preparing meals, doing housework, taking medicine properly, and
managing money (Exhibit 10–2). The IADLs may emphasize tasks traditionally performed by women, especially for the current cohort of
older persons.[54] This bias notwithstanding, these chores are required
daily activities for most persons, and if someone is unable to perform
them, the tasks must be performed by a caregiver.

The IADLs have been distilled into five items, which form a simple
screening test to determine who may require a more comprehensive
assessment.[23] The five items concern travel, shopping, meal preparation, housework, and handling money (Exhibit 10–3). The five-item
IADL scale has some interesting features.

First, as mentioned previously, the inability to perform these tasks is
correlated to mortality. Second, when the items are arranged verti-
cally, knowing a person can pass or perform one item indicates that
person can pass or perform all items below it on the scale but none of
the items listed above it. For example, when rated from the most difficult to the least difficult, the five items are ordered: housework, travel,
shopping, finances, and cooking.[23,55]

This five-item scale can demonstrate change as well, which may
identify who needs help, and might be administered on a scheduled
basis for all older patients in a primary care practice. For example, consider a 63-year-old woman presenting for routine examination and renewal of blood pressure medications. Last year she had no difficulties
getting places, shopping, preparing meals, doing housework, or handling money. Today she admits some recent trouble managing her
checkbook and reluctantly relates her worries about declining memory
and lack of concentration. The Folstein Mini-Mental State score is normal. On further questioning, vegetative symptoms of depression are
found. The items of ADLs and IADLs translate readily into services.
Knowledge of the ability of clients to perform various tasks becomes an
indicator of what services might be needed. For example, nursing care,
personal care, continuous supervision, meal preparation, or home-

**Exhibit 10–2** Instrumental Activities of Daily Living

1. *Telephone*
   I: able to look up numbers, dial, receive, and make calls without help
   A: able to answer phone or dial operator in an emergency, but needs special phone or help in getting number or dialing
   D: unable to use the telephone

2. *Traveling*
   I: able to drive own car or travel alone on bus or taxi
   A: able to travel, but not alone
   D: unable to travel

3. *Shopping*
   I: able to take care of all shopping with transportation provided
   A: able to shop, but not alone
   D: unable to shop

4. *Preparing meals*
   I: able to plan and cook full meals
   A: able to prepare light foods, but unable to cook full meals alone
   D: unable to prepare any meals

5. *Housework*
   I: able to do heavy housework (like scrub floors)
   A: able to do light housework, but needs help with heavy tasks
   D: unable to do any housework

6. *Medication*
   I: able to take medications in the right dose at the right time
   A: able to take medications, but needs reminding or someone to prepare it
   D: unable to take medications

7. *Money*
   I: able to manage buying needs, write checks, pay bills
   A: able to manage daily buying needs, but needs help managing checkbook, and paying bills
   D: unable to manage money

Abbreviations:  I, independent; A, assistance; D, dependent

*Source:* Adapted with permission from Duke University Center for the Study of Aging and Human Development, *The Multidimensional Functional Assessment Questionnaire*, ed. 2, pp. 154–156, 157–162, and 169–170. © 1978, Duke University at Durham, North Carolina.

**Exhibit 10–3** The Five-Item Instrumental Activities of Daily Living (IADL) Screening Questionnaire

---

1. Can you *get to places* out of walking distance:
   1  Without help (can travel alone on bus, taxi, or drive your own car)
   0  With some help (need someone to help you or go with you when travel-
      ing) or are you unable to travel unless emergency arrangements are made
      for a specialized vehicle such as an ambulance?
   –  Not answered

2. Can you *go shopping* for groceries or clothes (assuming you have transportation):
   1  Without help (taking care of all your shopping needs yourself, assuming
      you have transportation)
   0  With some help (need someone to go with you on all shopping trips), or
      are you completely unable to do any shopping?
   –  Not answered

3. Can you *prepare your own meals:*
   1  Without help (plan and cook meals yourself)
   0  With some help (can prepare some things but unable to cook full meals
      yourself), or are you completely unable to prepare any meals?
   –  Not answered

4. Can you do your *housework:*
   1  Without help (can scrub floors, etc.)
   0  With some help (can do light housework but need help with heavy work),
      or are you unable to do any housework?
   –  Not answered

5. Can you *handle your own money:*
   1  Without help (write checks, pay bills, etc.)
   0  With some help (manage day-to-day buying but need help with managing
      your checkbook and paying your bills), or are you completely unable to
      handle money?
   –  Not answered

*Source:* Adapted with permission from G Fillenbaum, Screening the Elderly: A Brief Instrumental Activities of Daily Living Measure, *Journal of the American Geriatric Society*, Vol. 33, pp. 683–706, © 1985, Lippincott Williams & Wilkins.

---

maker assistance may be required because of recent hospitalization or illness.[56]

## Combined IADL and ADL Assessments

Several instruments have been developed that combine both ADL and IADL domains. Although combined ADL and IADL instruments have generally been developed for specific purposes, they may have broader utility because the combined spectrum of behaviors is addressed. An instrument that combines both ADLs and IADLs in a single evaluation was developed by Paveza et al.[19,20] for use by persons working in community care settings. It has features that permit the practitioner to separate impairment on a behavior from the need for assistance with that same behavior. The developers of this instrument argue that not unlike the relationship of diagnosis to level of need for functional assistance, impairment in and of itself does not necessarily suggest the level of other personal assistance that an impaired older person may require. The need for assistance is based not only on impairment, but also on what assistive devices may be in use and what support systems may already be providing help.[19,20] The practitioner needs to consider help already in place when determining what additional assistance to request. Moreover, by focusing on the broad spectrum of behaviors, the evaluator can more easily place the older adult on a continuum of care and can even estimate the likelihood that he or she is at risk for institutionalization.[19,20]

## Determination of Need Assessment

The Determination of Need Assessment (DONA) is an ADL and IADL combined assessment designed by Paveza et al.[57] as part of a Medicaid waiver project (Exhibit 10–4). As such, this instrument was designed with the needs of the community-based practitioner in mind and approaches the assessment of functional status from a unique perspective. The DONA separates functional incapacity or impairment from the need for assistance. The authors argue that these are really separate phenomena, one dictated by the inability to perform a behavior based on some physical, emotional, or cognitive problem and the other by what assistance may already be in place or adaptations that the older adult may have already made to accommodate for the specific disability.

Furthermore, the scale defines levels of impairment on a multiple-point scale in which impairment can range from none to mild, moderate, or severe. The DONA also distinguishes these levels of impairment from the behaviors that the ratings are to evaluate. The need for assistance is placed on a similar 4-point scale that primarily asks the evaluator to consider the degree to which the person is at health risk if no additional help above the current level of functioning is provided.[19,20] The diversity in the construction of this scale allows the person doing

**Exhibit 10–4** Determination of Need Functional Assessment

| Function | Level of Impairment | Unmet Need for Care | Case Comments: Identify resources, and describe special needs and circumstances that should be taken into account when developing a care plan. |
|---|---|---|---|
| 1. Eating | 0 1 2 3 | 0 1 2 3 | |
| 2. Bathing | 0 1 2 3 | 0 1 2 3 | |
| 3. Grooming | 0 1 2 3 | 0 1 2 3 | |
| 4. Dressing | 0 1 2 3 | 0 1 2 3 | |
| 5. Transferring | 0 1 2 3 | 0 1 2 3 | |
| 6. Incontinence | 0 1 2 3 | 0 1 2 3 | |
| 7. Managing money | 0 1 2 3 | 0 1 2 3 | |
| 8. Telephoning | 0 1 2 3 | 0 1 2 3 | |
| 9. Preparing meals | 0 1 2 3 | 0 1 2 3 | |
| 10. Laundry | 0 1 2 3 | 0 1 2 3 | |

| | | | |
|---|---|---|---|
| 11. Housework | 0 1 2 3 | 0 1 2 3 | |
| 12. Outside home | 0 1 2 3 | 0 1 2 3 | |
| 13. Routine health | 0 1 2 3 | 0 1 2 3 | |
| 14. Special health | 0 1 2 3 | 0 1 2 3 | |
| 15. Being alone | 0 1 2 3 | 0 1 2 3 | |
| Box A: subtotal column A, items 1–6 | Box A | Box B | Box B: subtotal column B, items 1–6 |
| Box C: subtotal column A, items 7–15 | Box C | Box D | Box D: subtotal column B, items 7–15 |
| Box E: subtotal box A and box C | Box E | Box F | Box F: subtotal box B and box D |
| | | Box G | Box G: subtotal box E and box F |

*Source:* Paveza G, et al. A Brief Assessment Tool for Determining Eligibility and Need for Community-Based Long-Term Care Services. *Behav Health Aging.* Vol. 1, pp. 121–132, © 1990, Springer Publishing Company, Inc., New York 10012. Used by permission.

the evaluation to discuss both function and assistance on various levels from the behavior specific to a global combined assessment. Another important aspect of this instrument is that it was normed against
a Medicaid-supported institutional population. Thus, the authors
noted in their discussion of this instrument that if a person scores 15
or above on the impairment section of this instrument that he or she
is similar in level of functional impairment to the most disabled two
thirds of an institutional sample. Such a result suggests that the person
is at high risk for institutionalization and should definitely be considered for community-based services.[19,20] Because it was specifically developed for use in community-based, long-term care programs, its
qualities can be particularly useful when thinking about community
care for the older adult.

## Medical Outcomes Study Short Form 36

The Short Form 36 (SF-36) represents eight health concepts: physical
functioning, role disability caused by physical health problems, bodily
pain, general health perceptions, vitality, social functioning, role disability caused by emotional problems, and general mental health (Exhibit 10–5).[58] The scientific literature pertaining to the use of the SF-36
in studies of older adults was recently reviewed by McHorney,[59] who
concluded that, generally speaking, the SF-36 scales were predictive of
mortality and hospitalization over the course of a 2-year follow-up.
Correlation between SF-36 subscales was similar in cognitively impaired older subjects as in cognitively intact subjects. The SF-36 has
been employed in studies of outcome of patient care[58–62] and appears
to be reliable and valid even in frail older adults.[63]

## PERFORMANCE ASSESSMENT OF FUNCTION

Consider the source of information about functional impairment.[64]
Persons may perceive their level of functioning to be at a higher level
than the evaluation of nurses familiar with them would suggest. Assuming the nurses' evaluations were the most accurate, clients overrated
their functional status, whereas families underrated it.[65] Self-ratings
were found to reflect most closely the direct observations of research
staff.[66] Pincus et al.[67] found that self-reports on a simple questionnaire
of functional status were significantly correlated to objective measures
of physical impairment in rheumatoid arthritis. In the Framingham

**Exhibit 10–5** Medical Outcomes Study SF-36

**Instructions:** This survey asks for your views about your health. This information will help keep track of how you feel and how well you are able to do your usual activities. Answer every question by marking the answer as indicated. If you are unsure about how to answer a question, please give the best answer you can.

1. In general, would you say your health is:

(Circle one)

| | |
|---|---|
| Excellent | 1 |
| Very good | 2 |
| Good | 3 |
| Fair | 4 |
| Poor | 5 |

2. *Compared to 1 year ago,* how would you rate your health in general now?

(Circle one)

| | |
|---|---|
| Much better now than 1 year ago | 1 |
| Somewhat better now than 1 year ago | 2 |
| About the same now as 1 year ago | 3 |
| Somewhat worse now than 1 year ago | 4 |
| Much worse now than 1 year ago | 5 |

3. The following items are about activities you might do during a typical day. Does *your health* now limit you in these activities? If so, how much?

(Circle one number on each line)

| Activities | Yes, Limited a Lot | Yes, Limited a Little | No, Not Limited at All |
|---|---|---|---|
| a. Vigorous activities, such as running, lifting heavy objects, or participating in strenuous sports | 1 | 2 | 3 |
| b. Moderate activities, such as moving a table, pushing a vacuum cleaner, bowling, or playing golf | 1 | 2 | 3 |
| c. Lifting or carrying groceries | 1 | 2 | 3 |
| d. Climbing several flights of stairs | 1 | 2 | 3 |
| e. Climbing one flight of stairs | 1 | 2 | 3 |
| f. Bending, kneeling, or stooping | 1 | 2 | 3 |
| g. Walking more than a mile | 1 | 2 | 3 |
| h. Walking several blocks | 1 | 2 | 3 |
| i. Walking one block | 1 | 2 | 3 |
| j. Bathing or dressing yourself | 1 | 2 | 3 |

*continues*

**Exhibit 10–5** continued

4. During the *past 4 weeks,* have you had any of the following problems with your work or other regular daily activities *as a result of your physical health?*

(Circle one number on each line)

|  | Yes | No |
|---|---|---|
| a. Cut down on the amount of time you spent on work or other activities | 1 | 2 |
| b. Accomplished less than you would like | 1 | 2 |
| c. Were limited in the kind of work or other activities | 1 | 2 |
| d. Had difficulty performing the work or other activities (for example, it took extra effort) | 1 | 2 |

5. During the *past 4 weeks,* have you had any of the following problems with your work or other regular activities *as a result of any emotional problems* (such as feeling depressed or anxious)?

(Circle one number on each line)

|  | Yes | No |
|---|---|---|
| a. Cut down on the amount of time you spent on work or other activities | 1 | 2 |
| b. Accomplished less than you would like | 1 | 2 |
| c. Didn't do work or other activities as carefully as usual | 1 | 2 |

6. During the *past 4 weeks,* to what extent has your physical health or emotional problems interfered with your normal social activities with family, friends, neighbors, or groups?

(Circle one)

Not at all ................................................... .1
Slightly ..................................................... .2
Moderately .................................................. .3
Quite a bit .................................................. .4
Extremely ................................................... .5

7. How much *bodily* pain have you had during the *past 4 weeks?*

(Circle one)

None ....................................................... .1
Very mild .................................................. .2
Mild ....................................................... .3
Moderate ................................................... .4
Severe ..................................................... .5
Very severe ................................................ .6

8. During the *past 4 weeks,* how much did *pain* interfere with your normal work (including both work outside the home and housework)?

(Circle one)

Not at all . . . . . . . . . . . . . . . . . . . . . . . . . . . . . . . . . . . . . . . . . . . . . . . . . . . . .1
A little bit . . . . . . . . . . . . . . . . . . . . . . . . . . . . . . . . . . . . . . . . . . . . . . . . . . . .2
Moderately . . . . . . . . . . . . . . . . . . . . . . . . . . . . . . . . . . . . . . . . . . . . . . . . . . .3
Quite a bit . . . . . . . . . . . . . . . . . . . . . . . . . . . . . . . . . . . . . . . . . . . . . . . . . . . .4
Extremely . . . . . . . . . . . . . . . . . . . . . . . . . . . . . . . . . . . . . . . . . . . . . . . . . . . . .5

9. These questions are about how you feel and how things have been with you during the *past 4 weeks.* For each question, please give the one answer that comes closest to the way you have been feeling. How much of the time during the *past 4 weeks*

(Circle one number on each line)

| | All of the Time | Most of the Time | A Good Bit of the Time | Some of the Time | A Little of the Time | None of the Time |
|---|---|---|---|---|---|---|
| a. Did you feel full of pep? | 1 | 2 | 3 | 4 | 5 | 6 |
| b. Have you been a very nervous person? | 1 | 2 | 3 | 4 | 5 | 6 |
| c. Have you felt so down in the dumps that nothing could cheer you up? | 1 | 2 | 3 | 4 | 5 | 6 |
| d. Have you felt calm and peaceful? | 1 | 2 | 3 | 4 | 5 | 6 |
| e. Did you have a lot of energy? | 1 | 2 | 3 | 4 | 5 | 6 |
| f. Have you felt downhearted and blue? | 1 | 2 | 3 | 4 | 5 | 6 |
| g. Did you feel worn out? | 1 | 2 | 3 | 4 | 5 | 6 |
| h. Have you been a happy person? | 1 | 2 | 3 | 4 | 5 | 6 |
| i. Did you feel tired? | 1 | 2 | 3 | 4 | 5 | 6 |

10. During the *past 4 weeks,* how much of the time had your *physical health or emotional problems* interfered with your social activities (like visiting with friends, relatives, etc)?

(Circle one)

All of the time . . . . . . . . . . . . . . . . . . . . . . . . . . . . . . . . . . . . . . . . . . . . . . . . . .1
Most of the time . . . . . . . . . . . . . . . . . . . . . . . . . . . . . . . . . . . . . . . . . . . . . . . . .2
Some of the time . . . . . . . . . . . . . . . . . . . . . . . . . . . . . . . . . . . . . . . . . . . . . . . .3
A little of the time . . . . . . . . . . . . . . . . . . . . . . . . . . . . . . . . . . . . . . . . . . . . . . .4
None of the time . . . . . . . . . . . . . . . . . . . . . . . . . . . . . . . . . . . . . . . . . . . . . . . . .5

*continues*

**Exhibit 10–5** continued

11. How TRUE or FALSE is *each* of the following statements for you?
(Circle one number on each line)

|  | Definitely True | Mostly True | Don't Know | Mostly False | Definitely False |
|---|---|---|---|---|---|
| a. I seem to get sick a little easier than other people | 1 | 2 | 3 | 4 | 5 |
| b. I am as healthy as anybody I know | 1 | 2 | 3 | 4 | 5 |
| c. I expect my health to get worse | 1 | 2 | 3 | 4 | 5 |
| d. My health is excellent | 1 | 2 | 3 | 4 | 5 |

*Source:* Courtesy of Quality Metric, Inc., Lincoln, Rhode Island.

follow-up, older residents did not seem reluctant to assent to functional limitations when compared with limitations noted on observation.[68] In clinical settings, physicians should use information from both the client and the caregiver. Is the activity performed? Could the activity be performed if necessary? Because data from self-report of function predict mortality, it is obvious that self-report information is very valuable.

Because direct observation of the client is desirable to confirm information given by the client or caregiver about functional status, a number of instruments have been developed.[69–71] Measures that appear to be adequate for primary care practice, however, are few.[72] One early performance test used props much as does the Denver Developmental Screening Examination for children. Example items included drinking from a cup, lifting food on a spoon to the mouth (props: spoon and candy), making a telephone call, brushing teeth (prop: toothbrush), and telling the time.[73] Performance tests focusing on manual dexterity predict the need for formal support services and appear to be unaffected by age or educational level[74–77] but require specialized equipment.

Simple tests are sometimes used to assess functional status. In the "get up and go," the older person is timed while he or she rises from a chair, walks a given distance, turns, and sits down.[78,79] Impaired performance may identify older persons who are at risk of falling.[80] In functional reach, the distance that the person can extend the arm is measured.[81] The observation of performance may produce a more accurate assessment of capability than relying on report of function from the clients or caregivers. At the same time, the addition of performance measures increases the time required for assessment and may not tap all pertinent domains.[82]

## Physical Performance Test

The Physical Performance Test permits direct assessment of performance on a set of basic tasks that simulate the ADLs.[83,84] The Physical Performance Test consists of

1. Writing a sentence
2. Simulated eating
3. Lifting a book and putting it on a shelf
4. Putting on and removing a jacket
5. Picking up a penny from the floor
6. Turning 360 degrees
7. Walking
8. Climbing stairs

Explicit instructions for administrating and scoring are provided. Bed mobility, transfer skills, standing up from a chair, standing balance, stepping up one step with a handrail, and walking are the activities rated in another performance measure suitable for hospitalized older patients.[85]

## Direct Assessment of Functioning Scale

The utility of the Direct Assessment of Functioning Scale (DAFS)[69] is that it was developed specifically for use in working with persons who are demented. As such, it can assist with understanding what areas of behavior are affected by the dementia. Moreover, given the findings by Freels et al.[86] that for many demented persons the ADLs are not lost until well into the later stages of the disease, an instrument that is sensitive to early stages of dementia can help practitioners target interventions.

The DAFS was developed by Lowenstein et al.[69] out of concern that many of the functional assessment instruments rely on self-report rather than direct observation. As noted previously, there is some tendency when using self-report data for an impaired person to overestimate his or her functional abilities, but when the report is obtained from an informant, particularly a family member, the functional status is underestimated. The DAFS, as its name implies, re-

quires the direct measurement and observation of a number of behaviors, including ADLs and IADLs, as well as some measure of cognitive functioning.

Because this instrument requires the use of both props and observation by the examiner, the DAFS is best suited for an office environment. However, its unique aspects make it particularly suited for use
with demented persons, particularly those with Alzheimer's disease.
Indeed, it is the strong relationship to both the Blessed Dementia
Rating Scale and the Mini Blessed Dementia Rating Scale that makes
the DAFS a useful instrument when working with persons who have
already been diagnosed or are currently undergoing evaluation for
dementia. Moreover, the ability to distinguish nondepressed and
nondemented older adults from depressed or demented ones makes
the DAFS a practical assessment for inclusion in a diagnostic
workup.[69] Furthermore, the demonstrated ability to track changes
adequately in functioning over time suggests that, unlike some instruments, the DAFS does not have an appreciable ceiling or floor effect and can, therefore, assist the practitioner with monitoring
changes in older persons' functioning over time.

## CASE STUDY: ASSESSMENT OF ADLs

### History

Mrs. Jones was a 72-year-old white woman who was recently widowed. She had a history of hypertension, treated with an angiotensin-
converting enzyme inhibitor and a mild diuretic, and osteoarthritis,
especially of the lower back, treated intermittently with a non-
steroidal anti-inflammatory drug. She lived alone in her own home.
A 48-year-old working, married daughter lived in the same town and
visited on the weekends to run errands and do some light housekeeping. An unmarried son lived in a larger city some 400 miles
away.

Since her bereavement some 4 months ago, the woman, who did
not drive, had been socially isolated, especially because she was unable
to attend her usual functions, such as church meetings and bridge
club. Her daughter was quite concerned because of her mother's lack of
appetite and neglect of personal care. On questioning, Mrs. Jones admitted to early morning awakening, a lack of appetite, weight loss, and
crying spells. There was no prior history of depression, but the woman
was thought to be depressed as part of her grief reaction.

The daughter was able to rearrange her schedule in order to provide transportation to the bridge club and to church. Counseling was arranged to help her cope with the grieving process. Participating in Meals on Wheels was suggested as a means to increase her social contact, but Mrs. Jones refused. Overall, these efforts mitigated some of her feelings of depression, and she improved considerably over the next several months.

**Follow-Up**

She remained at the same functional level, receiving assistance from her daughter, with her son keeping in touch by phone and helping out financially, until, at the age of 77 years, Mrs. Jones sustained a hip fracture after slipping on the ice on the way to her mailbox. She was hospitalized with a fracture of the left femoral neck and made a good recovery after insertion of a pin to stabilize her hip. She spent 2 months in a nursing home receiving physical therapy and rehabilitation and kept her spirits up with the thought of returning home. She was discharged home where she ambulated with a walker.

To accommodate her, the bedroom was moved downstairs, a commode was placed at her bedside, nightlights were obtained, and a ramp to eliminate the need for stairs to the outside was installed. Her movement, however, was more severely limited. Her daughter continued to provide help with shopping and housework and was able to enlist the help of the postal carrier as a daily check on Mrs. Jones' well-being.

**Present Condition**

Three years later, Mrs. Jones is now 80 years old. Her daughter, at the age of 56 years, is hospitalized for a myocardial infarction and will not be able to keep up the same level of help. At least temporarily, she will no longer be available to assist her mother in shopping, housekeeping, laundry, meal planning and preparation, and bathing or to provide emotional support. Mrs. Jones does not wish to leave her home, but some of these activities are not getting done.

When her son visits, he is surprised and a little angry at the "condition Mom is in," although he keeps it to himself, considering his sister's recent heart attack. He believes Mrs. Jones should be immediately placed in a protective environment. Because Mrs. Jones is adamant about staying home, her son makes a compromise agreement with her to allow a live-in housekeeper. Although he tries to find a satisfactory live-in helper, he cannot find one who is satisfactory to both Mrs. Jones and him.

### Resolution

Because her son must return to work and the daughter is unable to care for her mother, Mrs. Jones reluctantly agrees to nursing home placement in an intermediate care facility, at least on a trial basis. The risk factors for nursing home placement in this case included living alone, old age, lack of a caregiver, and impaired mobility.

## DEMENTIA RATING SCALES

A combination of mental status questions, ADL, and IADL items are sometimes blended into a score used to quantify the severity of dementia, a common clinical problem in geriatric practice. The dementia rating scales may be considered a hybrid type of instrument. Dementia rating scales have been used not only to identify dementia but also to quantify it, that is, to assign a stage or degree of severity. One example is the Blessed Dementia Score (Exhibit 10–6), which can be correlated to pathologic changes seen in brains of demented older persons at autopsy.[87] Many of these scales might be used in clinical practice, particularly if the practice includes a significant number of demented patients. The ideal dementia rating scale should be short and easy to score, just like the mental status screening instruments, to facilitate its use in clinical practice. The rating instrument should allow some quantification of dementia with a few differentiating points to categorize the severity of dementia. It would also be helpful if the practitioner could use it to follow the progression of the dementing illness. Several of these instruments are discussed in this section.

### Functional Dementia Scale

A brief instrument to assess the severity of dementia is the Moore Functional Dementia Scale.[88] This questionnaire (Exhibit 10–7) can be

**Exhibit 10–6** Blessed Dementia Score

1. Inability to perform household tasks
2. Inability to cope with small sums of money
3. Inability to remember short lists of items
4. Inability to find way outdoors
5. Inability to find way about familiar streets
6. Inability to interpret surroundings
7. Inability to recall recent events
8. Tendency to dwell in the past
9. Eating:
   Messily, with spoon only
   Simple solids, such as biscuits (2 points)
   Has to be fed (3 points)
10. Dressing:
    Occasionally misplaced buttons, etc
    Wrong sequence, forgets items (2 points)
    Unable to dress (3 points)
11. Sphincter control:
    Occasional wet beds
    Frequent wet beds (2 points)
    Doubly incontinent (3 points)
12. Increased rigidity
13. Increased egocentricity
14. Impairment of regard for feelings of others
15. Coarsening of affect
16. Impairment of emotional control
17. Hilarity in inappropriate situations
18. Diminished emotional responsiveness
19. Sexual misdemeanor (de novo in old age)
20. Hobbies relinquished
21. Diminished initiative or growing apathy
22. Purposeless hyperactivity

Total score _____

Scores range from 0 to 27; the higher the score, the greater the degree of dementia. Each item scores 1 except the items noted. A second part, the Information Score, contains items testing orientation and memory.

*Source:* Adapted with permission from Blessed G, et al. The Association Between Quantitative Measures of Dementia and Senile Changes in the Cerebral Grey Matter of Elder Subjects. *Br J Psychiatry.* Vol. 114, pp. 797–811, © 1968, The Royal College of Psychiatrists.

given to family members in either written or oral form. The questionnaire gives results that quantify the dementia as well as provide a "review of systems" (or more accurately "review of symptoms") concerning the problems of dementia. No published guidelines on

**Exhibit 10–7** Functional Dementia Scale

1. Has difficulty in completing simple tasks on own, such as dressing, bathing, doing arithmetic
2. Spends time either sitting or in apparently purposeless activity
3. Wanders at night or needs to be restrained to prevent wandering
4. Hears things that are not there
5. Requires supervision or assistance in eating
6. Loses things
7. Appearance is disorderly if left to own devices
8. Moans
9. Cannot control bowel function
10. Threatens to harm others
11. Cannot control bladder function
12. Needs to be watched so does not injure self, such as by careless smoking, leaving the stove on, or falling
13. Destructive of materials within reach, such as breaks furniture, throws food trays, or tears up magazines
14. Shouts or yells
15. Accuses others of doing him or her bodily harm or stealing his or her possessions when you are sure the accusations are not true
16. Is unaware of limitations imposed by illness
17. Becomes confused and does not know where he or she is
18. Has trouble remembering
19. Has sudden changes of mood, such as gets upset, angered, or cries easily
20. If left alone, wanders aimlessly during the day or needs to be restrained to prevent wandering

Each item is rated by the caregiver as follows: none or little of the time, some of the time, a good part of the time, or most or all of the time.

*Source:* Moore J, et al. A Functional Dementia Scale, Vol. 16, p. 503, © 1983, Dowden Publishing Company, Inc. Reproduced with permission from *The Journal of Family Practice*.

whether the scale shows change with time are available. It would be of interest to know if, beyond a certain score, more persons require nursing home placement. Perhaps one would then give certain undesirable or difficult characteristics higher weight, such as incontinence, which is often an especially troublesome problem.

## Revised Memory and Behavior Problems Checklist

The Revised Memory and Behavior Problems Checklist assesses the frequency of observable problem behaviors and, on a separate dimension, the caregiver's response (Exhibit 10–8).[89–91] The frequency of the behavior is rated using the following phrases: (1) never, (2) not in the past week, (3) one to two times in the past week, (4) three to six times in the past week, or (5) daily. The degree to which each behavior upsets the caregiver is rated by the caregiver on a five-point scale: (1) not at all, (2) a little, (3) moderately, (4) very much, and (5) extremely. The assessment of caregiver distress is an advantage when considering disturbing behaviors sometimes associated with dementia. The development of depression in caregivers is predicted primarily by their subjective evaluations of circumstances rather than objective measures of function of the older person.[92]

## Functional Rating Scale for the Symptoms of Dementia

The Texas Tech Functional Rating Scale for the Symptoms of Dementia is a questionnaire devised to predict who may require nursing home placement.[18] According to the investigators, this is a brief dementia scale that measures severity, shows change, and may be valuable in predicting when nursing home placement is necessary (Exhibit 10–9). The concept that persons reaching a certain level of functional disability require nursing home placement is attractive because such objective measures are generally lacking in assessment for long-term care.

Scores on the Functional Rating Scale for the Symptoms of Dementia range from 0 (not demented) to 42. Persons were tested over a 2-year period every few months and were divided at the start of the study into two groups: (1) those with scores above 21 and (2) those with scores below 21. Persons with a score of greater than 21 had an average of 7 months until nursing home placement occurred, and those with scores of 21 or less did not require nursing home placement for an average of 18 months. Scores at the time of admission to the nursing home were about the same for both groups (i.e., about 32).[18]

Three items on the Functional Rating Scale for the Symptoms of Dementia were especially predictive of nursing home placement. If two of the three were present, 83% of these patients were in a nursing home before the next evaluation. The items were incontinence of bowel and bladder, inability to speak coherently, and inability to bathe and groom oneself. The investigators who developed this instrument suggested that scores above 30 may indicate a need for nurs-

**Exhibit 10–8** Revised Memory and Behavior Problems Checklist

The following is a list of problems patients sometimes have. Please indicate if any of these problems have occurred *during the past week*. If so, how much has this bothered or upset you when it happened? Use the following scales for the frequency of the problem and your reaction to it. Please read the description of the ratings carefully.

FREQUENCY RATINGS:
0 = never occurred
1 = not in the past week
2 = 1 to 2 times in the past week
3 = 3 to 6 times in the past week
4 = daily or more often
9 = don't know/not applicable

REACTION RATINGS:
0 = not at all
1 = a little
2 = moderately
3 = very much
4 = extremely
9 = don't know/not applicable

Please answer all the questions below. Please circle a number from 0–9 for both *frequency* and *reaction*.

| | Frequency | Reaction |
|---|---|---|
| 1. Asking the same question over and over. | 0 1 2 3 4 9 | 0 1 2 3 4 9 |
| 2. Trouble remembering recent events (e.g., items in the newspaper or on TV). | 0 1 2 3 4 9 | 0 1 2 3 4 9 |
| 3. Trouble remembering significant past events. | 0 1 2 3 4 9 | 0 1 2 3 4 9 |
| 4. Losing or misplacing things. | 0 1 2 3 4 9 | 0 1 2 3 4 9 |
| 5. Forgetting what day it is. | 0 1 2 3 4 9 | 0 1 2 3 4 9 |
| 6. Starting, but not finishing, things. | 0 1 2 3 4 9 | 0 1 2 3 4 9 |
| 7. Difficulty concentrating on a task. | 0 1 2 3 4 9 | 0 1 2 3 4 9 |
| 8. Destroying property. | 0 1 2 3 4 9 | 0 1 2 3 4 9 |
| 9. Doing things that embarrass you. | 0 1 2 3 4 9 | 0 1 2 3 4 9 |

| | | |
|---|---|---|
| 10. Waking you or other family members up at night. | 0 1 2 3 4 9 | 0 1 2 3 4 9 |
| 11. Talking loudly and rapidly. | 0 1 2 3 4 9 | 0 1 2 3 4 9 |
| 12. Appears anxious or worried. | 0 1 2 3 4 9 | 0 1 2 3 4 9 |
| 13. Engaging in behavior that is potentially dangerous to self or others. | 0 1 2 3 4 9 | 0 1 2 3 4 9 |
| 14. Threats to hurt oneself. | 0 1 2 3 4 9 | 0 1 2 3 4 9 |
| 15. Threats to hurt others. | 0 1 2 3 4 9 | 0 1 2 3 4 9 |
| 16. Aggressive to others verbally. | 0 1 2 3 4 9 | 0 1 2 3 4 9 |
| 17. Appears sad or depressed. | 0 1 2 3 4 9 | 0 1 2 3 4 9 |
| 18. Expressing feelings of hopelessness or sadness about the future (e.g., "Nothing worthwhile ever happens," "I never do anything right"). | 0 1 2 3 4 9 | 0 1 2 3 4 9 |
| 19. Crying and tearfulness. | 0 1 2 3 4 9 | 0 1 2 3 4 9 |
| 20. Commenting about death of self or others (e.g., "Life isn't worth living," "I'd be better off dead"). | 0 1 2 3 4 9 | 0 1 2 3 4 9 |
| 21. Talking about feeling lonely. | 0 1 2 3 4 9 | 0 1 2 3 4 9 |
| 22. Comments about feeling worthless or being a burden to others. | 0 1 2 3 4 9 | 0 1 2 3 4 9 |
| 23. Comments about feeling like a failure or about not having any worthwhile accomplishments in life. | 0 1 2 3 4 9 | 0 1 2 3 4 9 |
| 24. Arguing, irritability, and/or complaining. | 0 1 2 3 4 9 | 0 1 2 3 4 9 |

*Source:* Courtesy of Dr. L. Teri, © 1992, Seattle, Washington.

**Exhibit 10–9** Functional Rating Scale for the Symptoms of Dementia

**Instructions**
1. The scale must be administered to the most knowledgeable informant available. This usually is a spouse or close relative.
2. The scale should be read to the informant one category at a time. The informant is presented the description for behavior in each category. The informant is read each of the responses beginning with zero response. All responses should be read before the informant endorses the highest number response that best describes the behavior of the patient.
3. When responses have been obtained for each category, the circled numbers from each category are summed to give an overall score for functional rating of symptoms of dementia.

Circle the highest number of each category that best describes behavior during the past 3 months.

*Eating*
0 Eats neatly using appropriate utensils
1 Eats messily, has some difficulty with utensils
2 Able to eat solid foods (e.g., fruits, crackers, and cookies) with hands only
3 Has to be fed

*Dressing*
0 Able to dress appropriately without help
1 Able to dress self with occasionally mismatched socks, disarranged buttons, or laces
2 Dresses out of sequence, forgets items, or wears sleeping garments with street clothes, needs supervision
3 Unable to dress alone, appears undressed in inappropriate situations

*Continence*
0 Complete sphincter control
1 Occasional bed wetting
2 Frequent bed wetting or daytime urinary incontinence
3 Incontinent of both bladder and bowel

*Verbal communication*
0 Speaks normally
1 Minor difficulties with speech or word-finding difficulties
2 Able to carry out only simple, uncomplicated conversations
3 Unable to speak coherently

*Memory for names*
0 Usually remembers names of meaningful acquaintances
1 Cannot recall names of acquaintances or distant relatives
2 Cannot recall names of close friends of relatives
3 Cannot recall name of spouse or other living partner

*Memory for events*
0 Can recall details and sequences of recent experiences
1 Cannot recall details or sequences of recent events
2 Cannot recall entire events (e.g., recent outings or visits of relatives or friends) without prompting
3 Cannot recall entire events even with prompting

*Mental alertness*
0 Usually alert, attentive to environment
1 Easily distractible, mind wanders
2 Frequently asks the same questions over and over
3 Cannot maintain attention while watching television

*Global confusion*
0 Appropriately responsive to environment
1 Nocturnal confusion on awakening
2 Periodic confusion during daytime
3 Nearly always quite confused

*Spatial orientation*
0 Oriented, able to find and keep his or her bearings
1 Spatial confusion when driving or riding in local community
2 Gets lost when walking in neighborhood
3 Gets lost in own home or in hospital ward

*Facial recognition*
0 Can recognize faces of recent acquaintances
1 Cannot recognize faces of recent acquaintances
2 Cannot recognize faces of relatives or close friends
3 Cannot recognize spouse or other constant living companion

*Hygiene and grooming*
0 Generally neat and clean
1 Ignores grooming (e.g., does not brush teeth and hair, shave)
2 Does not bathe regularly
3 Has to be bathed and groomed

*Emotionality*
0 Unchanged from normal
1 Mild change in emotional responsiveness—slightly more irritable or more passive, diminished sense of humor, mild depression
2 Moderate change in emotional responsiveness—growing apathy, increased rigidity, despondent, angry outbursts, cries easily
3 Impaired emotional control—unstable, rapid cycling or laughing or crying in inappropriate situations, violent outbursts

*Social responsiveness*
0 Unchanged from previous, "normal"
1 Tendency to dwell in the past, lack of proper association for present situation
2 Lack of regard for feelings of others, quarrelsome, irritable
3 Inappropriate sexual acting out or antisocial behavior

*Sleep patterns*
0 Unchanged from previous, "normal"
1 Sleeps, noticeably more or less than normal
2 Restless, nightmares, disturbed sleep, increased awakenings
3 Up wandering for all or most of the night, inability to sleep

*Source:* Reprinted with permission of Hutton JT, et al. Predictors of Nursing Home Placement of Patients with Alzheimer's Disease. *Texas Med.* Vol. 7, No. 81, p. 41, © 1985 Texas Medical Association.

ing home placement.[18] If the physician can say that most persons reaching a certain level of disability require nursing home placement, it may help alleviate family guilt. Of course, such a scale should be used only in the context of other relevant medical, social, psychologic, and economic data.

## Global Deterioration Scale

Another approach to the problem of assessing the severity of cognitive impairment uses a clinical staging system. In Alzheimer's disease, three stages have been commonly recognized. First, a forgetfulness stage occurs, in which memory problems and impaired visuospatial skills predominate. Then a confusional stage ensues, in which language and calculations are affected, with some changes in personality. Finally, a dementia stage develops in which intellectual functions are severely deteriorated.[93]

The Global Deterioration Scale (GDS) for Primary Degenerative Dementia is one such staging system (Exhibit 10–10).[93] The person's stage is related to prognosis, and as expected, the more advanced the stage, the worse is the prognosis. For example, in the older adult with mild cognitive decline (stage 3), the prognosis is primarily benign, at least over a 4-year period. Persons in early stages may actually have aging-associated cognitive decline. On the other hand, when cognitive decline is severe (stage 6), one third of the persons have died after 4 years, and most have been placed in institutions.

The stages of the GDS correlate with results of the Mini-Mental State Examination (MMSE). Patients with GDS stage 4, indicating mild Alzheimer's disease, scored from 16 to 23 on the MMSE.[94] Independent validation of the MMSE set a cutoff score of 24 to detect dementia.[95–97] Persons at more impaired stages of the GDS had correspondingly lower scores on the MMSE.[94] Several recent articles have questioned the utility of this scale. These articles have noted that the functional deterioration proposed in the GDS is actually much more heterogeneous in the population than the scale suggests.[98,99] Some investigators contend that both families and practitioners may be better served by staying with the broader concepts of mild, moderate, and severe dementia based on neuropsychologic testing and then describing the actual levels of functional impairment and behavioral disturbance rather than trying to place a single value on the level of deterioration.[98,99]

**Exhibit 10–10** Global Deterioration Scale for Primary Degenerative Dementia with 4-Year Prognosis Data

*Stage 1:* No cognitive decline

*Stage 2:* Very mild cognitive decline

The patient complains of memory loss, especially forgetting where objects were placed or familiar names. There is no objective evidence of memory deficit in the clinical interview and no deficits in employment or social situations.

Prognosis: Benign in 95% over a 4-year period.*

*Stage 3:* Mild cognitive decline (early confusion)

Memory loss is evident on testing. Decreased ability to remember names of new acquaintances. Coworkers are aware of memory problems. Gets lost in travel. Associated anxiety or denial.

Prognosis: >80% show no further decline in 4 years.*

*Stage 4:* Moderate cognitive decline (late confusion)

Trouble concentrating on a task. Lessened knowledge of personal history, current events, and recent events. Trouble with travel and finances. Remains oriented to time and place. Denial is a prominent defense mechanism.

Prognosis: In 4 years, one fourth show no change, one fourth are worse but at home, one fourth are in institutions, and one fourth are dead.*

*Stage 5:* Moderately severe cognitive decline

The phase of dementia. Unable to recall major events of current life. Disoriented to time and place. Occasionally dresses improperly but feeds and toilets independently.

Prognosis: After 4 years, most are worse.*

*Stage 6:* Severe cognitive decline

Incontinent. Sleep-wake cycle disturbances. Personality changes. Forgets even the names of close relatives and spouse.

Prognosis: One third are dead in 4 years; two thirds are in institutions.*

*Stage 7:* Very severe cognitive decline

Late dementia, with no speech or psychomotor skills.

*The 4-year prognosis data are from *Psychiatric Annals* (1985;15:319–322), Copyright © 1985, Charles B Slack Inc.

Source: *American Journal of Psychiatry,* Vol. 139, pp. 1136–1139, 1982. Copyright © 1982, American Psychiatric Association. Reprinted by permission. *Psychiatric Annals,* Vol. 15, pp. 319–322, © 1985, Charles B. Slack Inc.

## Functional Assessment Staging of Alzheimer's Disease

The GDS has been expanded into a more elaborate staging system called the Functional Assessment Staging of Alzheimer's Disease (FAST).[100,101] Stages 1 through 5 of the FAST correspond exactly to stages 1 through 5 of the GDS. Stages 6 and 7 of the GDS have been subdivided into five and six substages, respectively, in the FAST (Exhibit 10–11).

This hierarchical arrangement accomplishes several objectives. First, when cognitive deficit yields only baseline or zero scores on a mental status examination, further delineation of severity is possible when stages are employed. Second, and more important clinically, when the patient experiences difficulty that seems to vary with the expected sequence for Alzheimer's disease, the clinician can consider a treatable condition in the differential diagnosis, rather than ascribing a new change to a progression of Alzheimer's disease.

Consider a 75-year-old man whose wife relates that he has trouble dressing but still picks out his clothes. Because picking the appropriate items should be lost before difficulty dressing (stage 5 vs. stage 6a), the clinician might consider superimposed depression or stroke as precipitating the trouble, rather than a worsening of the underlying dementia. Similarly, a 60-year-old woman who complains of inability to handle personal finances, but is able to function well in a demanding job may be depressed rather than have Alzheimer's disease. Here stage 4 (personal finances) appearing before stage 3 (working) is the clue to the diagnosis of depression. Another example of the clinical utility of FAST is premature development of urinary incontinence, suggesting the

**Exhibit 10–11** Functional Assessment Staging of Alzheimer's Disease Symptomatology and Differential Diagnostic Considerations

| FAST Characteristic | FAST Stage | Differential Diagnosis If FAST Stage Is Early |
|---|---|---|
| No functional decrement subjectively or objectively | 1 | |
| Complains of forgetting location of objects | 2 | Anxiety neurosis |
| Subjective work difficulties | | Depression |
| Decreased functioning in demanding work settings evident to coworkers | 3 | Depression Subtle manifestations of medical pathology |
| Difficulty traveling to new locations | | |

| | | |
|---|---|---|
| Decreased ability to perform complex tasks (e.g., planning dinner, shopping, or personal finances) | 4 | Depression<br>Psychosis<br>Focal process<br>(e.g., Gerstmann) |
| Requires assistance selecting attire<br>May require coaxing to bathe properly | 5 | Depression |
| Difficulty dressing properly | 6a | Arthritis<br>Sensory deficit<br>Stroke<br>Depression |
| Requires assistance bathing (fear of bathing) | b | Same as 6a |
| Difficulty with mechanics of toileting | c | Same as 6a |
| Urinary incontinence | d | Urinary tract infection<br>Other causes |
| Fecal incontinence | e | Infection<br>Malabsorption syndrome<br>Other causes |
| Vocabulary limited to one to five words | 7a | Stroke<br>Other dementing disorder<br>(e.g., space-occupying<br>lesion) |
| Intelligible vocabulary lost | b | Same as 7a |
| Ambulatory ability lost | c | Parkinsonism<br>Neuroleptic-induced or other<br>secondary extrapyramidal<br>syndrome<br>Creutzfeldt-Jakob disease<br>Normal pressure<br>hydrocephalus<br>Hyponatremic dementia<br>Stroke<br>Hip fracture<br>Arthritis<br>Overmedication |
| Ability to sit lost | d | Arthritis<br>Contractures |
| Ability to smile lost | e | Stroke |
| Ability to hold up head lost | f | Head trauma |
| Ultimately, stupor or coma | | Metabolic abnormality<br>Overmedication<br>Other causes |

**Exhibit 10–12** Clinical Dementia Rating Scale (CDR)

| | Healthy CDR 0 | Questionable Dementia CDR 0.5 | Mild Dementia CDR 1 | Moderate Dementia CDR 2 | Severe Dementia CDR 3 |
|---|---|---|---|---|---|
| *Memory* | No memory loss or slight inconsistant forgetfulness | Mild consistent forgetfulness; partial recollection of events; "benign" forgetfulness | Moderate memory loss, more marked for recent events; defect interferes with everyday activities | Severe memory loss; only highly learned material retained; new material rapidly lost | Severe memory loss; only fragments remain |
| *Orientation* | Fully oriented | | Some difficulty with time relationships, oriented for place and person at examination, but may have geographic disorientation | Usually disoriented in time, often to place | Orientation to person only |
| *Judgment, problem solving* | Solves everyday problems well, judgment good in relation to past performance | Only doubtful impairment in solving problems, similarities, differences | Moderate difficulty in handling complex problems; social judgment usually maintained | Severely impaired in handling problems, similarities, differences; social judgment usually impaired | Unable to make judgments or solve problems |

| | | | | | |
|---|---|---|---|---|---|
| *Community affairs* | Independent function at usual level in job, shopping, business and financial affairs, volunteer and social groups | Only doubtful or mild impairment, if any, in these activities | Unable to function independently at these activities though may still be engaged in some; may still appear normal to casual inspection | | No pretense of independent function outside home |
| *Home, hobbies* | Life at home, hobbies, intellectual interests well maintained | Life at home, hobbies, intellectual interests well maintained or only slightly impaired | Mild, but definite impairment of function at home; more difficult chores abandoned; more complicated hobbies and interests abandoned | Only simple chores preserved; very restricted interests, poorly sustained | No significant function in home outside of own room |
| *Personal care* | Fully capable of self-care | | Needs occasional prompting | Requires assistance in dressing, hygiene, keeping of personal effects | Requires much help with personal care; often incontinent |

*Note:* Score each item as 0.5, 1, 2, or 3 only if impairment is due to cognitive loss.

*Source:* Adapted with permission from *The British Journal of Psychiatry*, Vol. 140, pp. 566–572, © 1982, The Royal College of Psychiatrists.

presence of a urinary tract infection. Finally, premature loss of speech in an otherwise uncomplicated setting of Alzheimer's disease may suggest focal cerebral pathology such as an infarction.[100,101]

## Clinical Dementia Rating Scale

The Clinical Dementia Rating Scale (CDR) was found to correlate to results of the SPMSQ and to the Blessed Dementia Score, but the CDR was able to differentiate a greater number of degrees of severity over the range of dementia (Exhibit 10–12). For example, persons in CDR 2 scored 8.4 on the SPMSQ and in CDR 3 an indistinguishable 8.7.[102] The CDR correlates with screening tests of cognitive function such as the SPMSQ[103] and has good reliability.[104] The CDR correlates more strongly than do tests of mental status with functional impairment.[12,105]

The clinical stage assigned depends on the pattern of the answers to the questions on the rating scale form (Figure 10–1). The best description of the patient in each of six domains is checked off or circled on the rating scale form. The six areas to be evaluated are memory, orientation, judgment and problem solving, community affairs, home and hobbies, and personal care. The CDR scale can be employed for the assessment of older demented patients in primary care practice to have a standard form to use to assess severity of dementia.

The shaded areas in Figure 10–1 show the defined range into which the scores must fall in order to be assigned a specific CDR stage. Memory is considered the primary category, and if at least three other categories are given the same score as memory, then the rating is the same as the rating that describes the memory function. Otherwise, if three or more secondary categories are given a score greater or less than the memory score, the rating is the score of the majority of the secondary categories. If the secondary assessments lie to either side of the memory score, the rating is the same as the memory score.[102] Alternative algorithms for scoring the CDR have been devised to diminish the influence that the memory assessment has on the final CDR score.[106]

## ASSESSMENT FOR LONG-TERM CARE

Various facets of assessment and instruments whose use helps maintain consistency and a systematic approach are reviewed in this book. It is hoped that assessment of areas such as performance of

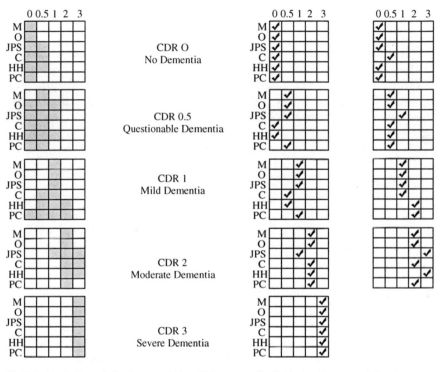

Shaded areas indicate defined range within which scores of individual subjects must fall to be assigned a given CDR.

M = Memory; O = Orientation; JPS = Judgment and problem solving; C = Community affairs; HH = Home, hobbies; PC = Personal care.

Instructions for assigning the CDR are as follows:

Use all information and make the best judgment. Score each category (M, O, JPS, C, HH, PC) as independently as possible. Mark in only one box, rating each according to subject's cognitive function. For determining the CDR, memory is considered the primary category; all others are secondary. If at least three secondary categories are given the same numerical score as memory, then CDR = M. If three or more secondary categories are given a score greater or less than the memory score, CDR = score of majority of secondary categories, unless three secondary categories are scored on one side of M and two secondary categories are scored on the other side of M. In this last circumstance, CDR = M.

When M = 0.5, CDR = 1 if at least three of certain others (O, JPS, C, HH) are scored 1 or greater (PC not influential here). If M = 0.5, CDR cannot be 0; CDR can only be 0.5 or 1. If M = 0, CDR = 0 unless there is slight impairment in two or more secondary categories, in which case CDR = 0.5.

**Figure 10–1** How to determine level of dementia using the CDR scale.
*Source:* Adapted with permission from *The British Journal of Psychiatry,* Vol. 140, pp. 566–572, © 1982, The Royal College of Psychiatrists.

ADLs helps achieve some congruity between needs and resources. An algorithm that provides an overview of long-term care assessment has been suggested by Williams and Williams (Exhibit 10–13).[107]

Levels of care to be provided depend on the amount of medical, ADL, or social help required. There is a continuum from acute hospitalization to the skilled nursing facility to the intermediate care facility to domiciliary care to the person's own home. The algorithm is essentially a hierarchy based on mental state and the ability to perform ADLs and IADLs, as well as the need for special medical interventions, such as provision of oxygen.

If the issue is nursing home placement, precipitating factors should be kept in mind.[108,109] Why is nursing home placement being considered at this time? If a precipitating factor is relieved, can the person be cared for at home? Is the precipitating factor a change in the person's functioning in a specific ADL? Has the coping ability of a key caregiver become diminished? Thorough physical assessment and documentation of mental status are essential. Issues of guilt and the restructuring of family roles should not be neglected if the decision is finally made that nursing home placement is the most appropriate course of action.[109]

The primary care practitioner is in an excellent position to assess the older person's mental status and ability to perform ADLs and IADLs. When decline is noted, it alerts the practitioner to search for a cause. Perhaps help is no longer available to perform some necessary function.

Recommendations about resources prescribed or changes in routine can be made to accommodate the loss. The line may be crossed when it is no longer possible to provide enough assistance to keep the person functioning adequately at home, and then alternative arrangements such as nursing home placement can be recommended.

## CASE STUDY: ASSESSMENT FOR LONG-TERM CARE

### History

Mr. Smith was a fit 78-year-old white man who lived with his 67-year-old wife in their own home. He exhibited considerable memory impairment thought to be Alzheimer's disease, scoring 5 of 10 on the SPMSQ. He had no major physical problems. He performed ADLs with some coaxing from his wife (e.g., bathing, dressing when she lays out his clothes, and feeding himself). He had occasional lapses in judgment, such as wandering and urinating at inappropriate places or

**Exhibit 10–13** Algorithm for Deciding Need for Long-Term Care

---

I.  1. Is the patient medically unstable?
    2. Is the patient mentally unstable to the extent of being a danger to himself or herself or others?

    NO (continue below)              YES → ACUTE HOSPITAL

II. 1. Is the patient totally disoriented chronically?
    2. Is the patient immobile (i.e., always requires human assistance in locomotion)?
    3. Does the patient have need of special therapy (e.g., intravenous line, tracheostomy, oxygen, or ostomy)?
    4. Does the patient require total supervision?
    5. Does the patient require total ADL care?

    NO (continue below)              YES → SKILLED NURSING
                                           FACILITY
                                              or
                                     HOME IF SUPPORT
                                         AVAILABLE

III. 1. Does the patient have intermittent disorientation or wandering?
     2. Does the patient fluctuate in ADL ability?
     3. Does the patient require a structured environment—some supervision?
     4. Does the patient require special therapeutics (e.g., complex diet, complex medication schedule, close monitoring)?

    NO (continue below)              YES → INTERMEDIATE LEVEL
                                           FACILITY
                                              or
                                     HOME IF SUPPORT
                                         AVAILABLE

IV. Can the patient do all of the following:
    1. Feed self                    7. Plan meals
    2. Bathe                        8. Use transportation
    3. Dress                        9. Use telephone
    4. Use the toilet without help  10. Handle finances
    5. Change position              11. Manage medications
    6. Shop

    NO (continue below)              YES → HOME

V. Are resources available to meet these needs?

    NO → DOMICILIARY CARE           YES → HOME WITH SUPPORT

*Source:* Reprinted with permission from the *Journal of the American Geriatric Society,* Vol. 30, No. 7, p. 73, Lippincott Williams & Wilkins.

---

times. The couple had no children. The man's sister-in-law lived several blocks away. A next-door neighbor provided assistance with shopping and transportation to the physician's office for years. In addition, the neighbor had been a source of social interaction for the man's wife. Mr. Smith's behavior made it difficult for Mrs. Smith to do some of the things that she used to do for relaxation. She found a woman in the neighborhood to sit with Mr. Smith so that she could run errands and obtain some time for herself for respite.

## Follow-Up

Over the years, Mr. Smith's memory worsened, and catastrophic reactions increased in frequency and intensity. He hallucinated and talked to himself in the mirror. He frequently did not recognize his wife, which of course disturbed her. Mr. Smith's physician helped Mrs. Smith realize that she had become socially isolated, depressed, and even more preoccupied with her husband's care than in years past. Interviewing Mrs. Smith, the physician rates Mr. Smith's behavior according to the Texas Tech Functional Rating Scale for the Symptoms of Dementia. His score was 30. On occasion, the physician in similar circumstances has used the Moore Functional Dementia Scale as a questionnaire for the family member while the patient was being examined.

## Resolution

Because of Mr. Smith's deteriorating ability to perform ADLs, increasing confusion, and catastrophic reactions, including wandering, the physician recommends nursing home placement. The physician anticipates guilt and depression in Mrs. Smith and plans to counsel her to deal with the loss of the husband she knew.

## CONCLUSION

The use of instruments to assess the functional status of older persons is an area that physicians frequently neglect. For the older adults, however, functional assessment is critical because the ability to remain independent may hinge on the ability to perform ADLs.[1,9] The focus on functional needs puts the emphasis on what is important to the person. How can the person maximize functioning at home and in the community? The functional status directs attention to the health and support services required and the possible alternative settings or levels of care.[110]

A systematic approach to functional assessment is helpful because it provides a task-specific framework to check that the person can perform (or has help performing) the tasks that are required to live independently, such as toileting or preparing meals. In fact, problems found in these areas should be listed alongside the patient's medical problems, thereby yielding a clear picture of his or her difficulties, which can then be organized to find a solution. As Weed suggested, creating such a problem list may help the clinician find hitherto unrecognized correlations among physical, mental, and functional spheres.[111] The comprehensive problem-oriented medical record keeps the constellation of medical diagnoses, undiagnosed conditions, and problems of daily living to the fore.

**REFERENCES**

1. Applegate WB, Blass JP, Williams TF. Instruments for the functional assessment of older patients. *N Engl J Med.* 1990;322:1207–1214.

2. Department of Health and Human Services. *Healthy People 2000: National Health Promotion and Disease Prevention Objectives.* Washington, DC: US Government Printing Office; 1991. DHHS Publication No. PHS 91–50213.

3. Fried LP, Bush TL. Morbidity as a focus of preventive health care in the elderly. *Epidemiol Rev.* 1988;10:48–64.

4. Hadley EC, Ory MG, Suzman R, Weindruch R, Fried L. Physical frailty: A treatable cause of dependence in old age. *J Gerontol.* 1993;48:1–88.

5. Katz S, Branch LG, Branson MH, et al. Active life expectancy. *N Engl J Med.* 1983; 309:1218–1224.

6. George LK, Bearon LB. *Quality of Life in Older Persons: Meaning and Measurement.* New York: Human Sciences Press; 1980.

7. Rubenstein LV, Calkins DR, Greenfield S, et al. Health status assessment for elderly patients: Report of the Society of General Internal Medicine Task Force on Health Assessment. *J Am Geriatr Soc.* 1988;37:562–569.

8. Granger CV, Gresham GE. *Functional Assessment in Rehabilitation Medicine.* Baltimore: Williams & Wilkins; 1984.

9. Mosqueda LA. Assessment of rehabilitation potential. *Clin Geriatr Med.* 1993;9: 689–703.

10. Heath JM. Comprehensive functional assessment of the elderly. *Primary Care.* 1989;16:305–327.

11. Guralnik JM, Simonsick EM. Physical disability in older Americans. *J Gerontol.* 1993;48:3–10.

12. Skurla E, Rogers JC, Sunderland T. Direct assessment of activities of daily living in Alzheimer's disease: A controlled study. *J Am Geriatr Soc.* 1988;36:97–103.

13. Reed BR, Jagust WJ, Seab J. Mental status as a predictor of daily function in progressive dementia. *Gerontologist.* 1989;29:804–807.

14. Brink TL, Capri D, DeNeeve V, et al. Senile confusion: Limitations of assessment by the Face–Hand Test, Mental Status Questionnaire, and staff ratings. *J Am Geriatr Soc.* 1978;26:380–382.

15. Barberger-Gateau P, Commenges D, Gagnon M, Letenneur L, Sauvel C, Dartigues JF. Instrumental activities of daily living as a screening tool for cognitive impairment and dementia in elderly community dwellers. *J Am Geriatr Soc.* 1992;40:1129–1134.

16. Iliffe S, Tai SS, Haines A, et al. Assessment of elderly people in general practice: 4: Depression, functional ability and contact with services. *Br J Gen Pract.* 1993;43: 371–374.

17. Keene JS, Anderson CA. Hip fractures in the elderly. *JAMA.* 1982;248:564–567.

18. Hutton JT, Dippel RL, Loewenson RB, et al. Predictors of nursing home placement of patients with Alzheimer's disease. *Tex Med.* 1985;81:40–43.

19. Paveza GJ, Cohen D, Hagopian M, Prohaska T, Blaser CJ, Brauner D. A brief assessment tool for determining eligibility and need for community-based long-term care services. *Behav Health Aging.* 1990;1:121–132.

20. Paveza GJ, Cohen D, Blaser CJ, Hagopian M. A brief form of the Mini-Mental State Examination for use in community care settings. *Behav Health Aging.* 1990;1:133–139.

21. Lichtenstein MJ, Federspiel CF, Shaffner W. Factors associated with early demise in nursing home residents: a case control study. *J Am Geriatr Soc.* 1985;33:315–319.

22. Incalzi AR, Capparella O, Gemmo A, Porcedda P, Raccis G. A simple method of recognizing geriatric patients at risk for death and disability. *J Am Geriatr Soc.* 1992;40: 34–38.

23. Fillenbaum G. Screening the elderly: A brief instrumental activities of daily living measure. *J Am Geriatr Soc.* 1985;33:698–706.

24. Koyano W, Shibata H, Nakazato K, Haga H, Suyama Y, Matsuzaki T. Mortality in relation to instrumental activities of daily living: One year follow-up in a Japanese urban community. *J Gerontol.* 1989;44:S107–S109.

25. Mor V, Murphy J, Masterson-Allen S, Willey C, Razmpour A. Risk of functional decline among frail elders. *J Clin Epidemiol.* 1989;42:895–904.

26. Mor V, Wilcox V, Rakowski W, Hiris J. Functional transitions among the elderly: Patterns, predictors, and related hospital use. *Am J Public Health.* 1994;84:1274–1280.

27. Burton JR. The house call: An important service for the frail elderly. *J Am Geriatr Soc.* 1985;33:291–293.

28. Levy MT. Psychiatric assessment of elderly patients in the home. *J Am Geriatr Soc.* 1985;33:9–12.

29. Reuben DB, Solomon DH. Assessment in geriatrics: Of caveats and names. *J Am Geriatr Soc.* 1989;37:570–572.

30. Fried LP, Ettinger WH, Lind B, Newman AB, Gardin J. Physical disability in older adults: A physiological approach. *J Clin Epidemiol.* 1994;47:747–760.

31. Yurick AG, Spier BE, Robb SS, et al. *The Aged Person and the Nursing Process,* 2nd ed. Norwalk, CT: Appleton-Century-Crofts; 1984.

32. Carnevali DL, Patrick M. *Nursing Management for the Elderly,* 2nd ed. Philadelphia: JB Lippincott Company; 1986.

33. Applegate WB. Use of assessment instruments in clinical settings. *J Am Geriatr Soc.* 1987;35:45–50.

34. Siu AL, Reuben DB, Hays RD. Hierarchical measures of physical function in ambulatory geriatrics. *J Am Geriatr Soc.* 1990;38:1113–1119.

35. Blazer D, Siegler IC. *A Family Approach to Health Care of the Elderly.* Menlo Park, CA: Addison-Wesley Publishing; 1984.

36. Woodhouse K, Wynne H, Baillie S, et al. Who are the frail elderly? *Q J Med.* 1988; 28:505–506.

37. Schulz R, Williamson GM. Psychosocial and behavioral dimensions of physical frailty. *J Gerontol.* 1993;48:39–43.

38. Rockwood K, Fox RA, Stolee P, Robertson D, Beattie BL. Frailty in elderly people: An evolving concept. *Can Med Assoc J.* 1994;150:489–495.

39. Feinstein AR. An additional basic science for clinical medicine: IV: The development of clinometrics. *Ann Intern Med.* 1983;99:843–848.

40. Feinstein AR, Josephy BR, Wells CK. Scientific and clinical problems in indexes of functional disability. *Ann Intern Med.* 1986;105:413–420.

41. Becker PM, Cohen HJ. The functional approach to the care of the elderly: A conceptual framework. *J Am Geriatr Soc.* 1984;32:923–929.

42. Granger CV, Albrecht GL, Hamilton BB. Outcome of comprehensive medical rehabilitation: Measurement by PULSES profile and the Barthel index. *Arch Phys Med Rehabil.* 1979;60:145–154.

43. Kane RA, Kane RL. *Assessing the Elderly: A Practical Guide to Measurement.* Lexington, MA: Lexington Books; 1981.

44. Pope AM, Tarlov AR. *Disability in America: Toward a National Agenda for Prevention.* Washington, DC: National Academy Press; 1991.

45. Katz S, Ford AB, Moskowitz RW, et al. Studies of illness in the aged: The index of ADL. *JAMA.* 1963;185:914–919.

46. Bruett TL, Overs RP. A critical review of 12 ADL scales. *Phys Ther.* 1969;49: 857–862.

47. Katz PR, Dube DH, Calkins E. Use of a structured functional assessment format in a geriatric consultative service. *J Am Geriatr Soc.* 1985;33:681–686.

48. Katz S, Downs TD, Cash HR, et al. Progress in development of the index ADL. *Gerontologist.* 1970;10(1)Pt 1:20–30.

49. Kelly JF, Winograd CH. A functional approach to stroke management in elderly patients. *J Am Geriatr Soc.* 1985;33:48–60.

50. Mahoney FI, Barthel DW. Functional evaluation: The Barthel index. *Md State Med J.* 1965;14:61–65.

51. Fortinsky RH, Granger CV, Seltzer GB. The use of functional assessment in understanding home care needs. *Med Care.* 1981;19:489–497.

52. Lawton MP, Brody EM. Assessment of older people: Self-maintaining and instrumental activities of daily living. *Gerontologist.* 1969;9:179–186.

53. The Older American Resources and Services (OARS) Methodology. *Multidimensional Functional Assessment Questionnaire,* 2nd ed. Durham, NC: Duke University Center for the Study of Aging and Human Development; 1978:169–170.

54. Teresi JA, Cross PS, Golden RR. Some applications of latent trait analysis to the measurement of ADL. *J Gerontol.* 1989;44:196–204.

55. Suurmeijer TPBM, Doeglas DM, Moum T, et al. The Groningen Activity Restriction Scale for measuring disability: Its utility in international comparisons. *Am J Public Health.* 1994;84:1270–1273.

56. Gallo JJ, Franch MS, Reichel W. Dementing illness: The patient, caregiver, and community. *Am Fam Phys.* 1991;43:1669–1675.

57. Paveza GJ, Prohaska T, Hagopian M, Cohen D. *Determination of Need Revision: Final Report,* vol 1. Chicago: Gerontology Center, University of Illinois at Chicago; 1989.

58. Stewart AL, Ware JE. *Measuring Functioning and Well-Being.* Durham, NC: Duke University Press; 1993.

59. McHorney CA. Measuring and monitoring general health status in elderly persons: Practical and methodological issues in using the SF-36 health survey. *Gerontologist.* 1996;36:571–583.

60. Wells KB, Stewart A, Hays RD, et al. The functioning and well-being of depressed patients: Results from the Medical Outcomes Study. *JAMA.* 1989;262:914–919.

61. Stewart AL, Greenfield S, Hays RD, et al. Functional status and well-being of patients with chronic conditions: Results from the Medical Outcomes Study. *JAMA.* 1989; 262:907–913.

62. Stewart AL, Hays RD, Ware JE. The MOS Short-Form General Health Survey: Reliability and validity in a patient population. *Med Care.* 1988;26:724–735.

63. Stadnyk K, Calder J, Rockwood K. Testing the measurement properties of the Short Form-36 health survey in a frail elderly population. *J Clin Epidemiol.* 1998;51:827–835.

64. Branch LG, Meyers AR. Assessing physical function in the elderly. *Clin Geriatr Med.* 1987;3:29–51.

65. Rubenstein LZ, Schairer C, Willard GD, et al. Systematic biases in functional status assessment of elderly adults. *J Gerontol.* 1984;39:686–691.

66. Dorevitch MI, Cossar RM, Bailey FJ, et al. The accuracy of self and informant ratings of physical functional capacity in the elderly. *J Clin Epidemiol.* 1992;45:791–798.

67. Pincus T, Callahan LF, Brooks RH, Fuchs HA, Olsen NJ, Kaye JJ. Self-report questionnaire scores in rheumatoid arthritis compared with traditional physical, radiographic, and laboratory measures. *Ann Intern Med.* 1989;110:259–266.

68. Kelly-Hayes M, Jette AM, Wolf PA, D'Agostino RB, Odell PM. Functional limitations and disability among elders in the Framingham study. *Am J Public Health.* 1992; 82:841–845.

69. Lowenstein DA, Amigo E, Duara R, et al. A new scale for the assessment of functional status in Alzheimer's disease and related disorders. *J Gerontol Psychol Sci.* 1989; 44:P114–P121.

70. Marsiske M, Willis SL. Dimensionality of everyday problem solving in older adults. *Psychol Aging.* 1995;10:269–282.

71. Diehl M, Willis SL, Schaie KW. Practical problem solving in older adults: Observational assessment and cognitive correlates. *Psychol Aging.* 1995;10:478–491.

72. Guralnik JM, Branch LG, Cummings SR, Curb JD. Physical performance measures in aging research. *J Gerontol.* 1989;44:M141–M146.

73. Kuriansky J, Gurland B. The Performance Test of Activities of Daily Living. *Int J Aging Hum Dev.* 1976;7:343–352.

74. Williams ME, Hadler NM, Earp JAL. Manual ability as a marker of dependency in geriatric women. *J Chronic Dis.* 1982;35:115–122.

75. Williams ME. Identifying the older person likely to require long-term care. *J Am Geriatr Soc.* 1987;35:761–766.

76. Williams ME, Gaylord SA, McGaghie WC. Timed manual performance in a community elderly population. *J Am Geriatr Soc.* 1990;38:1120–1126.

77. Williams ME, Gaylord SA, Gerrity MS. The timed manual performance test as a predictor of hospitalization and death in a community-based elderly population. *J Am Geriatr Soc.* 1994;42:21–27.

78. Tinetti M. Performance-oriented assessment of mobility problems in elderly patients. *J Am Geriatr Soc.* 1986;34:119–126.

79. Mathias S, Nayak USL, Isaacs B. Balance in elderly patients: The "get up and go" test. *Arch Phys Med Rehabil.* 1986;67:387–389.

80. Salgado R, Lord SR, Packer J, Ehrlich F. Factors associated with falling in elderly hospital patients. *Gerontology.* 1994;40:325–331.

81. Duncan PW, Weiner DK, Chandler J, Studentski S. Functional reach: A new clinical measure of balance. *J Gerontol Med Sci.* 1990;45:192–197.

82. Guralnik JM, Reuben DB, Buchner DM, Ferrucci L. Performance measures of physical function in comprehensive geriatric assessment. In: Rubenstein LZ, Wieland D, Bernabei R, eds. *Geriatric Assessment Technology: The State of the Art.* New York: Springer Publishing; 1995:59–74.

83. Reuben DB, Siu AL. An objective measure of physical function of elderly outpatients: The Physical Performance Test. *J Am Geriatr Soc.* 1990;38:1105–1112.

84. Rozzini R, Frisoni GB, Bianchetti A, et al. Physical Performance Test and activities of daily living scales in the assessment of health status in elderly people. *J Am Geriatr Soc.* 1993;41:1109–1113.

85. Winograd CH, Lemsky CM, Nevitt MC, et al. Development of a physical performance and mobility examination. *J Am Geriatr Soc.* 1994;42:743–749.

86. Freels S, Cohen D, Eisdorfer C, et al. Functional status and clinical findings in patients with Alzheimer's disease. *J Gerontol Med Sci.* 1992;47:M177–M182.

87. Blessed G, Tomlinson BE, Roth M. The association between quantitative measures of dementia and of senile changes in the cerebral grey matter of elderly subjects. *Br J Psychiatry.* 1968;114:797–811.

88. Moore J, Bobula JA, Short TB, et al. A functional dementia scale. *J Fam Pract.* 1983;16:499–503.

89. Teri L, Truax P, Logsdon R, Uomoto J, Zarit S, Vitaliano PP. Assessment of behavioral problems in dementia: The revised Memory and Behavior Problems checklist. *Psychol Aging.* 1992;7:622–631.

90. Zarit SH, Todd PA, Zarit J. Subjective burden of husbands and wives as caregivers: A longitudinal study. *Gerontologist.* 1986;26:260–266.

91. Zarit SH, Anthony CR, Boutselis M. Interventions with care givers of dementia patients: Comparison of two approaches. *Psychol Aging.* 1987;2:225–232.

92. Gallo JJ. The effect of social support on depression in caregivers of the elderly. *J Fam Pract.* 1990;30:430–436.

93. Reisberg B, Ferris SH, DeLeon MJ, et al. The global deterioration scale for assessment of primary degenerative dementia. *Am J Psychiatry.* 1982;139:1136–1139.

94. Reisberg B, Ferris SH, Borenstein J, et al. Assessment of presenting symptoms. In: Poon LW, ed. *Clinical Memory Assessment of Older Adults.* Washington, DC: American Psychological Association; 1986.

95. Smyer MA, Hofland BF, Jonas EA. Validity study of the Short Portable Mental Status Questionnaire for the elderly. *J Am Geriatr Soc.* 1979;27:263–269.

96. Shuttleworth EC. Memory function and the clinical differentiation of dementing disorders. *J Am Geriatr Soc.* 1982;30:363–366.

97. Fillenbaum G. Comparison of two brief tests of organic brain impairment, the MSQ and the Short Portable MSQ. *J Am Geriatr Soc.* 1980;28:381–384.

98. Eisdorfer C, Cohen D, Paveza GJ, et al. An empirical evaluation of the Global Deterioration Scale for staging Alzheimer's disease. *Am J Psychiatry.* 1992;149:190–194.

99. Paveza GJ, Cohen D, Jankowski LM, Freels S. An analysis of the Global Deterioration Scale in older persons applying for community care services. *J Ment Health Aging.* 1995;1:35–45.

100. Reisberg B. Dementia: A systematic approach to identifying reversible causes. *Geriatrics.* 1986;41:30–46.

101. Reisberg B, Ferris SH, Franssen E. An ordinal functional assessment tool for Alzheimer-type dementia. *Hosp Community Psychiatry.* 1985;36:593–595.

102. Hughes CP, Berg L, Danziger WL, et al. A new clinical scale for the staging of dementia. *Br J Psychiatry.* 1982;140:566–572.

103. Davis PB, Morris JC, Grant E. Brief screening tests versus clinical staging in senile dementia of the Alzheimer type. *J Am Geriatr Soc.* 1990;38:129–135.

104. Burke WJ, Miller JP, Rubin EH, et al. Reliability of the Washington University clinical dementia rating. *Arch Neurol.* 1988;45:31–32.

105. Winograd CH. Mental status tests and the capacity for self care. *J Am Geriatr Soc.* 1984;32:49–53.

106. Gelb DJ, St. Laurent RT. Alternative calculation of the Global Clinical Dementia Rating. *Alzheimer Dis Assoc Disord.* 1993;7:202–211.

107. Williams TF, Williams ME. Assessment of the elderly for long-term care. *J Am Geriatr Soc.* 1982;30:71–75.

108. Rabins P, Mace NL, Lucas MJ. The impact of dementia on the family. *JAMA.* 1982;248:333–335.

109. Pace WD, Anstett RE. Placement decisions for the elderly: A family crisis. *J Fam Pract.* 1984;18:31–46.

110. Williams TF. Assessment of the geriatric patient in relation to needs for services and facilities. In: Reichel W, ed. *Clinical Aspects of Aging,* 2nd ed. Baltimore: Williams & Wilkins; 1983:543–548.

111. Weed L. *Medical Records, Medical Education, and Patient Care.* Cleveland, OH: Case Western Reserve Press; 1970.

# 11

## Social Assessment

Carmen Morano and Barbara Morano

Social assessment, like medical, mental health, and functional assessment, is a critical element of any comprehensive geriatric assessment.[1] Social assessment for older patients has multiple dimensions that include but are not limited to the sources of formal and informal help available to the older person from their social networks. With more than 80% of all care delivered by family caregivers,[2] the social assessment will frequently require an assessment of the older person and his or her caregivers.

In addition to assessing the social support of the client and the primary caregiver, the financial, environmental, and spiritual dimensions must be assessed, as well as the client's health and long-term care coverage. By using a multidimensional assessment, the practitioner will be able to identify potential risks or issues ranging from older person neglect and mistreatment to premature or unnecessary institutionalization.

Social assessment is essential to a comprehensive assessment because it provides information that is vital to understanding the contextual reality of the client's life. This permits either the individual assessor or the geriatric assessment team to develop an effective and appropriate care plan that addresses current and future risks to the geriatric client and his or her caregiver. However, although the importance of the social assessment is well established, great inconsistency exists in the exact dimensions that should be included, who performs this part of the assessment, and how the information is gathered.

The social assessment may be the most time-consuming element of a comprehensive assessment. It may easily take the team or independent practitioner as long or longer to complete the social part of the assessment as it does to complete the medical or functional assessment. However, without such a complete assessment, the capacity to plan for care will be adversely affected. Although there is no special sequence that needs to be followed in conducting a social assessment, it is important that it is completed in a standardized way. The needs of the client, family, agency, and practitioner will dictate how it is conducted. All of the information discussed in this chapter constitutes the basics of a comprehensive social assessment.

## ASSESSMENT OF SOCIAL SUPPORT

For many older adults, life is immeasurably enhanced by their relationship with their families. Similarly, the life of many families is immeasurably enhanced by their involvement with an older parent, grandparent, and great-grandparent. The benefits of this type of intergenerational relationship are reciprocal. Older members of the family may give gifts and financial aid or assist with domestic chores such as housekeeping or regular or intermittent child care. Currently, more than 2.5 million grandparents are raising their grandchildren.[3] In addition to assisting with a variety of tasks, older family members also provide a sense of membership and connectedness[4] as well as a sense of life cycle to younger members.

On the other hand, younger family members provide companionship, care management, nursing, transportation, and a source of pride to older members. The current cohort of adult children who find themselves caring for older parents can be actively engaged with their own family and work responsibilities, to those in the growing cohort who are themselves at retirement age or older. One fourth of all caregivers are 65 to 74 years of age, and 10% are over the age of 75 years.[3] One in 10 persons over the age of 65 years has a child who is at least 65 years of age.[5] Not uncommonly, the caregiver is a woman in her 60s caring for a mother in her 90s. Trends toward smaller families and, hence, fewer adult children to serve as caregivers, as well as the increasing participation of women in the workplace, further strain the support system for the older person.

The assessment of the social situation, particularly of the support available to the person unable to perform independently all of the activities of daily living (ADLs), is significantly intertwined with the issues surrounding nursing home placement. Numerous studies indicate that the presence of a caregiver is the most important factor in the disposition of older patients from the hospital.[6-12] A clinic at the University of Wisconsin assessed persons with Alzheimer's disease who were living in the community at the time of assessment. Those who eventually had to be placed in a nursing home did not differ from the others in their ability to perform ADLs or in health status. The major precipitating reason for placement was the lack of a willing caregiver.[8] Despite myths to the contrary, families continue to provide help for their older members, sometimes stretching financial and emotional resources to the limit.

The support system of older adults is comprised of three components: the informal network, the semiformal support system, and formal supports.[13,14] Informal supports are provided by family and friends; semiformal support refers to the support provided by neighborhood organizations such as churches or senior citizen centers.[13] Formal supports include financial (Social Security, Supplemental Social Security), medical (Medicare, Medicaid), as well as social welfare agencies and private fee-for-service providers.

*Informal supports* are generally accessed by the older persons themselves and are often based on a number of factors. Proximity to the care receiver, cultural beliefs about who is the most appropriate person to help, prior relationships, and the availability of the caregiver are just a few of the determining factors. The informal network is traditionally thought of as the constellation of social relationships that provide not only social interaction and discourse, such as daily phone contact, but also assistance with chores such as transportation to the physician's office or to the grocery store. Although the informal social network is the constellation of a person's social relationships, social support is the actual help (i.e., financial, emotional, or otherwise) that the social network provides.[15] Persons in the social network may or may not be helpful (i.e., provide social support).

For example, although a son lives nearby to a parent, this does not ensure that adequate support is being provided for an older widowed mother. Neighbors who deal with the older person on a daily basis may form the helping network that performs chores or errands for her. At times, the family may be unaware of the extent of the help provided by this natural helper network; indeed, the older person may not fully comprehend it.[16] The postal carrier who sees to it that the mail is picked up, the grocery clerk who helps with bags, and neighbors who bake and share their cooking and company are examples of natural helpers. In rural communities, informal helpers may acquire considerable importance because of geographic isolation and reluctance to participate in formal programs.[17] Some rural older persons are not comfortable receiving even informal assistance unless they have accumulated social credit, that is, they have helped others.[18]

Semiformal supports such as church groups, neighborhood organizations, and clubs are also important sources of social support for older adults. For many of these kinds of support, the older adult will usually have had some prior relationship with the organization and must take the initiative to gain access to services and might require encouragement or assistance to do so from health professionals or family members. Unfortunately, some older adults resist using this type of support because of a genuine concern for how their need for assistance will be perceived.

Finally, there is the formal support system that consists of public and private social welfare and social service agencies and the public and private health care delivery agencies. These programs play an important role in the social and physical well-being of older persons, especially in a mobile, industrialized society in which children move far from their parents. Unfortunately, the adequate funding of these formal public support programs is becoming more and more problematic for local, state, and federal agencies. A large body of evidence indicates that there is significant variation in the availability of these services from one region to another, as well as variation in who uses them. Race, ethnicity, gender, and the availability of an informal caregiver are just a few of the factors that have been found to predict use of formal services. Although the use of private fee-for-service social service models (i.e., private geriatric care management) is limited to those with adequate resources, their use will continue to grow in importance as more consumers purchase long-term care insurance.

Professionals who are providing care for older people should familiarize themselves with the available support and get a sense of what informal, formal, and semiformal help the older persons have employed in the past and what the experience was like. This latter question will help to explain the client's willingness or resistance to accessing needed support.

The assessment of social support can be conducted in a structured manner through the use of a variety of instruments that have been tested over time or through a more informal means by asking a series of questions aimed at gathering information about who provides help and support to both the older adult and the caregiver. The most fruitful method for providing the practitioner with the desired information may be a combination of a structured assessment instrument and open-ended questions.

If the practitioner believes that the use of a formal scale would either be too time consuming or inappropriate, a number of options are available. Kane[19] has recently suggested that the minimum assessment of a person's social network should consist of three questions: (1) whether the person has anyone he or she can contact when the person needs help and who that person is, (2) how many relatives other than children the person feels close to and with whom he or she has contact at least once a month, and (3) how many friends the person feels close to and has contact with at least once a month. Although these questions certainly would provide some sense of the size of the social network and whether at least one person could be counted on for assistance, social support might more critically be seen as not only the numbers of persons, but also the willingness of those persons to provide assistance when needed.[19,20]

One scale that can be considered for assessment of social support is the Lubben Social Network Scale (Exhibit 11–1).[21] This scale, through a series of 10 questions representing five categories (family network, friends network, confidant relationships, helping others, and living arrangements), seeks information about the nature of the client's social support system. The score is obtained by adding up the scores on each of the 10 items, with a possible range of scores from 0 to 50. A score below 20 indicates a risk for limited social network. An especially low score in any of the five categories will also provide important information that could be explored further with the client. This instrument can be used equally well with the client and the caregiver to provide a broad-based picture about the size of the support network and its availability to assist with care and decision making.

Another formal assessment instrument is the Norbeck Social Support Questionnaire,[20,22] which has been shown to have strong construct validity. Moreover, it has been demonstrated to have utility for measuring social support not only with caregivers, but also for the clients themselves. This instrument's subscales likewise permit the determination of the areas in which a person perceives adequate social support and those areas in which the person perceives social support is lacking. The scale permits the ascertainment of information about complex social networks, including the actual perceived sources of support. Furthermore, this measure of social support has

**Exhibit 11–1** Lubben Social Network Scale (LSNS)

---

**FAMILY NETWORKS**

1. How many relatives do you see or hear from at least once a month (note: include in-laws with relatives)?

|  |  |
|---|---|
| 0 = zero | 3 = three or four |
| 1 = one | 4 = five to eight |
| 2 = two | 5 = nine or more    _____ |

2. Tell me about the relative with whom you have the most contact. How often do you see or hear from that person?

|  |  |
|---|---|
| 0 = zero | 3 = three or four |
| 1 = one | 4 = five to eight |
| 2 = two | 5 = nine or more    _____ |

3. How many relatives do you feel close to? That is, how many of them do you feel at ease with, can talk to about private matters, or can call for help?

|  |  |
|---|---|
| 0 = zero | 3 = three or four |
| 1 = one | 4 = five to eight |
| 2 = two | 5 = nine or more    _____ |

**FRIENDS NETWORKS**

4. Do you have any close friends? That is, do you any friends with whom you feel at ease, can talk to about private matters, or can call on for help? If so how many?

|  |  |
|---|---|
| 0 = zero | 3 = three or four |
| 1 = one | 4 = five to eight |
| 2 = two | 5 = nine or more    _____ |

5. How many of these friends do you see or hear from at least once a month?

|  |  |
|---|---|
| 0 = zero | 3 = three or four |
| 1 = one | 4 = five to eight |
| 2 = two | 5 = nine or more    _____ |

6. Tell me about the friend with whom you have the most contact. How often do you see or hear from that person?

|  |  |
|---|---|
| 0 = < monthly | 3 = weekly |
| 1 = monthly | 4 = a few times a week |
| 2 = a few times a month | 5 = daily    _____ |

## CONFIDANT RELATIONSHIPS

7. When you have an important decision to make, do you have someone you can talk to about it?

| Always | Very Often | Often | Sometimes | Seldom | Never | |
|---|---|---|---|---|---|---|
| 5 | 4 | 3 | 2 | 1 | 0 | _____ |

8. When other people you know have an important decision to make, do they talk to you about it?

| Always | Very Often | Often | Sometimes | Seldom | Never | |
|---|---|---|---|---|---|---|
| 5 | 4 | 3 | 2 | 1 | 0 | _____ |

## HELPING OTHERS

9a. Does anybody rely on you to do something from them each day (e.g., shopping, cooking dinner, doing repairs, cleaning house, providing child care, etc.)?

NO—if no, go on to 9b.
YES—if yes, 9 is scored 5 and skip to 10                          _____

9b. Do you help anybody with things like shopping, filling out forms, doing repairs, and providing child care?

| Always | Very Often | Often | Sometimes | Seldom | Never | |
|---|---|---|---|---|---|---|
| 5 | 4 | 3 | 2 | 1 | 0 | _____ |

## LIVING ARRANGEMENTS

10. Do you live alone or with other people (note: include in-laws with the relatives)?

5 Live with spouse
4 Live with other relatives or friends
1 Live with other unrelated individuals (e.g., paid help)
0 live alone                                                      _____

TOTAL LSNS SCORE    _____

SCORING
The total LSNS score is obtained by adding up scores from each of the 10 individual items. Thus, total LSNS scores can range from 0 to 50. Scores on each item were anchored between 0 to 5 in order to permit equal weighting of the 10 items. It is suggested that a score below 20 indicates risk for limited social networks.

been linked to life stress indicators, suggesting that the low social support scores are likely to be predictive of high stress and high scores low stress. As has already been noted, it is this stress that puts many older adults at risk for institutionalization. Also, as is discussed in detail later in this chapter, stress has been linked to older person mistreatment as well.[23]

## ASSESSMENT OF CAREGIVER BURDEN AND SATISFACTION

Ample research has found that the task of caregiving can be demanding and onerous to the caregiver and results in both negative and positive outcomes. Research suggests a clear link between the caregiver's perceived burden and the risk of depression among caregivers.[24,25] Furthermore, caregiver depression, particularly among those caring for family members with Alzheimer's disease, has been linked to increased risk of older person abuse.[26] These risks suggest that it is crucial for the practitioner to assess carefully for caregiver perception of burden in addition to the actual tasks being provided.

Caregiver burden has long been recognized as a mulitdimensional construct.[25,27,28] The potential sources of caregiver burden have also been conceptualized into three primary components.[29] The first deals with the impairment of the older adult, including assessing the ability to perform ADLs, sociability, disruptive behavior, and mental status. Second, the tasks that correspond to the older adult's needs are rated as difficult, tiring, or upsetting. Dealing with bowel or bladder incontinence, for example, would probably be considered more difficult, tiring, and upsetting than assisting with meals. Finally, the impact of the behaviors and associated tasks on the caregiver's life is assessed. For example, having to care for an older family member may result in a change of job, quitting or turning down a promotion, or redefined family relationships.[29]

Although the severity of symptoms, degree of impairment, and the length of time one has been providing care alone may be a poor predictor of the degree of caregiver stress,[30] the occurrence of problematic behaviors by the care receiver and the caregivers perception or appraisal of his or her situation are two of the prime predictors of caregiver burden.[31]

A number of instruments can be used to assess the caregiver's burden, as well as the caregiver's appraisal of the situation. Instruments such as the Caregiving Hassles Scale[32] and the Zarit Burden Interview[33] can be used to assess the degree or amount of care the caregiver provides. One of the most often used scales to measure the caregivers perception of burden is the Lawton Scale of Appraised Burden.[27,34] The Caregiver Burden inventory[28] is a multidimensional scale that measures five domains (time, developmental, physical, social, and emotional) of burden that can be especially helpful in completing a comprehensive assessment of caregiver burden. Each domain includes five items (except physical burden, which has four) that enable the practitioner to assess specific sources of potential burden, as well as an overall measure of caregiver burden (Exhibit 11–2).

For many caregivers, the provision of care to a loved one can result in feelings of life satisfaction,[35] uplifts,[36] and mastery.[37] The caregiver's perceived satisfaction, or what is termed caregiving gain,[38] has been linked with positive outcomes.[35] Just as burden is a risk factor to burnout and older person maltreatment, satisfaction is an important protective factor that can mediate the effects of burden. The scale developed by Lawton[27] is a short 5-item scale that can be used to measure appraisal of satisfaction.

Both caregiver burden and satisfaction are often linked with the caregiver's coping capabilities and perception of mechanisms he or she can use to assist in handling the stresses inherent in the caregiving situation.[39] Ample evidence suggests that a caregiver who uses a problem-focused type of coping style will fare significantly better than those caregivers who use an emotion-focused coping style. It is useful for the clinician to seek information about the coping style, including the use of a variety of techniques that have been described by Pearlin and Schooler,[40] Pearlin and Skaff,[41] and Stephens et al.[42] Although not always recognized as part of the social assessment, a number of scales can identify the caregivers type of coping style.

Given the increased physical burden of caregiving and that many caregivers are over the age of 65 years,[5] assessing the physical well-being of the caregiver has practical value as well. The caregiver with cardiovascular problems, arthritis, or chronic back problems cannot be expected to do heavy lifting in the course of caring for an impaired older person. This emphasizes again the need to consider the functional status of older caregivers. In one survey, one third of caregivers rated their health as fair or poor.[5] Other investigators showed that caregivers had three times as many stress-related symptoms and used more psychoactive drugs than similar control subjects.[25]

In addition to assessing burden and coping styles, the clinician might wish to expand the caregiver assessment into other areas that are likely to affect the caregiver's ability to provide useful care. Although this may

**Exhibit 11–2** Novak and Guest Caregiver Burden Inventory

Please circle the number that best reflects your experience.

| | |
|---|---|
| **Not at all descriptive** | **0** |
| **Somewhat descriptive** | **1** |
| **Descriptive** | **2** |
| **Somewhat descriptive** | **3** |
| **Very descriptive** | **4** |

| | | *Score* |
|---|---|---|
| 1. My care receiver needs my help to perform many daily tasks. | 0  1  2  3  4 | |
| 2. My care receiver is dependent on me. | 0  1  2  3  4 | |
| 3. I have to watch my care receiver constantly. | 0  1  2  3  4 | |
| 4. I have to spend to help my care receiver with many basic functions. | 0  1  2  3  4 | |
| 5. I don't have a minute's break from my caregiving chores. | 0  1  2  3  4 | |
| **Time Dependence Burden Score** | | *Score* |
| 1. I feel that I am missing out on life. | 0  1  2  3  4 | |
| 2. I wish I could escape from this situation. | 0  1  2  3  4 | |
| 3. My social life has suffered. | 0  1  2  3  4 | |
| 4. I feel emotionally drained because of caring for my care receiver. | 0  1  2  3  4 | |
| 5. I expected that things would be different at this point in my life. | 0  1  2  3  4 | |
| **Developmental Burden Score** | | *Score* |
| 1. I'm not getting enough sleep. | 0  1  2  3  4 | |
| 2. My health has suffered. | 0  1  2  3  4 | |
| 3. Caregiving has made me physically weak. | 0  1  2  3  4 | |
| 4. I'm physically tired. | 0  1  2  3  4 | |
| **Physical Burden Score** | | *Score*\* |

Please circle the number that best reflects your experience.

| | |
|---|---|
| **Not at all descriptive** | **0** |
| **Somewhat descriptive** | **1** |
| **Descriptive** | **2** |
| **Somewhat descriptive** | **3** |
| **Very descriptive** | **4** |

| | | *Score* |
|---|---|---|
| 1. I don't get along with other family members as I used to. | 0  1  2  3  4 | |
| 2. My caregiving efforts aren't appreciated by others in my family. | 0  1  2  3  4 | |
| 3. I've had problems with my marriage. | 0  1  2  3  4 | |
| 4. I don't do as good a job at work as I used to. | 0  1  2  3  4 | |
| 5. I feel resentful of other relatives who could but do not help. | 0  1  2  3  4 | |
| **Social Burden Score** | | *Score* |
| 1. I feel embarrassed over my care receiver's behavior. | 0  1  2  3  4 | |
| 2. I feel ashamed of my care receiver. | 0  1  2  3  4 | |
| 3. I resent my care receiver. | 0  1  2  3  4 | |
| 4. I feel uncomfortable when I have friends over. | 0  1  2  3  4 | |
| 5. I feel angry about my interactions with my care receiver. | 0  1  2  3  4 | |
| **Emotional Burden Score** | | *Score* |
| **Total Burden Score** | | —— |

*Because this subscale only has four items, use a multiplier of 1.5 to determine a raw score that is equivalent to the other five-item subscales.

A score of greater than or equal to 10 on any subscale indicates a potential area of caregiver burden.

lengthen the process, if conducted by a coworker or ancillary worker, this part of the assessment may be conducted while the physician is completing other parts of the assessment. Areas of caregiver assessment that should also be considered included a formal assessment for depression, as well as one of the caregiver's social support system, mental status, and functional status. Caregiver depression can increase the caregiver's sense of hopelessness in coping with the caregiving experience. It is also possible that while the primary client may describe a reasonable support system, the caregiver may describe a very different one. When this is the case, the physician needs to view the caregiver as fragile and in need of strengthening through the infusion of external services. Of equal importance is taking the time to check the mental and functional status of the caregiver. Clinical experience with caregivers of persons with Alzheimer's has shown caregivers who are as cognitively impaired as and sometimes more than the family members diagnosed with the disease. Such a caregiver, particularly when a spouse, is often simply better at hiding the problem than the diagnosed family member. This kind of caregiving situation could easily result in both persons suffering from lack of care. A similar possibility exists if the clinician fails to assess the functional ability of the caregiver. Again, clinical experience has demonstrated that it is not unusual to have a caregiver that has equal or greater functional impairment than the primary client.

Although the need for assessing these may appear obvious, clinical experience suggests that these areas are often overlooked. Unaddressed, these issues may affect the ability of the caregiver to provide care, thereby resulting in a more rapid institutionalization of the primary client and medical compromise and premature placement of the caregiver.

## ASSESSMENT OF OLDER PERSON MISTREATMENT

Although it is likely that older persons have been mistreated throughout history, only recently have health and mental health providers and the legal system teamed up in an effort to heighten social awareness of the problem of older person abuse and neglect.[43] Accounting for this change in the last half of the 20th century is not only the increased numbers of the older population, but also a willingness by providers and society to intervene within the privacy of the family. Older adults are vulnerable to mistreatment because they are more likely to be suffering from physical and cognitive impairments, which necessitate a reliance on caregivers and family members for basic needs.

It is critical that the health care provider understand the extent and seriousness of older person mistreatment. The National Elder Abuse Incidence Study (NEAIS)[44] indicated that approximately 450,000 older adults living in noninstitutional settings were abused or neglected in 1996. The study also suggests that if the number of older adults who self-neglect are included the number increases to over 500,000, an increase of 150% since 1986. The most common form of older person maltreatment that is reported and substantiated is neglect, which comprises almost one half of all reported cases.[44] Although these numbers may seem to suggest that abuse is a rare event, the NEAIS suggests that many older adults who are abused and neglected never come to the attention of the authorities.[44] It is estimated that less then one fifth of all cases of older person mistreatment are reported and that less than half of those cases are substantiated.[44] This study also found that only 16% of the abusive situations are referred for help—84% remain hidden. Although a few studies estimate that between 3% and 5% of the older population has been abused, the Senate Special Committee on Aging estimates that there may be as many as 5 million victims every year.[44]

Currently, all 50 states and most US territories have either adult protection statutes or older person abuse statutes. However, reporting is not mandated in every state, with seven states relying on voluntary reporting to identify cases of older person mistreatment.[43] These laws are specifically designed to assist with providing needed social services to older adults who are the victims of mistreatment. Although it is true that in some states these statutes are part of the criminal code in which punishment of the abuser is of equal concern, in almost all states in which there are criminal protective statutes, there are also statutes whose purpose is to help provide needed assistance to the older adult who may be the victim of such mistreatment.

Another problem facing reporting is the lack of uniform definitions of older person abuse and neglect. Although physical abuse is more clearly defined, emotional and/or psychologic abuse is more subjective. Many professionals question whether self-neglect should be included in the estimates of the problem. The definitions established by the 1987 amendments to the Older Americans Act include the following in defining maltreatment: physical abuse (including sexual abuse), emotional or psychologic abuse, financial exploitation, neglect by others, and self-neglect.

Although still in its infancy, research in the field of older person abuse and neglect has provided useful information regarding how to identify those at risk for abuse and neglect. Most often, those at risk are among the more physically vulnerable who are often dependent on family members for physical care.[45] Other studies suggest that the most vulnerable are women[36] and that abuse is equally divided between spouse caregivers and child caregivers.[23,46] More recently, several studies have suggested that the prevalence of violence may be greater in families providing care to a member with Alzheimer's disease.[26,47,48] Moreover, these articles also suggest there are some unique factors that place persons suffering from Alzheimer's at greater risk for violence. These included depression, living arrangement, burden, years of care, hours of care per day, and whether the caregiver was the object of violence from the primary client.[26,47,48] It is important to remember that this work focuses on those older adults who are living in the general community. Little work has been done on the presence of violence and neglect in institutional settings. Yet many of the older adults that health care providers see are living in just such situations.

As with other aspects of social assessment, assessment of older person mistreatment may be accomplished with the use of formal instruments or modifications of formal instruments. The abuse assessment instrument developed by Fulmer and Wetle[49] quickly assesses patients presenting in an emergency department setting. This instrument provides the health care provider with the types and range of questions that he or she needs to ask.

The importance of completing some type of older person mistreatment screening is no less important in settings other than the emergency room (i.e., home health, social service, and care management). The Elder Abuse Screen (see Exhibit 11–3) is a short questionnaire that can be administered by social workers and other nonhealth providers that will help to identify an increased potential for current and future older person maltreatment.

Assessment of older person mistreatment for many health providers constitutes a number of ethical dilemmas. Because state laws require reporting suspected older person mistreatment, providers are concerned that doing so may damage the doctor–patient bond. Although this concern is understandable, failure to assess for older person mistreatment increases the risk of premature institutionalization and in some cases premature death. Additionally, although the state has the responsibility to offer an intervention to prevent future abuse, the older adult is not required under law to accept those services. The ethical dilemma faced by a provider when an older adult refuses services is determining whether that older adult is capable of making decisions to refuse services. If the patient has the cognitive ability to make

**Exhibit 11–3** The Elder Abuse Screen

---

1. Is the client alert and oriented?
2. What is the physical appearance of the client and caregiver?
   a. Personal hygiene
   b. Clothing
3. How does the client interact with the identified caregiver?
   a. Observe verbal and nonverbal communication between the client and identified caregiver.
   b. Does the client exhibit anxiety when the caregiver is present?
   c. Are the verbal statements of the caregiver consistent with what you are observing?
4. Does the caregiver appear anxious about your visit/meeting?
5. Does the caregiver cooperate with your request to have some private time with the client?
6. What type of supports does the caregiver have?
7. How often does the caregiver get a break from his or her caregiving responsibilities?
8. How often does the client get out of the home to attend doctors' appointments or other activities?
9. How are the finances of the client managed?
10. Are there other persons who regularly come in contact with the client?

---

an informed choice and refuses services, the older person's decision must stand. However, if there is some question about capacity, additional action must be taken.

Regardless of the setting, the practitioner must ensure that adequate and appropriate referral is made to either adult protective services or another social service agency capable of providing the needed interventions. The health care provider must understand, just like the victim, that mistreatment rarely just stops, nor does it stop with some counseling.[50,51] Bringing an end to maltreatment requires consistent and ongoing intervention in almost all cases.

## ECONOMIC ASSESSMENT

Complaints that a patient brings to the physician's office can be a direct result of economic factors. Weight loss may occur when a patient cannot afford proper nutrition or dentures that fit. Medical compromise can occur when an older person fails to take prescribed medication or alters the dose because of financial considerations. The clinician may or may not use formal screening instruments; however, without assessing financial factors, the care plan or recommended therapy may be impractical. This part of the geriatric assessment deserves attention to prevent financial exploitation and the unintentional dissipation of assets as well as minimizing future barriers to accessing long-term care.

An economic assessment needs to include an evaluation of personal income and assets, as well as health insurance. The clinician may feel uncomfortable asking clients about financial status. Clues, such as the condition of the clothing, personal hygiene, as well as the condition of teeth, could indicate that economic difficulty is sometimes overlooked or attributed to other causes. A home visit may provide a more comprehensive picture of the economic status of the older adult than is possible elsewhere. Although the focus and depth of the questions that need to be asked will vary depending on the presenting situation, the instrument developed by Fillenbaum[52] (Exhibit 11–4) provides a useful guide to complete an economic assessment.

A rough indication of the adequacy of financial resources is the ability to spend money on small luxuries. Living on fixed incomes makes it difficult to juggle unexpected expenses. Out-of-pocket expenses for health care may cut significantly into the older adult's ability to use money for other purposes. As public long-term care supports diminish, self-paid health care, including chronic care in the home, will become much more common. According to Campsi et al. (p. 12),[53] "The amount of cash spent on care is higher now than it was before the enactment of Medicare and Medicaid." Although the total assets of the older person, such as a paid-for house, may be substantial, these assets may not be available to pay day-to-day bills. A home may have fallen into disrepair because taxes and maintenance costs have increased. If income is low, the older adult may choose deprivation rather than sell a familiar house. Consequently, what the older person once thought was an adequate savings for his or her later years may no longer even pay the bills.

Many older persons who need financial help do not receive it simply because they are unaware of where or how to receive it. In addition to a bureaucracy that can be overwhelming, some older persons may be poorly educated, even illiterate, or have such a poor command of the English language that they lack knowledge of or the ability to access available assistance. For those who might have the knowledge and ability to access assistance, the stigma of public assistance keeps some older people from even making an inquiry about accessing it.

**Exhibit 11–4** Economic Resources Assessment Scale of the Older Americans Resources and Services Multidimensional Functional Assessment Questionnaire

1. Are you presently employed full-time, part-time, retired, retired on disability, not employed and seeking work, or not employed and not seeking work? Or are you a full-time student or a part-time student?
2. What kind of work have you done most of your life?
3. Does your spouse work or did he or she ever work?
4. Where does your income (money) come from (i.e., yours and your spouse's)?
   Earnings from employment
   Income from rental, interest from investments, etc.
   Social Security (but not Supplemental Security Income)
   Veterans Administration Benefit
   Disability payments not covered by Social Security, Supplemental Security Income, or the Veterans Administration
   Unemployment compensation
   Retirement pension from job
   Alimony or child support
   Scholarships or stipends
   Regular assistance from family members
   Regular financial aid from private organizations and churches
   Welfare payments
   Other
5. How much income do you and your spouse have in a year?
6. How many persons live on this income (i.e., it provides at least half their income)?
7. Do you own your own home?
8. Are your assets and financial resources sufficient to meet emergencies?
9. Are your expenses so heavy that you cannot meet the payments? Can you barely meet the payments, or are your payments no problem to you?
10. Is your financial situation such that you believe you need financial assistance or help beyond what you are already getting?
11. Do you pay for your own food, or do you get any regular help with costs of food or meals?
12. Do you believe that you need food stamps?
13. Are you covered by any kinds of health or medical insurance?
14. Please tell me how well you think you and your family are now doing financially as compared with other persons your age—better, about the same, or worse.
15. How well does the amount of money you have take care of your needs—very well, fairly well, or poorly?
16. Do you usually have enough to buy little extras, that is, those small luxuries?
17. Do you believe that you will have enough for your needs in the future?

*Source:* Reprinted with permission from Fillenbaum G, *Multidimensional Functional Assessment of Older Adults: The Duke Older Americans Resources and Services Procedures.* Hillsdale, NJ: Lawrence Erlbaum Associates; 1988:130–135.

Health insurance is both a long-term care planning resource and an immediate defense against the high cost of health care. There are four categories of health insurance in the United States: Medicare, Medicaid, private health insurance, and long-term care insurance.

## MEDICARE

Medicare, the government health insurance program for the older person and the disabled, is primarily an acute-care coverage system. Medicare pays about 75% of hospital bills, 55% of physician bills, and only 2% of nursing home bills. Part A of Medicare pays for 90 days of hospitalization and the first 20 days of skilled nursing facility care. The next 80 days of rehabilitative care are partially covered. After that, the resident uses personal resources, which at current nursing home costs would rapidly deplete all but the most wealthy person's resources.

Part B pays for physician services up to 80% of "reasonable charges" as determined by the program (after an annual deductible). Physicians who accept "assignment" are paid directly by the program and agree to accept the sum as final payment.[54] Medicare is not a provider of long-term coverage.

Medicare Part D, which is legislated to go into effect in 2006, will provide limited coverage of medications for Medicare beneficiaries. Unfortunately, as this text is going to press, it is still not certain whether this legislation will remain as originally drafted or undergo substantial changes before taking effect. As the legislation was crafted, Medicare beneficiaries will become eligible to participate in a variety of plans that would cover approximately $1,400 of the consumer's first $5,000 in medication expenses. The projected monthly premium for this coverage will be approximately $35.00.

## MEDICAID

Medicaid is a joint federal and state means tested health care and long-term care insurance available to those who fall within certain income and asset limitations. Many states also allow middle-income citizens to acquire Medicaid in community settings under "Medicaid Waiver" home and community-based programs. Eligibility requirements differ from state to state. More recently, many states have attempted to control the costs of the various Medicaid programs by moving those covered by Medicaid into a number of managed care programs. The success and the future of this trend remain less than clear.

## PRIVATE HEALTH INSURANCE

Many older patients are also covered by a supplemental policy through a private company. The supplement, also known as a Medigap policy, may pay for health care costs not covered by Medicare. These policies cover some or all of the charges not paid for by Medicare, depending on the type of policy selected. As would be expected, the more coverage provided, the higher the monthly premiums are. Private insurers, including Health Maintenance Organizations (HMOs) and Preferred Provider Organizations (PPOs), may also be the primary payer for those Medicare beneficiaries who have elected coverage under the Medicare+Choice program. This has come to be known as "Managed Care Medicare." Private health insurance, whether managed care or fee-for-service/indemnity plans, is not long-term care insurance, but rather a subsidy for medical treatment and acute care.

## LONG-TERM CARE INSURANCE

Long-term care insurance is the newest type of health insurance that specifically provides benefits for chronic care services, including personal care assistance, nursing home care, or assisted living. Policies differ with respect to coverage limits and options. Premiums are calculated based on policy choice and age of applicant. Typically, those over 80 years old may find the premiums prohibitive and not a good investment.

Planning for retirement and ensuring that appropriate arrangements are made are each a field in their own right.[55] For most persons, income falls after retirement, but at the same time, retirees expect that their standard of living will not change. Indeed, this is the desirable goal toward which retirement planning strives. It is estimated that about 64% of preretirement income would be needed from interest and dividend income, pensions, and Social Security in order to maintain the same living standard as before retirement.[56]

Older adults constitute a largely untapped resource. This is true from an economic perspective as well as from a personal and societal one. The care of some frail older adults might be partially provided by healthy older people with special training. Teachers' aides and foster grandparent are other roles for retirees. Retired adults might choose to continue working, performing tasks (not yet paying full market wages).[57] Because many older adults can expect to live 1 to 2 decades after retirement, such options could provide more opportunities for the productive use of time.

Retirement in the future will reflect changing careers, mobility of the workforce, flexible work hours, shortened workweeks, and favorable attitudes toward work and retirement. In some settings, retirement is gradually phased in, as the older adult has a shorter and shorter workweek. Some older workers may remain as temporary consultants. Mental and physical functioning may be maintained through the pursuit of volunteer activities and hobbies, which health professionals should actively encourage.

Anticipatory guidance with regard to the use of time, maintaining self-esteem, attitudes toward household tasks, and the moderate use of alcohol and tobacco may be useful to the retiree. Dr. Gene Cohen, former Director of the National Institute on Aging, suggested that older adults develop a "social portfolio" containing four compartments: (1) group active (activities that involve others actively, such as tennis or travel), (2) group passive (such as discussion groups centered around movies or books), (3) individual active (walking and gardening are examples), and (4) individual passive (such as reading, woodworking, or knitting). Then when occupational roles wane, the older adult is ready with a portfolio of other activities that keep the mind and body active.

## ASSESSMENT OF THE ENVIRONMENT

A health care provider needs to be aware of problems in the client's environment that may limit his or her ability to carry out a care plan. The goals of the environmental assessment are to promote mobility, reduce the likelihood of falling, ensure continued independence, and improve the quality of life. In many cases, the assessment of the home brings out problems that are not readily apparent during an office interview.[58] A thorough environmental assessment should include such issues as the condition of the living arrangements, the nature of the neighborhood, including the physical infrastructure, and the transportation system.

It is well established that when given a choice, most older adults would prefer to remain in their home.[59] Yet for someone whose mobility is compromised and whose sight and hearing may be impaired, the home environment can be a help or a hindrance. "The architecture of chronic care brings new meaning to the famed Chicago architect Louis Sullivan's dictum that 'form follows function.'"[60] Environmental assessment and modification can promote mobility and reduce the likelihood of falling. Falling is the leading cause of death in women and the fourth leading cause of death in men between 65 and 85 years of age. It is the leading cause of death for men and women over the age of 85 years.[61] The percentage of falls among community-dwelling older adults increases from 25% at the age of 70 years to 35% after the age of 75 years.[61] One fourth of older adults who sustain a hip fracture die within a year.[61] These and other statistics have resulted in the *Elder Fall Prevention Act of 2003,* sponsored by US Senators Michael B. Enzi and Barbara A. Mikulski, which seeks to reduce falls among older Americans.

Steel et al.[58] noted that there is a prima facie belief that understanding the environment is critical when working with older adults. At the same time, they noted that little attention has been paid to best implement such an evaluation. Using a checklist is a time-efficient and comprehensive method for assessing environmental needs. The Home Safety Checklist (Exhibit 11–5) is one tool that can be used to ascertain potential hazards.[62] Moreover, although several instruments are available for assessment of the home,[58] few instruments cover such issues as the physical infrastructure of the house, its foundation, and the sidewalks around the home, as well as available transportation systems. Several environmental modifications are an important but complex issue that may be tied to finances, personal preferences, adaptations, and the ability to get the work completed. Other practical matters to consider include whether the older community dwelling adult takes a bus for transportation, carries heavy objects, or has pets.

## SPIRITUAL ASSESSMENT

A systematic approach to spiritual assessment can be a key feature to understanding the overall well-being of an older adult. In that the aging process is often accompanied by a time of introspective reflection, an evaluation of one's accomplishments, meaning, and purpose, spiritual assessment could take on added importance. Recent literature related to spirituality and aging also noted the associations between intrinsic religiosity and spiritual well-being with hope and

**Exhibit 11–5** Home Safety Checklist

This checklist is used to identify fall hazards in the house. After identification, hazards should be eliminated or reduced. One point is allowed for every no answer. A score of 1 to 7 is excellent, 8 to 14 is good, 15 or higher is hazardous.

| Housekeeping | Yes | No |
| --- | --- | --- |
| 1. Do you clean up spills as soon as they occur? | — | — |
| 2. Do you keep the floors and stairways clean and free of clutter? | — | — |
| 3. Do you put away books, magazines, sewing supplies, and other objects as soon as you are through using them? | — | — |
| 4. Do you store frequently used items on shelves and never leave them on the floor or stairways? | — | — |

| Floors | | |
| --- | --- | --- |
| 5. Do you keep everyone from walking on freshly washed floors before they are dry? | — | — |
| 6. If you wax floors do you apply 2 thin coats and buff each thoroughly or else use a self-polishing, nonskid wax? | — | — |
| 7. Do all nonsmall rugs have nonskid backings? | — | — |
| 8. Have you eliminated small rugs and carpets at the tops and bottoms of stairways? | — | — |
| 9. Are all carpet edges tacked down? | — | — |
| 10. Are rugs and carpets free of curled edges, worn spots, and rips? | — | — |
| 11. Have you chosen rugs and carpets with short, dense pile? | — | — |
| 12. Are rugs and carpets installed over good-quality, medium-thick pads? | — | — |

| Bathroom | | |
| --- | --- | --- |
| 13. Do you use a rubber mat or nonslip decals on the tub or shower? | — | — |
| 14. Do you have a grab bar securely anchored over the tub or on the shower wall? | — | — |
| 15. Do you have a nonskid rug on the bathroom floor? | — | — |
| 16. Do you keep soap in an easy-to-reach receptacle? | — | — |

| Traffic Lanes | | |
| --- | --- | --- |
| 17. Can you walk across every room in your home and from one room to another without detouring around furniture? | — | — |
| 18. Is the traffic lane from your bedroom to the bathroom free of obstacles? | — | — |
| 19. Are telephone and appliance cords kept away from areas where people walk? | — | — |

|                                                                                                   | Yes  | No   |
|---------------------------------------------------------------------------------------------------|------|------|
| Lighting                                                                                          |      |      |
| 20. Do you have light switches near every doorway?                                                | ___  | ___  |
| 21. Do you have enough good lighting to eliminate shadowy areas?                                  | ___  | ___  |
| 22. Do you have a lamp or light switch within easy reach from your bed?                           | ___  | ___  |
| 23. Do you have night-lights in your bedroom and in the hallway leading from your bedroom to your bathroom? | ___  | ___  |
| 24. Are all stairways well lighted?                                                               | ___  | ___  |
| 25. Do you have a light switches at both the tops and bottoms of stairways?                       | ___  | ___  |
| Stairways                                                                                         |      |      |
| 26. Do securely fastened handrails extend the full length of the stairs on each side of stairway? | ___  | ___  |
| 27. Do rails stand out from the walls so that you can get a good grip?                            | ___  | ___  |
| 28. Are rails distinctly shaped so you are alerted when you reach the end of the stairway?        | ___  | ___  |
| 29. Are all stairways in good condition, with no broken, sagging, or sloping steps?               | ___  | ___  |
| 30. Are all stairway carpeting and metal edges securely fastened and in good condition?           | ___  | ___  |
| 31. Have you replaced any single-level steps with gradually rising ramps and made sure such steps are well lighted? | ___  | ___  |
| Ladders and Step Stools                                                                           |      |      |
| 32. Do you have a sturdy step stool that you use to reach high cupboard and closet shelves?       | ___  | ___  |
| 33. Are all ladders and step stools in good condition?                                            | ___  | ___  |
| 34. Do you always use a step stool or ladder that is tall enough for the job?                     | ___  | ___  |
| 35. Do you always set up your step stool or ladder in a firm, level base that is free of clutter? | ___  | ___  |
| 36. Before you climb a ladder or step stool, do you always make sure that it is fully open and that the stepladder spreaders are locked? | ___  | ___  |
| 37. When you use a ladder or step stool, do you face the steps and keep your body between the side rails? | ___  | ___  |
| 38. Do you avoid standing on top of a step or climbing beyond the second step from the top of the ladder? | ___  | ___  |

*continues*

**Exhibit 11–5** continued

|  | Yes | No |
|---|---|---|
| **Outdoor Areas** | | |
| 39. Are the walks and driveways in your yard and other areas free of breaks? | — | — |
| 40. Are lawns and gardens free of holes? | — | — |
| 41. Do you put away garden tools and hoses when they're not in use? | — | — |
| 42. Are outdoor areas kept free of rocks, loose boards, and other tripping hazards? | — | — |
| 43. Do you keep outdoor walkways, steps, and porches free of wet leaves and snow? | — | — |
| 44. Do you sprinkle icy outdoor areas with de-icers as soon as possible after a snowfall? | — | |
| 45. Do you have mats at doorways for people to wipe their feet? | | |
| 46. Do you know the safest way of walking when you can't avoid walking on a slippery surface? | — | — |
| **Footwear** | | |
| 47. Do your shoes have soles and heels that provide good traction? | — | — |
| 48. Do you wear house slippers that fit well and don't fall off? | — | — |
| 49. Do you avoid walking in stocking feet? | — | — |
| 50. Do you wear low-heeled oxfords, loafers, or good-quality sneakers when you work in your house or garden? | — | — |
| 51. Do you replace boots or galoshes when their soles or heels are worn too smooth to keep you from slipping on wet or icy surfaces? | — | — |
| **Personal Precautions** | | |
| 52. Are you always alert for unexpected hazards, such as out-of-place furniture? | — | — |
| 53. If young grandchildren visit, are you alert for children playing on the floor and toys left in your path? | — | — |
| 54. If you have pets, are you alert for sudden movements across your path and pets getting underfoot? | — | — |
| 55. When you carry bulky packages, do you make sure that they don't obstruct your vision? | — | — |
| 56. Do you divide large loads into smaller loads whenever possible? | — | — |

|  | Yes | No |
|---|---|---|
| 57. When you reach or bend, do you hold onto a firm support and avoid throwing your head back or turning it too far? | — | — |
| 58. Do you always use a ladder or step stool to reach high places and never stand on a chair? | — | — |
| 59. Do you always move deliberately and avoid rushing to answer the phone or doorbell? | — | — |
| 60. Do you take time to get your balance when you change position from lying down to sitting to standing? | — | — |
| 61. Do you hold onto grab bars when you change position in the tub or shower? | — | — |
| 62. Do you keep yourself in good condition with moderate exercise, good diet, adequate rest, and regular medical check-ups? | — | — |
| 63. If you wear glasses, is your prescription up-to-date? | — | — |
| 64. Do you know how to reduce injury in a fall? | — | — |
| 65. If you live alone, do you have daily contact with a friend or neighbor? | — | — |

positive mood states[63] and the positive correlation between religious well-being with social support and hope.[64] Gerwood et al.[65] noted that spirituality is also related to positive high scores on the Purpose-in-Life Test, which may therefore be a clinically useful indicator for spiritual well-being.

Spiritual assessment encompasses a broad range of concepts that has different meanings as well as different degrees of importance. Consequently, it is important to obtain from the older adult what spirituality means to him or her. Maas et al.[66] have proposed a definition for spiritual distress as well as summarized ideologic factors and defining characteristics that can help guide the clinician in conducting a spiritual assessment. Kelly[67] has defined spiritual distress as a feeling of despair or alienation related to religious, moral, or other beliefs/values. Possible reasons for spiritual distress noted in that work include the following:

- Disruption in usual religious activity
- Personal and family disasters
- Loss of significant others
- Behaviors in contrast to society/cultural norms

**Exhibit 11–6** Spiritual Assessment Scale

|  | Strongly Agree | Agree | Neutral | Disagree | Strongly Disagree |
|---|---|---|---|---|---|
| 1. In the future, science will be able to explain everything. | 1 | 2 | 3 | 4 | 5 |
| 2. I can find meaning in times of hardship. | 1 | 2 | 3 | 4 | 5 |
| 3. A person can be fulfilled without pursuing an active spiritual life. | 1 | 2 | 3 | 4 | 5 |
| 4. I am thankful for all that has happened to me. | 1 | 2 | 3 | 4 | 5 |
| 5. Spiritual activities have not helped me become closer to other people. | 1 | 2 | 3 | 4 | 5 |
| 6. Some experiences can be understood through one's spiritual beliefs. | 1 | 2 | 3 | 4 | 5 |
| 7. A spiritual force influences the events in my life. | 1 | 2 | 3 | 4 | 5 |
| 8. My life has a purpose. | 1 | 2 | 3 | 4 | 5 |
| 9. Prayers do not really change what happens. | 1 | 2 | 3 | 4 | 5 |
| 10. Participating in spiritual activities helps me forgive other people. | 1 | 2 | 3 | 4 | 5 |
| 11. My spiritual beliefs continue to evolve. | 1 | 2 | 3 | 4 | 5 |
| 12. I believe there is a power greater than myself. | 1 | 2 | 3 | 4 | 5 |
| 13. I probably will not re-examine my spiritual beliefs. | 1 | 2 | 3 | 4 | 5 |
| 14. My spiritual life fulfills me in ways that material possessions do not. | 1 | 2 | 3 | 4 | 5 |
| 15. Spiritual activities have not helped me develop my identity. | 1 | 2 | 3 | 4 | 5 |
| 16. Meditation does not help me feel more in touch with my inner spirit. | 1 | 2 | 3 | 4 | 5 |

| | Strongly Agree | Agree | Neutral | Disagree | Strongly Disagree |
|---|---|---|---|---|---|
| 17. I have a personal relationship with a power greater than myself. | 1 | 2 | 3 | 4 | 5 |
| 18. I have felt pressure to accept spiritual beliefs that I do not agree with. | 1 | 2 | 3 | 4 | 5 |
| 19. Spiritual activities help me draw closer to a power greater than myself. | 1 | 2 | 3 | 4 | 5 |
| 20. When I wrong someone, I make an effort to apologize. | 1 | 2 | 3 | 4 | 5 |
| 21. When I am ashamed of something I have done, I tell someone about it. | 1 | 2 | 3 | 4 | 5 |
| 22. I solve my problems without using spiritual resources. | 1 | 2 | 3 | 4 | 5 |
| 23  I examine my actions to see whether they reflect my values. | 1 | 2 | 3 | 4 | 5 |

24. During the last week I prayed (check one)
  ☐ 10 or more times
  ☐ 7 times
  ☐ 4 times
  ☐ 1–3 times
  ☐ 0 times

25. During the last week I meditated (check one)
  ☐ 10 or more times
  ☐ 7 times
  ☐ 4 times
  ☐ 1–3 times
  ☐ 0 times

26. Last month I participated in spiritual activities with at least one other person (check one)
  ☐ more than 15 times
  ☐ 11–15 times
  ☐ 6–10 times
  ☐ 1–5 times
  ☐ 0 times

*Source:* Hatch RL, et al. The Spiritual Involvement and Beliefs Scale, Development and Testing of a New Instrument, Vol. 46, No. 6, pp. 476–486, © 1988, Dowden Publishing Company, Inc. Reproduced with permission from *The Journal of Family Practice.*

Defining characteristics of spiritual distress are noted to be

1. Feeling separated or alienated from the deity
2. Dissatisfaction with personal past or present
3. Depression
4. Crying
5. Self-destructive behavior or threats
6. Fear
7. Feelings of abandonment
8. Feelings of hopelessness[67]

A number of spiritual assessment instruments are available in the literature.[68] An example is shown in Exhibit 11–6. Assessment tools elicit information related to the following key concepts:[66]

1. The older person's concept of God or deity
2. Religious practices
3. Beliefs about spirit and hell
4. Values and meaning of life

---

**REFERENCES**

1. Paveza GJ. Social services and the Alzheimer's disease patient: An overview. *Neurology.* 1993;43(8 Suppl 4):11–15.

2. Stone R, Cafferata GL, Sangl J. Caregivers of the frail elderly: A national profile. *Gerontologist.* 1987;27;616–626.

3. Child Welfare League of America. (2003). *Fact Sheet: Grandparents and Other Relatives Raising Children.* Washington, DC: Child Welfare League of America.

4. Falck HS. *The Membership Perspective.* New York, NY: Springer Publications; 1988.

5. US Senate Special Committee on Aging. *Developments in Aging,* vol 1. Washington, DC: US Government Printing Office; 1988.

6. Berkman L. The assessment of social networks and social support in the elderly. *J Am Geriatr Soc.* 1983;31:743–749.

7. Brown LJ, Potter JF, Foster BG. Caregiver burden should be evaluated during geriatric assessment. *J Am Geriatr Soc.* 1990;38:455–460.

8. Fisk AA, Pannill FC. Assessment of the elderly for long-term care. *J Am Geriatr Soc.* 1987;35:307–311.

9. Lindsey AM, Hughes EM. Social support and alternatives to institutionalization for the at-risk elderly. *J Am Geriatr Soc.* 1981;29:308–315.

10. Sloane PD. Nursing home candidates: Hospital inpatient trial to identify those appropriately assignable to less intensive care. *J Am Geriatr Soc.* 1980;28:511–514.

11. Wachtel TJ, Fulton JP, Goldfarb J. Early prediction of discharge disposition after hospitalization. *Gerontologist.* 1987;27:98–103.

12. Williams TF, Williams ME. Assessment of the elderly for long-term care. *J Am Geriatr Soc.* 1982;30:71–75.

13. Rzetelny H, Mellor J. *Support Groups for Caregivers of the Aged.* New York: Community Service Society; 1981.

14. Zarit SH, Pearlin LI, Schaie KW, eds. *Caregiving Systems: Informal and Formal Helpers.* Hillsdale, NJ: Lawrence Erlbaum Associates; 1993.

15. Gallo JJ, Franch MS, Reichel W. Dementing illness: The patient, caregiver, and community. *Am Fam Phys.* 1991;43:1669–1675.

16. Hooyman NR, Lustbader W. *Taking Care: Supporting Older People and Their Families.* New York: Free Press; 1986.

17. Reichel W. Care of the elderly in rural America. *Md Med J.* May 1980:75.

18. Lozier J, Althouse R. Retirement to the porch in rural Appalachia. *Int J Aging Hum Dev.* 1975;6:7–15.

19. Kane RA. Assessment of social functioning: Recommendations for comprehensive geriatric assessment. In: Rubenstein LZ, Wieland D, Bernabei R, eds. *Geriatric Assessment Technology: The State of the Art.* New York: Springer Publishing; 1995:91–110.

20. Norbeck JS, Lindsey AM, Carrieri VL. The development of an instrument to measure social support. *Nurs Res.* 1981;30:264–269.

21. Lubben JE. Assessing social networks among elderly populations. *Fam Community Health.* 1988;11:45–52.

22. Norbeck JS, Lindsey AM, Carrieri VL. Further development of the Norbeck Social Support Questionnaire: Normative data and validity testing. *Nurs Res.* 1983;32:4–9.

23. Pillemer KA, Wolf RS, eds. *Elder Abuse: Conflict in the Family.* Dover, MA: Auburn House; 1986.

24. George LK, Blazer DG, Hughes DC, Fowler N. Social support and the outcome of major depression. *Br J Psychiatry.* 1989;154:478–485.

25. George LK, Gwyther LP. Caregiver well-being: A multidimensional examination of family caregivers of demented adults. *Gerontologist.* 1986;26:253–259.

26. Paveza GJ, Cohen D, Eisdorfer C, et al. Severe family violence and Alzheimer's disease: Prevalence and risk factors. *Gerontologist.* 1992;32:493–497.

27. Lawton MP, Kleban MH, Moss M, Rovine M, Glicksman A. Measuring caregiving appraisal. *J Gerontol.* 1989;44:P61–P71.

28. Novak M, Guest C. Application of a Multidimensional Caregiver Burden Inventory. *The Gerontologist.* 1989;29:798–803.

29. Poulshock SW, Deimling GT. Families caring for elders in residence: Issues in the measurement of burden. *J Gerontol.* 1984;39:230–239.

30. Zarit SH, Orr NK. *Working with Families of Dementia Victims: A Treatment Manual.* Washington, DC: US Government Printing Office; 1984. Publication No. 84–20816.

31. Schulz R, O'Brien AT, Bookwala J, Fleissner K. Psychiatric and physical morbidity effects of dementia caregiving: Prevalence, correlates, and causes. *The Gerontologist.* 1995;35:771-791.

32. Kinney JM, Stephens MA. *The Caregiving Hassles Scale: Administration, Reliability, and Validity.* Kent, OH: Psychology Department, Kent State University; 1987.

33. Zarit SH, Rever K, Bach-Peterson J. Relatives of impaired elderly: Correlates of feelings of burden. *The Gerontologist.* 1980;20:649–655.

34. Lawton MP, Moss M, Kleban MH, Glicksman A, Rovine M. A two-factor model of caregiving appraisal and psychological well-being. *J Gerontol*. 1991;46:P181–P189.

35. Morano C. Appraisal and coping: Moderators or mediators of stress. *Social Work Res*. 2003;27:116–128.

36. Kinney JM, Stephens MA. Hassles and uplifts of giving care to a family member with dementia. *Gerontologist*. 1989;29:402–408.

37. Picot SJ, Debanne SM, Namazi KH, Wykle ML. Religiosity and perceived rewards of black and white caregivers. *The Gerontologist*. 1997;37:89–101.

38. Kramer BJ. Gain in the caregiving experience: Where are we? What next? *The Gerontologist*. 1997;37:218–232.

39. Kiyak HA. *Coping with Alzheimer's Disease: Patient and Family Responses* (Paper presentation). Chicago: Gerontological Society of America; November 11, 1986.

40. Pearlin LI, Schooler C. The structure of coping. *J Health Soc Behav*. 1978;18:2–21.

41. Pearlin LI, Skaff MM. Stressors and adaptation in late life. In: Gatz M, ed. *Emerging Issues in Mental Health and Aging*. Washington, DC: American Psychological Association; 1995:97–123.

42. Stephens MAP, Crowther JH, Hobfoll SE, Tennenbaum DL, eds. *Stress and Coping in Later-Life Families*. New York: Hemisphere Publishing; 1990.

43. McInnis-Dittrich, K. *Social Work with Elders*, 2nd ed. Boston: Allyn & Bacon; 2002.

44. The National Center on Elder Abuse at the American Public Human Services Association in collaboration with Westat I. The National Elder Abuse Incidence Study–Final Report. Washington, DC: The Administration on Aging; 1998.

45. Steinmetz SK. *Duty Bound: Elder Abuse and Family Care*. vol. 166. Newbury Park, CA: Sage Publications; 1988.

46. Pillemer K, Finkelhor D. The prevalence of elder abuse: A random sample survey. *Gerontologist*. 1988;8:51–57.

47. Coyne AC, Reichman WE, Berbig LJ. The relationship between dementia and elder abuse. *Am J Psychiatry*. 1993;150:643–646.

48. Pillemer K, Suitor JJ. Violence and violent feelings: What causes them among family caregivers? *J Gerontol Soc Sci*. 1992;47:S165–S172.

49. Fulmer T, Wetle T. Elder abuse screening and intervention. *Nurse Pract*. 1986; 11:33–38.

50. Pritchard J. *Working with Elder Abuse: A Training Manual for Home Care, Residential and Day Care Staff*. London: Jessica Kingsley Publishers; 1996.

51. Quinn MJ, Tomita SK. *Elder Abuse and Neglect*, 2nd ed. New York: Springer Publishing; 1997.

52. Fillenbaum GG. The OARS multidimensional functional assessment questionnaire. In: *Multidimensional Functional Assessment of Older Adults: The Duke Older Americans Resources and Services Procedures*, 2nd ed. Durham, NC: Duke University Center for the Study of Aging and Human Development; 1978:7–12.

53. Campsi L, Cook S, Moore F, Marson D, Parker MW. Legal insurance financial tasks associated with parent care. *Geriatr Care Manage J*. 2003;13:1, 7–15.

54. Schulz JH. *The Economics of Aging*. Belmont, CA: Wadsworth Publishing Co.; 1985.

55. Dennis H, ed. *Retirement Preparation: What Retirement Specialists Need To Know*. Lexington, MA: Lexington Books; 1984.

56. England R. Greener era for gray America. *Insight.* 1987;3:8–11.

57. Morris R, Bass SA. The elderly as surplus people: Is there a role for higher education? *Gerontologist.* 1986;26:12–18.

58. Steel K, Musliner M, Berg K. Assessment of the home environment. In: Rubenstein LZ, Wieland D, Bernabei R, eds. *Geriatric Assessment Technology: The State of the Art.* New York: Springer Publishing; 1995:135–145.

59. Braun JA. Home safe home: Preventing falls through environmental assessment and modification. *Geriatr Care Manage J.* 2003;13:2, 8–12.

60. Jackson JA. *Health Care Without Medicare.* Lenox, MA: Solarian Press; 2000.

61. Braun JA. Federal legislation seeks to reduce falls among older Americans. *Geriatr Care Manage J.* 2000;13:2, 4–6.

62. Barber C. Geriatric Assessment. In: Cress C, ed. *Handbook of Geriatric Care Management.* Gaithersburg, MD: Aspen Press; 2001.

63. Fehring RJ, Miller J, Shaw C. Spiritual well-being, religiosity, hope, depression, and other mood states in elderly people coping with cancer. *Oncol Nurs Forum.* 1997; 24:663–671.

64. Zorn CR, Johnson M. Religious well-being in noninstitutional elderly women. *Health Care Women Int.* 1997;18:209–219.

65. Gerwood JB, Le Blanc LM, Piazza N. The Purpose-in-Life Test and religious denomination: Protestant and Catholic scores in an elderly population. *J Clin Psychol.* 1998;54:49–53.

66. Maas M, Buckwalter KC, Hardy MA, eds. *Nursing Diagnoses and Interventions for the Elderly.* Redwood City, CA: Addison-Wesley Publishing; 1991.

67. Kelly MA. *Nursing Diagnosis Source Book: Guidelines for Clinical Application.* Norwalk, CT: Appleton-Century-Crofts; 1985.

68. Fehring RJ, Rantz M. Spiritual distress. In: BK, Maas M, Hardy MA, eds. *Nursing Diagnoses and Interventions for the Elderly.* Redwood City, CA: Addison-Wesley Publishing; 1991:598–609.

# 12

# Physical Assessment

David Nicklin

The earlier chapters have discussed comprehensive history taking, including considerations of ethnicity and cultural sensitivity by the clinician and mental status assessment, functional assessment, social assessment, and values assessment. In addition, the traditional medical history would include a chief complaint, any primary difficulties or symptoms that are troubling the patient at the time of the visit. A history of present illness would follow, documenting the time course and evolution of the symptoms. A family health history for heritable risks and a social history for occupational (e.g., asbestos) and behavioral (e.g., tobacco, alcohol, sexuality) health exposure would also be included. Finally, a concise but comprehensive head-to-toe review of body systems would follow to identify additional symptoms.

A comprehensive history is essential, as it helps focus the physical examination. A complete, exhaustive physical examination would take over an hour to perform. For example, a neurologic exam (which formally assessed judgment and cognition; the 12 cranial nerves individually; sensation, including sharp, soft touch and temperature over all extremities, trunk and face; strength of all extensor and flexor muscles as well as trunk, neck, and face muscles; evaluation of nystagmus; a thorough funduscopic exam, etc.) alone could take an hour. Therefore, the examiner must perform a brief examination of each body system, with more in-depth examination of those systems where the history has focused attention. The same would be true of additional diagnostic testing (blood tests, x-rays and scans, electrocardiogram (EKG), electroencephalogram (EEG), and many others) where the physician faces almost limitless choices for further evaluation. Such testing is focused and directed by the finding on history and further on physical examination. However, a brief examination of all body parts and systems is necessary.

Increasing rates of disease and infirmity with advancing age require a greater vigilance on the part of the examiner to discover abnormalities and to judge the relevance for a particular patient (separating pathologic processes from aging processes). The assessment process is complicated because the presenting symptom in the older person is often nonspecific—a signal that something is amiss somewhere but not necessarily in the system expected. Dysfunction in any organ system may manifest as deteriorating mental status, for example, so that pneumonia (respiratory), appendicitis (gastrointestinal), or congestive heart failure (cardiac) cause confusion (central nervous system). The physical examination of the older person therefore needs to be as complete and systematic as time allows, particularly at the time of admission to the hospital or nursing home or before surgery.[1,2]

Frequently, the precise sequence and timing of the examination must be modified when dealing with an older person because of impaired hearing, sight, comprehension, or mobility. Rather than rush through the history and physical examination, it may be better to complete the entire process over two or more visits, along with an assessment of other domains. Unfortunately, physicians, if anything, may spend less time with older patients than with younger ones.[3]

What makes examination of older persons different, then, is not the content of the examination, but rather the need to develop an approach that does the older adult justice without undue discomfort or embarrassment. The approach must patiently take into account the older adult's impaired special senses or diminished mobility and must consider his or her slowed response time in answering questions. The physician must respectfully allow concerns that the person thinks are most important to be expressed. Caregivers and family may have concerns that need to be addressed within this context as well. Indeed, the chief complaint may be formulated by the family rather than by the person being examined.

## COMMUNICATION AND RAPPORT

The clinician must use the information obtained in the history telling about cultural background, cognitive, sensory, and other physical disabilities to perform a culturally sensitive physical examination. Because older persons frequently have impaired communication skills as a result of illness or lack of schooling, the examiner must pay special attention to communication issues in history taking and physical examination. When introducing himself or herself, the physician must take special note of communication problems. For many older adults, English may be a second language; consequently, the examiner must keep in mind that the person may have difficulty in providing or understanding information during the interview. A hearing problem may be easily disguised and can result in misunderstanding if not recognized. Someone who is hearing impaired may respond to questions inappropriately, and an erroneous evaluation could result. If the individual uses a hearing aid, the volume of both the hearing aid and the examiner's voice must be adjusted. The physician should speak clearly and articulate rather than shout.

Eye contact, handshake, the use of last name, and physical contact are the rudiments of good communication with all persons but particularly for older adults. Eye contact is important to establish a relationship. Prolonged eye contact can seem like staring, however, and in some cultures, eye contact is believed to be inappropriate. Addressing the individual by the last name is a sign of respect. Most of today's older adults grew up in a time when one would not think of addressing an older person or the physician by his or her first name. Using the last name is no barrier to friendliness; professional caregiving relationships are not less loving and warm as a result of using the last name. Many older persons appreciate a touch on the hand or shoulder. Done in a sincere and caring manner, a touch may allay some of the anxiety associated with a trip to the physician's office or with a home visit by a nurse or social worker.

Speak to the older adult directly, not through others who may have accompanied him or her to the visit. For all but the most cognitively impaired, the clinician should talk to the caregiver only with the permission of the individual. The family members may appreciate some time alone with the practitioner to express their concerns without feeling embarrassed by the older person's presence. A natural time for this to occur is while the person undresses in preparation for the physical examination. The environment of the encounter must be comfortable with a minimum of noise, distractions, and interruptions. Provide the patient and family with a brief explanation and description of what is to be accomplished during the visit and subsequent visits (if the evaluation is to be spread out over several visits).

The writings of Viktor Frankl and others suggested that having meaning and purpose in life contributes to a healthy life.[4-6] At times when older persons experience loss of health, family and friends, vocation, or home, they are more apt to succumb to depression, alcoholism, hypochondriasis, or other disorders. The physician can contribute to hope by asking about what offers meaning in the patient's life. Meaning may derive from seeing a grandchild get married or to be assured that an adult child's marriage is stabilized. Feeling connected to family, neighborhood, or a faith community can support meaningfulness. In assessing older patients, the physician can discreetly and noncoercively enter these areas. By raising hope related to certain circumstances (i.e., that with appropriate social supports the person may be able to remain at home rather than be admitted to a nursing home), the physician may facilitate healing and increase motivation to improve. Practitioners rarely enter the areas of religious or spiritual beliefs, which are often thought to be taboo. However, in completing the history, practitioners might ask the older person the following questions (avoiding a coercive or intrusive tone):[7-9] What role does religion play in your life? Are you a member of a faith community? Do you participate actively with this community? Spirituality is discussed in more detail in Chapter 11. Asking questions pertaining to meaning and purpose, as well as spiritual and religious issues, can open up a dialog that will benefit the patient and enhance his or her relationship with the doctor.

## EXAMINATION OF OLDER ADULTS WITH DEMENTIA

The physical examination of the person with Alzheimer's disease poses special challenges because the person may not be able to pinpoint what is wrong. Mental impairment severely limits the ability of many to express themselves. One danger is that mental deterioration will be automatically ascribed to Alzheimer's disease, and a reversible superimposed factor might consequently be overlooked. Therefore, the physical examination of the older person with mental impairment needs to be particularly thorough. Not only may a person with Alzheimer's disease have communication difficulties, but he or she may not be cooperative. Because of memory difficulties, the individual may need to be gently but firmly reminded of what is expected. These persons may be extraordinarily restless. A firm and reassuring touch, such as in holding the hand or a shoulder, giving clear and simple, one-step requests, and maintaining eye contact, may forge the necessary links to communication and cooperation. Often, the presence of a family member or friend can have a calming, orienting effect on the person being examined.

## HISTORY TAKING

During the initial examination, an older person might present to the practitioner a barrage of complaints and difficulties. The family might inform the practitioner of problems of which their relative is unaware. The physical and laboratory evaluation may uncover yet other undisclosed problems. The practitioner could easily begin to feel frustrated and overwhelmed. Where to begin? What is important to address now, and what can wait? Just collecting adequate data with which to make a decision, let alone implementing a treatment plan, can be difficult within the time constraints of a primary care practice. At the initial interview, it is probably best to attend to the specific problem, if there is one, be it medical or social, that prompted the evaluation,[10] with careful listing of other problems that may be addressed at subsequent visits.

Although some older persons are reluctant to give information to the interviewer, others are more than willing to share, at length, numerous irrelevant incidents that happened long ago. Without showing disinterest or disrespect, the interviewer must strive to help the person focus on the issues at hand. Functional assessment helps to direct the clinician's initial efforts to the solution of the problems that have a direct impact on the ability to perform the tasks of daily living.

The trouble is that there often are multiple chief complaints or the chief complaint is unclear (e.g., "Mom just doesn't seem herself"), or the chief complaint does not fit the usual mold (e.g., "Mom just doesn't cook anymore"). The physician should use good problem-oriented medical records to help sort things out over time. Although not all of the "problems" recorded will be addressed in a single visit, spelling them out, even if expressed as undifferentiated medical problems or functional difficulties, helps to organize the problems. For older people, this is particularly important because the "parsimony of diagnosis" rule may not apply—several diseases (and their treatments) may coexist and interact. By keeping track of diagnosed and undifferentiated medical, social, and functional problems in this way, each visit will build on the information and rapport obtained in previous encounters. The physician should negotiate with the patient and family regarding which problems are the most salient to be addressed at each visit.

Although it is generally a good idea to use open-ended questions to obtain information (and older adults are no exception), it is sometimes necessary to supply the older person with specific words to choose from to help describe the problem. For example, "Describe your chest pain" is open-ended; "Was the pain sharp, stabbing, dull, or crushing?" may help the older individual to describe the pain. Older adults have the reputation of answering yes to all of the questions in the review of systems. Still, there are problems that may otherwise remain hidden unless specifically asked about by the examiner. Ham[11] has identified several: sexual dysfunction, depression, incontinence, musculoskeletal stiffness, alcoholism, hearing loss, and dementia. A suggested review of systems is presented in Exhibit 12–1. Some problems such as dyspnea may not be new, but rather altered in quality or frequency. The older person may always have had trouble on the stairs with shortness of breath, but now must rest three times instead of negotiating the stairs without resting.[12] Such a change in the degree of disability will be discovered by the careful interviewer.

Trying to confirm the diagnosis of every abnormality in every case may not be in the patient's best interest. The physician–patient rela-

---

**Exhibit 12–1** Geriatric Review of Systems

| | | | |
|---|---|---|---|
| General | Weight change | Genitourinary | Incontinence |
| | Fatigue | | Dysuria |
| | Falls | | Nocturia |
| | Anorexia | | Hematuria |
| | Anemia | | Sexual |
| | Poor nutrition | | functioning |
| Special senses | Visual changes | Musculoskeletal | Morning |
| | Cataract | | stiffness |
| | Hearing changes | | Joint pain |
| | Imbalance | | Joint swelling |
| | Vertigo | | Limitation of |
| Mouth and teeth | Dentures | | movement |
| | Denture discomfort | Neurology | Memory |
| | Dry mouth | | problems |
| Respiratory | Cough | | Headaches |
| | Hemoptysis | | Syncope |
| | Dyspnea | | Gait |
| Cardiovascular | Chest pain on exertion | | Sensory |
| | Orthopnea | | function |
| | Ankle edema | | Sleep disorders |
| | Claudication | | Transient focal |
| Gastrointestinal | Dysphagia | | symptoms |
| | Melena | | Voice changes |
| | Change in stool caliber | Psychiatric | Depression |
| | Laxative use | | Alcoholism |
| | Constipation | | Anxiety |

*Source:* Reprinted from J. Gallo, Ed., Physical Assessment, *Handbook of Geriatric Assessment,* 2nd ed., pp. 151, © 1994, Aspen Publishers, Inc.

tionship may be undermined if it depends solely on discovering reversible disease, rather than on optimal management of chronic disorders. Older adults often have multiple chronic illnesses that, although incurable, have aspects that can be modified to enhance function and limit discomfort.[13,14] Of course, a balance must be struck. The clinician must not be too quick to assume the symptoms are fully explained by the most serious, advanced, or chronic disease. Less serious but treatable conditions may contribute to disability. Blind pessimism is unwarranted and can be counterproductive.

## OVERVIEW OF THE PHYSICAL EXAMINATION

The physical assessment really begins when the physician first meets the patient and observes how he or she behaves and how well the patient is dressed and groomed. Much information is taken in during the first 10 seconds in the room with the patient. Does the person seem well nourished or thin and emaciated? Does he or she move about easily or unsteadily and unbalanced? How easily does the person arise from a chair to the examining table? During the history taking, the physician should observe the patient for involuntary movement, cranial nerve dysfunctions, and difficult respiration. The physician should also listen for the pace and clarity of speech.

The examination should require as few changes in position as possible. With the patient seated, the head, eyes, ears, nose, throat, neck, heart, lungs, joints, and neurologic examinations follow in turn. The patient is then positioned supine for examination of the abdomen, peripheral pulses, breasts, genitalia, and inguinal regions. The patient can then be turned to the lateral decubitus position for rectal examination. Finally, the patient is brought to a standing position so that orthostatic blood pressure and pulse changes can be detected. Balance and gait can then also be tested.

## COMPONENTS OF THE EXAMINATION

### Pulse

The measurement of vital signs, temperature, and height and weight has been basic to physical assessment for centuries. The Chinese methods of diagnosis, thousands of years old, include questioning, feeling the pulse, and observing the voice and body. The radial artery is convenient for determining the heart rate. When the pulse is irregular, it is further characterized as regularly irregular or irregularly irregular. A regularly irregular pulse may indicate consistently dropped beats, as in a second-degree atrio-ventricular (A-V) block, or added beats, such as with premature ventricular contractions. An irregularly irregular pattern often represents atrial fibrillation but can also be caused by very frequent premature ventricular or atrial contractions. Palpation of the carotid pulse with simultaneous auscultation of the heart is helpful in timing murmurs or other sounds emanating from the heart.

## Blood Pressure

Blood pressure is ideally taken with the patient both supine and standing, especially if he or she is taking medication for hypertension. Some fall in the systolic blood pressure is fairly common in older persons, particularly in those with chronic disease or those on medication.[15] In one study of orthostatic blood pressure, after 1 minute of quiet standing, 24% of 494 persons over the age of 65 years sustained a fall of 20 mm Hg or more in systolic blood pressure. Five percent had decreases of 40 mm Hg or more.[16] When older patients without risk factors for postural hypotension (such as chronic disease or medication use) were tested, only 8 of 125 persons (6.4%) had a 20 mm Hg or greater fall in systolic blood pressure on standing.[17]

The fall in blood pressure on standing can be exaggerated if the blood volume is low or if the reflex orthostatic mechanisms are impaired because of age or medication. Even mild volume depletion secondary to diuretics can result in marked postural hypotension in older adults, although no such change occurs in younger subjects.[18]

The balloon of the blood pressure cuff should encircle about two thirds of the arm's circumference. If the person is obese, a wide cuff is used because a smaller cuff may overestimate the blood pressure. Palpation of the cuff pressure at which the radial pulse disappears is a way to check the accuracy of the auscultated systolic blood pressure.

The Korotkoff sounds are listened for with the bell of the stethoscope pressed lightly over the brachial artery. The pressure at which the sounds are first heard is the systolic pressure. The sounds may become muffled before they disappear, but the point at which the sounds are no longer heard is the diastolic pressure. Occasionally, an auscultatory gap is found, in which the sounds disappear only to reappear again at a lower pressure. If the auscultatory gap is not recognized, the diastolic pressure may be erroneously recorded as higher than its true value, or the systolic pressure may be erroneously recorded as lower than its true value. Cuffs should be inflated to at least 200 mm Hg, and the examiner should continue to listen until a pressure of 50 is reached to avoid this error.

Atherosclerosis may result in misleading blood pressure readings. The blood pressure reading may vary from one arm to the other because atherosclerosis involvement may be slightly asymmetrical. Stiff peripheral arteries may result in spuriously high readings. William Osler used a simple maneuver to detect its presence. Osler's maneuver is performed by inflating the blood pressure cuff above systolic pressure and then palpating the radial or brachial artery. If the pulseless artery is palpable, the true intra-arterial blood pressure reading may be lower than the blood pressure obtained by auscultation. Persons whose arteries remained palpable (Osler positive) when the cuff was inflated above systolic pressure had a blood pressure reading taken by auscultatory methods that was 20% higher than the intra-arterial measured pressure.[19] Some subjects had a diastolic cuff reading of 120 or 100 mm Hg while a simultaneous intra-arterial pressure was 80 mm Hg. Such persons with pseudohypertension might be erroneously diagnosed as hypertensive. Perhaps older hypertensive persons are particularly susceptible to the adverse effects of antihypertensive drugs because this overestimation and overtreatment of blood pressure occur.[19]

Antihypertensive drugs can sometimes be withdrawn from older adults without the return of hypertension. For example, of 169 patients withdrawn from therapy in one study, 51 patients had blood pressure increases immediately, and medication was reinstituted. Of the 118 remaining patients, 43 (25% of the original group) were still normotensive 1 year later, 16 required treatment for hypertension, 34 were treated with diuretics for congestive heart failure or angina pectoris, and 12 were lost to follow-up.[20] This evidence should not deter appropriate treatment of hypertension in older adults. Studies of older subjects have demonstrated reduction in cardiovascular mortality and stroke with treatment.[21-24]

Isolated systolic hypertension is defined as a blood pressure of greater than 160 mm Hg systolic, whereas the diastolic blood pressure remains less than 90 mm Hg. Isolated systolic hypertension is quite common and is estimated to be present in 20% of persons over the age of 80 years and in about 13% of those aged 70 to 79 years.[25] Isolated systolic hypertension will not be found in up to one third of cases when the blood pressure measurement is repeated.[26] Although believed by many in the past to represent a normal phenomenon in older adults, sustained isolated systolic hypertension is associated with an increased risk of stroke and cardiovascular risk, even in the older population.[27-31] Reduction of the cardiovascular risk may not be the only benefit of hypertension control. When the systolic blood pressure was controlled so that the measurement fell between a window of 135 to 150 mm Hg, cognitive improvement was noted in persons with vascular dementia.[32]

Low blood pressure may be associated with some additional risk in older people,[30] namely, exposing the older person to falling hazard and injury. The condition may be only evident if the person is examined for orthostatic changes in blood pressure. Low blood pressure should prompt a search for a remedial condition such as overmedication, heart failure, or Addison's disease.[33]

## Respirations

After assessment of the pulse and blood pressure, the respirations are observed and counted to assess their rate and depth. Observe for use of accessory muscles of respiration and for retraction in the supraclavicular fossae. During the history taking, does the person have to interrupt speaking to catch his or her breath? The usual rate in adults is about 12 to 18 breaths per minute.

## Temperature

Older adults are less able to maintain normal body temperature when stressed by heat or cold. Also, older adults frequently do not have a normal febrile response to infections. Pneumonia may present without fever, for example, as was observed by Osler, who remarked, "In old age, pneumonia may be latent, coming on without chill." Indeed, older persons are prone to hypothermia even from mildly cool ambient temperatures. Body temperatures of less than 95°F may not be readable on some thermometers, and those caring for older adults ideally use special thermometers that register the lower temperatures. Medications that interfere with the thermoregulatory mechanism, such as tranquilizers, antihypertensives, vasodilators, and antidepressants, as well as ingestion of alcohol, put the older person, who may already have numerous predisposing chronic conditions, at increased risk for hypothermia.

## Height, Weight, and Nutrition

Older persons are at increased risk of malnutrition because of inappropriate food intake, social isolation, disability, and chronic medical conditions and medications.[34] Good nutritional status underlies adequate functioning and a sense of well-being. Height and weight are initial elements of the nutritional assessment. Four components of the nutritional assessment can be remembered as ABCD: A for anthropometric measurement such as height and weight, B for biochemical parameters such as serum albumin and the hemoglobin, C for clinical assessment (medical history, physical examination, and other domains discussed in this book), and D for dietary history, such as the content and adequacy of the diet and the use of nutritional supplements.

Although measurement of weight is standard for every patient encounter, measuring the height is not. Measurement of height is necessary to interpret the person's weight. Height may be estimated using landmark measurements on arms and legs.[35] Serial height measurements may be useful. Recording serial height measurements in an aging woman who has a vertebral compression fracture due to osteoporosis may reveal loss of height and kyphosis from other asymptomatic fractures or bone loss. Therapy might then become more aggressive to prevent further bone loss (e.g., hormonal therapy). Serial height measurements may also increase the person's awareness of osteoporosis and improve compliance with regimens of calcium, vitamin D, and, if prescribed, hormonal replacement.

The body mass index (BMI) can be calculated to improve interpretation of the height and weight. To calculate BMI, divide the weight of the person in kilograms by the square of the height in meters. Because 1 kg is equivalent to 2.2 lb, the person's weight in pounds must be divided by 2.2 to convert the weight to kilograms. Similarly, because 1 m equals 39.4 in, the person's height in inches must be divided by 39.4 to convert the height to meters. For example, a 72-year-old woman weighs 154 lb and is 5 ft 6 in (66 in). Her weight is 70 kg (154/2.2), and her height is 1.68 m (66/39.4). Her BMI is then calculated as 70/(1.68 × 1.68) = 24.8. Clinical Guidelines of the National Heart, Lung, and Blood Institute in cooperation with the National Institute of Diabetes and Digestive and Kidney Diseases, working with many other professional organizations, defined overweight as a BMI between 25 to 29.9 and obesity as 30 and higher.[36]

Biochemical parameters that are useful for assessing nutritional status include the hemoglobin count, serum albumin, and serum cholesterol level. A reduced serum albumin (lower than 4 g/dL) may be a significant indicator of malnutrition. Clinical assessment of nutrition includes notation of changes in weight. Change in weight is an important parameter to follow in hospitalized or institutionalized patients who may be at increased risk of malnutrition.[37] Loss of subcutaneous fat, muscle wasting, and edema on physical examination may signal chronic malnourishment.[38]

The last component of the nutritional assessment is signified by a "D," the dietary history.[34,36] How does the person obtain and prepare meals? Does the daily diet contain appropriate proportions of food from the Food Guide Pyramid's five food groups: bread, cereal, rice, and pasta (6 to 11 servings); vegetables (3 to 5 servings); fruit (2 to 4 servings); milk, yogurt, and cheese (2 to 3 servings); and meat, poultry, fish, dried beans, eggs, and nuts (2 to 3 servings); fats, oils, and sweets (sparingly)? Does the person take any nutritional supplements, such as multivitamins? Does he or she take any medication that affects appetite or nutrients? Does he or she have a special diet, such as a diabetic diet, or does the person's diet contain an unusual amount of alcohol, sweets, or fried foods? Consider the ABCD components when assessing nutritional status.

## Skin

Assessment of the skin should occur as other areas are examined, and the patient is disrobed. Changes in skin condition are generally believed to constitute the quintessential mark of aging itself. Older adults generally have less subcutaneous fat, and consequently, the skin is thinner, especially on the dorsa of the hands and on the forearms. Elasticity is lost, and the skin turgor is routinely diminished, even in patients who are adequately hydrated. Wrinkling and creasing occur, resulting in "crow's feet" at the corners of the eyes and lines on the forehead. Because older adults often have decreased sweat and sebaceous gland production, dry skin is a common finding. The tendency toward dryness can be exaggerated by disease (hypothyroidism) or medication (such as antidepressants with significant anticholinergic effects). Dry skin contributes to conditions such as nummular eczema and "winter itch."

The normal skin changes that occur in aging include the development of hyperpigmented macular lesions called senile freckles or lentigines, sometimes called age or liver spots. Cherry hemangiomas, small red or violet growths, are most often seen on the trunk or extremities and are very common. Skin tags are fleshy soft growths, typically with a pedicle, and are frequently ignored unless injured by clothing or jewelry.

*Seborrheic keratoses* are pigmented lesions with a waxy or greasy surface that have a stuck-on appearance and generally occur on the trunk and face. Seborrheic keratoses may become secondarily infected. Early lesions could resemble melanoma or other conditions.

*Solar lentigo* is a brown, flat lesion that is believed to be related to chronic exposure to sunlight. Solar lentigo is to be distinguished from *lentigo maligna,* which is an insidious flat lesion with irregular borders and a distinct variegated color that may include flecks of black. It is believed to represent melanoma in situ; raised areas may represent invasion into the dermis. Doubt about the nature of any lesion should be resolved by biopsy or excision.

*Actinic keratoses* occur on sun-exposed areas of the skin. The lesions are usually multiple and scaly, enlarging slowly over many years. Some can develop into squamous cell carcinoma, and a sudden spurt of growth in a senile keratosis should raise that possibility. A cutaneous horn is a very proliferative hyperkeratotic form of senile keratosis in which the hyperkeratosis resembles a horn. Such lesions can become quite large.

*Basal cell carcinoma* is the most common cancer of the skin. Fortunately, basal cell carcinomas only rarely metastasize. Over 90% occur on the head and neck and may take the form of an ulcer or a nodule. A characteristic feature of the ulcerative type is a firm, rolled border. One 65-year-old woman had such a lesion behind her ear for 6 months that she ascribed to irritation from her glasses. *Squamous cell carinoma* has the potential for metastasis, and sometimes regional lymphadenopathy is found. Typically, these lesions arise on sun-exposed areas, especially the face, and are hard and fixed. The lesion eventually becomes erythematous and scaling, initially resembling an actinic keratosis. Unchecked, however, squamous cell carcinoma and basal cell carcinoma, although eminently treatable, may be devastating and curative excision may be disfiguring. Early diagnosis and treatment are essential.

*Nummular eczema* is generally seen in the winter and is characterized by coin-shaped areas, resembling ringworm, on the arms and legs that may become secondarily infected. The lesions are intensely pruritic and chronic. The etiology of nummular eczema is unknown, but the low indoor humidity of winter dries the skin and intensifies the itch.

*Seborrheic dermatitis* also affects older adults. Seborrhea symmetrically involves the scalp, face, and body folds with scaly indistinct macules and papules. These lesions are often greasy and sometimes pruritic. Seborrheic dermatitis is particularly common in persons with Parkinson's disease. Psoriasis affects all age groups. The characteristic lesions in psoriasis are the scaly patches that typically involve the scalp, elbows, and knees. Psoriasis may also cause pitting of the nails and may be associated with arthritis.

*Herpes zoster* causes a painful eruption in the distribution of a peripheral nerve. After a primary infection that causes chickenpox, the virus remains dormant, possibly for decades, until it erupts as shingles. The pain may precede the rash, causing confusion with other conditions. The classic rash of grouped vesicles on an erythematous base in a dermatomal distribution is diagnostic. Herpes zoster involving the first branch of the trigeminal nerve can involve the eye, resulting in corneal scarring. A clue that this is occurring is the presence of vesicles at the tip of the nose. Unfortunately, pain often persists in the involved area even after the lesions have resolved.

Clues to physical abuse of an older adult may come from the examination of the skin. Bruises and welts on the chest, shoulders, back, arms, or legs, perhaps in various stages of healing, can be found in such cases. Unusual patterns, such as bruises that are clustered, might reflect the use of an instrument or a hand or even biting. Lacerations and abrasions on the lips, eyes, or parts of the face may be associated with infection. Hemorrhages beneath the scalp may have resulted from hair pulling. Of course, frail older persons will be more prone to injuries from falls as well, making detection of real abuse more difficult. In addition, many older persons also bruise easily due to capillary fragility or poor nutrition. In any case, the possibility that such abuse is occurring should be considered when the pattern of injury does not fit the history obtained.[39-42]

## Decubitus Ulcers

Impaired mobility puts the older adult at risk for the development of decubitus ulcers, or pressure sores. Other risk factors include malnutrition, dehydration, anemia, cardiovascular disease, edema, and urinary or fecal incontinence.[43] A pressure ulcer can develop over a short period of time (e.g., as a result of several hours of surgery). Constant vigilance is required to prevent the development of pressure ulcers in institutionalized or hospitalized older adults.[44] Recurrent or extensive decubiti in older adults might signal abuse or neglect. Patients with decreased mobility, especially older patients admitted to the hospital or nursing home, should be evaluated for risk of decubiti using a standard assessment tool such as that shown in Exhibit 12–2.[45] Once present, treatment should be based on stage of ulceration, and measures to prevent further development of pressure sores should be instituted.[43] Removing pressure from the involved area is essential. Adequate nutrition and vitamin supplements, along with excellent wound care, are also required.

## Hair and Nails

Among the most notable indicators of age are changes in the color and distribution of hair. Hair color becomes gray or whitened. Progressive thinning of all body hair, including hair of the axillae and pubis, occurs with age. The growth of facial hair in older women can sometimes be quite distressing, but measures to reduce the problem, such as depilatory agents, can be recommended. A lack of hair on the lower extremities may indicate diminished peripheral circulation but is often a normal finding in older adults. The nails are frequently afflicted by onychomycosis, a chronic fungal condition of the nail. The thickened, brittle, and crumbling nail is difficult to treat and is a common problem for neglected persons living alone.

## Head

The patient is examined in the sitting position starting with the head and working down. The head and skull should be examined for evidence of trauma, especially in cases of delirium or sudden changes in level of consciousness. Besides palpation for tenderness and deformity of the skull, the temporal artery is examined for tenderness. Changes in the skull that are characteristic of Paget's disease should be sought, such as frontal bossing or an increase in hat size. Temporal arteritis (or giant cell arteritis) is a condition in which the temporal arteries become tender and may lose their pulsations. This disorder may present as a headache that is unilateral and classically temporal. There may be dimness of vision. Temporal arteritis is an important condition to recognize because if untreated it can lead to blindness. Fever and elevated white blood cell count may occur. The sedimentation rate is markedly increased in advanced cases. Symmetrical pain and weakness of shoulders and hips can accompany temporal arteritis (polymyalgia rheumatica).

**Exhibit 12-2** Braden Scale for Predicting Risk of Pressure Ulcers

Patient's Name _____   Evaluator's Name _____   Date of Assessment _____

| | | | | |
| --- | --- | --- | --- | --- |
| | | | | |
| | | | | |
| | | | | |
| | | | | |

|  | | | | |
| --- | --- | --- | --- | --- |
| **Sensory perception**<br>Ability to respond meaningfully to pressure-related discomfort | 1. *Completely limited:*<br>a. Unresponsive (does not moan, flinch, or gasp) to painful stimuli, due to diminished level of consciousness or sedation,<br>OR<br>b. Limited ability to feel pain over most of body surface. | 2. *Very limited:*<br>a. Responds only to painful stimuli. Cannot communicate discomfort except by moaning or restlessness,<br>OR<br>b. Has a sensory impairment that limits the ability to feel pain or discomfort over ½ of body. | 3. *Slightly limited:*<br>a. Responds to verbal commands but cannot always communicate discomfort or need to be turned,<br>OR<br>b. Has some sensory impairment that limits ability to feel pain or discomfort in 1 or 2 extremities. | 4. *No impairment:*<br>Responds to verbal commands. Has no sensory deficit that would limit ability to feel or voice pain or discomfort. |
| **Moisture**<br>Degree to which skin is exposed to moisture | 1. *Constantly moist:*<br>Skin is kept moist almost constantly by perspiration, urine, etc. Dampness is detected every time patient is moved or turned. | 2. *Moist:*<br>Skin is often but not always moist. Linen must be changed at least once a shift. | 3. *Occasionally moist:*<br>Skin is occasionally moist, requiring an extra linen change approximately once a day. | 4. *Rarely moist:*<br>Skin is usually dry; linen requires changing only at routine intervals. |
| **Activity**<br>Degree of physical activity | 1. *Bedfast:*<br>Confined to bed. | 2. *Chairfast:*<br>Ability to walk severely limited or nonexistent. Cannot bear own weight and/or must be assisted into chair or wheelchair. | 3. *Walks occasionally:*<br>Walks occasionally during day but for very short distances, with or without assistance. Spends majority of each shift in bed or chair. | 4. *Walks frequently:*<br>Walks outside the room at least twice a day and inside room at least once every 2 hours during waking hours. |

| | 1 | 2 | 3 | 4 |
|---|---|---|---|---|
| *Mobility* Ability to change and control body position | 1. *Completely immobile:* Does not make even slight changes in body or extremity position without assistance. | 2. *Very limited:* Makes occasional slight changes in body or extremity position but unable to make frequent or significant changes independently. | 3. *Slightly limited:* Makes frequent though slight changes in body or extremity position independently. | 4. *No limitations:* Makes major and frequent changes in position without assistance. |
| *Nutrition* Usual food intake pattern | 1. *Very poor:* a. Never eats a complete meal. Rarely eats more than ⅓ of any food offered. Eats 2 servings or less of protein (meat or dairy products) per day. Takes fluids poorly. Does not take a liquid dietary supplement, OR b. Is NPO[1] and/or maintained on clear liquids or IV[2] for more than 5 days. | 2. *Probably inadequate:* a. Rarely eats a complete meal and generally eats only ½ of any food offered. Protein intake includes only 3 servings of meat or dairy products per day. Occasionally will take a dietary supplement, OR b. Receives less than optimum amount of liquid or tube feeding. | 3. *Adequate:* a. Eats over ½ of most meals. Eats a total of 4 servings of protein (meat, dairy products) each day. Occasionally will refuse a meal, but will usually take a supplement if offered, OR b. Is on a tube feeding or TPN[3] regimen, which probably meets most nutritional requirements. | 4. *Excellent:* Eats most of every meal. Never refuses a meal. Usually eats a total of 4 or more servings of meat and dairy products. Occasionally eats between meals. Does not require supplementation. |
| *Friction and shear* | 1. *Problem:* Requires moderate to maximum assistance in moving. Complete lifting without sliding against sheets is impossible. Frequently slides down in bed or chair, requiring frequent repositioning with maximum assistance. Spasticity, contractures, or agitation lead to almost constant friction. | 2. *Potential problem:* Moves feebly or requires minimum assistance. During a move, skin probably slides to some extent against sheets, chair, restraints, or other devices. Maintains relatively good position in chair or bed most of the time but occasionally slides down. | 3. *No apparent problem:* Moves in bed and in chair independently and has sufficient muscle strength to lift up completely during move. Maintains good position in bed or chair at all times. | |

Total score

[1]NPO: Nothing by mouth.   [2]IV: Intravenously.   [3]TPN: Total parenteral nutrition.
*Source:* Courtesy of Barbara Braden and Nancy Bergstrom. Copyright © 1988. Reprinted with permission.

## Eyes

After the cranium is assessed, the eyes are examined. Age-related changes in the eyes include darkening of the skin around the orbits, crow's feet, slower pupillary light reflex (which still, however, ought to be equal bilaterally), decreased tearing, and decreased adaptation to the dark. The older person, perhaps because of diminished pupil size and increased thickness and opacity of the lens, needs more illumination to compensate than someone younger.

The structures surrounding the eye itself are inspected first. Xanthomas are fat deposits sometimes seen in the skin near the eyes and may be associated with elevated levels of blood lipids. Loss of the lateral third of the eyebrows, although a classic sign of hypothyroidism, may be a normal finding in some older persons. On each eyelid, the examiner will find a central, relatively rigid tarsal plate that, in advancing age, may become lax, leading to ectropion (eversion of the lids), thereby exposing the eyes to drying and infection. The margin of the lid may roll backward toward the eye as well so that eyelashes brush against the cornea, causing entropion.

The sclera is normally white but is uniformly yellow in patients with jaundice. In older persons, the periphery of the sclera may be yellow because of deposits of fat showing through thinned scleral membranes. Pingueculae are thin fatty structures that usually lie laterally on the eyeball. They may increase in size with advancing age but are benign and generally cause no problem with vision. The conjunctiva, or lining of the eye, can become inflamed or infected. This is a common eye problem in older adults, particularly because they are prone to having dry eyes. Such drying may predispose them to infection of the conjunctiva by bacterial or viral agents. Conjunctivitis is associated with a red eye and purulent discharge, but discomfort is minimal. A painful red eye may signal iritis, glaucoma, or an abrasion.

Arcus senilis is a striking finding in some older persons. Initially a thin line that is limited to the upper portion of the eye, it becomes thicker and denser and completely encircles the cornea. Although arcus is found with other stigmata in persons with familial hypercholesterolemia, many persons with arcus will have normal cholesterol levels. Arcus senilis is a very common finding in persons 65 years old and older.

The lens of the eye produces new fibers throughout life, but none is lost. These accumulate in the center of the lens, increasing its density and contributing to the development of senile cataracts that are generally bilateral. The lens loses its elasticity with advanced age so that the eye is more farsighted (presbyopia). Before ophthalmoscopy, the person's visual acuity is checked for reading and distance, with and without glasses. The pupils may react more sluggishly to light but should be equal in size. Many disorders may cause asymmetry of the pupils, including central nervous system lesions and diabetes; drugs can have this effect as well. After iridectomy, the pupil is irregular. The extraocular muscles are checked for full range of motion: up and down, left and right.

Ophthalmoscopic examination of each eye should begin by focusing on the most anterior structures first and then working back to the retina. A cataract may be best visualized by focusing on the lens with an ophthalmoscope. A cataract appears as an opaque or a black area against the orange reflection from the retina. The precise significance of the cataract depends on how much it interferes with the person's vision, function, and work.

Increased lens opacity with advancing age allows less light to pass to the retina than at younger ages. The 60-year-old retina receives only a fraction of the amount of light as the 20-year-old retina. Improved lighting may be all that is required to allow an older person to read small print, such as that in a telephone directory or the newspaper. Provision of excellent lighting in waiting and examination rooms is essential.

Examination of the retina with the ophthalmoscope requires some practice. The normal fundus reveals the optic disc, the macula, and arteries and veins. Pigment in the retina usually corresponds to skin pigmentation. The normal optic disc is frequently outlined by pigment. In older adults with hypertension or arteriosclerosis and sometimes in normal older adults, so-called copper-wire changes caused by thickening of the arteriolar walls may be seen. As the vessel walls become more thickened, the vessels appear white or silver. Nicking, or narrowing, of venules by crossing arterioles becomes evident as the process continues. Exudates, hemorrhages, and cotton-wool spots may also be seen on the retina as a result of hypertension or diabetes.

Macular degeneration is a major cause of visual disability in older persons. The macula, the region of the retina with the sharpest acuity, is affected. Visual acuity is decreased, but peripheral vision is preserved. Special studies by an ophthalmologist may be required to make the diagnosis of senile macular degeneration.

In glaucoma, the intraocular pressure is elevated, and there is contraction of the visual field. On ophthalmoscopic examination, the optic cup, which is a depression in the optic nerve as it emerges on the retina, is accentuated. The visual field of the person with Alzheimer's disease is contracted when compared with that of persons who were demented from other causes. This may significantly alter the demented person's perception of the environment.[46]

## Ears

After the practitioner examines the eyes, the otoscope is used to examine the ears. Painless nodules on the pinnae of the ears could be basal cell carcinomas, rheumatoid nodules, or even gouty tophi. Common changes seen with age include increased ear lobe length, hair growth in the canal, and accumulation of cerumen. Loss of hearing that is due to problems with the external ear includes impacted cerumen, external otitis, or a foreign body. External otitis can be due to allergic reactions or irritation due to hearing aids. Malignant otitis externa is a *Pseudomonas* infection that involves the ear canal and presents as granulation tissue at the juncture of bone and cartilage.

The normal tympanic membrane is gray or pink with a light reflex produced by its cone shape. The malleus, which is the first of the three small bones in the inner ear, can be seen indenting the membrane, pointing posteriorly. The tympanic membrane may be thickened in the older person (tympanosclerosis), possibly as a result of scarring from prior infections. Effusions occur in relationship to eustachian tube dysfunction, as in allergy or upper respiratory tract infection.

Hearing is assessed during the history-taking session but can be grossly gauged by such techniques as whispering words in the person's ear. Hearing loss may, for the sake of simplicity, be divided into conductive loss and sensorineural loss. Conductive hearing loss implies interference in the conduct of sound energy into the inner ear. It can be due to foreign bodies, cerumen, abnormalities of the tympanic membrane, otitis media or externa, or involvement of the ossicles with Paget's disease, rheumatoid arthritis, or otosclerosis (in which the stapes becomes fixed to the oval window of the cochlea).[47] Cerumen in the canal may be the primary or a contributing cause of hearing loss that is easily remedied.

Sensorineural hearing loss means disease anywhere from the organ of Corti to the brain. The cells within the organ of Corti are not replaced; thus, there is a gradual loss as the person ages. The result is high-tone hearing loss because it is hair cells in the basal turn of the organ of Corti, those sensitive to high tone, that are lost. Presbycusis is sensorineural hearing loss caused by aging of the inner ear.[47] Often both conductive and sensorineural hearing losses are present simultaneously, and the precise nature of the defect requires sophisticated audiometric testing. The ability to hear high-frequency sounds is affected first so that certain consonants and sibilants become unintelligible (e.g., f, s, th, ch, and sh). Understanding speech depends in large measure on the clear perception of these high-frequency consonants rather than low-frequency vowel sounds. Sensorineural hearing loss can be due to toxic damage to the hair cells of the organ of Corti from aspirin, aminoglycoside antibiotics, or diuretics; from trauma; and from a wide variety of disorders from vascular insufficiency (the inner ear is dependent on a single end artery for its blood supply) to central nervous system disease.

The combination of hearing loss and cognitive impairment can lead to social isolation and paranoia and may make mental status testing a real challenge. Three simple clinical tests using a tuning fork may help sort out the type of hearing loss. These are the Rinne test, Weber's test, and Schwabach's test. To perform the Rinne test, the tuning fork is struck and applied to the mastoid prominence behind the ear. When the person indicates that he or she no longer hears the sound, the vibrating fork is immediately put near the external canal. Normally, the sound is then heard and the test is said to be positive. Put another way, air conduction is better than bone conduction. A negative test, one in which the person does not hear the tuning fork in air, suggests that there is a conduction loss in that ear. Whether there is a conductive hearing loss in one ear can then be confirmed by *Weber's test*. A vibrating tuning fork is placed on the vertex of the head and the patient is asked whether the sound is heard better in one ear than the other. Normally, the sound appears to come from above, that is, in the middle. If a conductive defect is present in one ear, the sound is heard best in that ear (bone conduction makes up for the defect). On the other hand, if deafness in an ear is due to neural problems, that ear will not sense any sound, and sound will only be heard in the contralateral or good ear.

*Schwabach's test* confirms a diagnosis of sensorineural deafness by comparing the person's hearing with the examiner's. The vibrating tuning fork is put on the person's mastoid process. When the sound is no longer heard by the patient, the fork is put on the examiner's mastoid. If the sound is heard by the examiner, then a sensorineural deficit in the person is confirmed.

## Nose

The otoscope can be used to examine the nasal mucosa and the internal nasal architecture. Nasal patency should be tested by occluding one nostril. Nasal congestion due to vasomotor rhinitis, characterized by postnasal drip, little sneezing, and no eosinophils on nasal smear, can be particularly disturbing and interfere with sleep.

Rhinophyma of the nose starts as a diffuse redness, followed by papules, pustules, and later, dilated venules. Excess ingestion of alcohol may be associated. The paranasal sinuses may be palpated for tenderness. Any chronic drainage from the nose that does not respond to therapy should be investigated because chronic drainage can be a symptom of cancer in the sinuses.

The sense of smell decreases with age, and the decrease in smell is often experienced as a loss of taste. The loss of the sense of smell can be significant for nutrition and safety. Many older persons cannot enjoy the pleasant smell of food cooking—smells that stimulate the appetite and make eating enjoyable. The inability to smell leaking natural gas creates a risk of serious accident. With age, the anterior taste buds, which are sensitive to sweet and salt, deteriorate before the posterior taste buds, which are sensitive to bitter and sour; thus, older adult patients frequently complain that food tastes bitter or sour. When cooking, older people may add undesirable amounts of salt to food to compensate for the loss of taste. Progressive loss of the senses of smell and taste means that, for older persons, the appearance of consistency of food plays a proportionately greater role in food's appeal.

## Mouth

Cheilosis, or fissures at the angles of the mouth, may be a sign of poor nutrition and vitamin deficiency. Carcinomatous lesions may occur on the lips, which are highly exposed to sunlight. The oral mucosa may be dry because of diminished sputum production or due to drugs the individual is taking, particularly those with anticholinergic side effects. The oral mucosa should be carefully inspected for lesions by using the tongue blade to move the buccal mucosa away from the teeth. Leukoplakia is a white patch or plaque on any of the mucous membranes of the mouth that may appear to be painted on the surface. These patches may be present for years and represent a premalignant condition. Such lesions should be biopsied for definitive diagnosis. Other lesions with a similar appearance are Candida (thrush) and lichen planus. Traumatic injury, in particular from ill-fitting dentures, may damage the oral mucosa, producing erythematous tissue changes. In addition to inspection, a moistened glove may be used to palpate the buccal cavity, including the lips and floor of the mouth, for areas of induration. Palpation is particularly important to evaluate complaints related to the oral region, to assess suspicious areas, or to evaluate persons at risk of oral cancer (e.g., those with a history of tobacco or alcohol use).

A lesion of the hard palate with no particular clinical significance except that it be recognized as benign is the torus palatinus. It must be reiterated, however, that any masses not in the midline are suspect as neoplasms. A slowly growing asymptomatic lesion with a rough surface, irregular margin, and firm consistency should be biopsied, no matter how long it has been there.

The examination of the tongue should not be neglected. A sore, red inflamed tongue may be found in persons with vitamin B12 or iron deficiency. Hairy or black tongue is a condition in which it looks as if the tongue is growing short hairs. It is symptomless and appears during treatment with antibiotics that inhibit normal bacteria and permit fungal overgrowth. The tongue may also be observed for fasciculations, which indicate lower motor neuron disease, and for abnormal movements such as tardive dyskinesia.

**Teeth**

Tooth loss and periodontal disease are extremely common in older persons. As many as half of all persons over the age of 65 years are edentulous. Older persons are likely to see their physician more frequently than their dentist.[48,49] For this reason, it is particularly important to remove the dentures and inspect the mouth surfaces for areas of irritation and for suspicious lesions. The upper and lower lips are examined, including hidden surfaces. Poorly fitting dentures can have far-reaching consequences, such as malnutrition, and result in numerous problems, such as traumatic ulcers, denture stomatitis, and possibly even cancer.

Any dental malocclusion, as well as abnormal speech sounds, such as slurred "s," clicks, or whistles, which signal improperly fitting dentures, should be recognized. The person may fail to realize that a misfitting of dentures has developed. Older adults should be encouraged to visit the dentist every year or two so that dentures can be adjusted to account for changing mandibular bone structure.

Older persons who retain teeth need to have their oral hygiene assessed. Dental caries may appear as soft white, yellow, or brown areas on the tooth. The person may complain of sensitivity to extremes of temperature. Periodontal disease, a major cause of tooth loss, involves inflammation and destruction of the supporting structures of the teeth.[49] Foul breath odor is common with dental infections, retention of food particles in the teeth or dentures, or chronic periodontal disease. It can also result from sinusitis or pulmonary infection.

## Neck

The neck presents several important structures for examination: the lymph nodes, the trachea, the thyroid gland, the carotid arteries, and jugular veins. The posterior and anterior cervical lymph node chains as well as the supraclavicular area should be carefully palpated. Virchow's node, enlargement of the lymph node in the left supraclavicular fossa, is a classic sign of metastatic gastrointestinal carcinoma. The trachea should be checked for lateral deviation and a search made for jugular venous distention, which could be a sign of heart failure. Prominent pulsations above the clavicle may represent kinking of a carotid artery or prominence of the innominate artery.

The carotids should be gently palpated. The pulses should be symmetrical. A bounding or collapsing pulse, in which the upstroke of the pulse wave is very sharp and the downstroke falls rapidly, may be present in a person with essential hypertension, thyrotoxicosis, aortic regurgitation, or an extreme emotional state. The carotids may be auscultated using the bell of the stethoscope, listening for bruits that signify turbulent blood flow (and not necessarily hemodynamically significant narrowing). The presence of bruits may be a clue to atherosclerosis and could be an important finding in an individual with a history of syncope, stroke, or transient ischemic attack. In asymptomatic persons, bruits are probably more indicative of coronary artery disease than of cerebrovascular disease, at least in older men.[50]

Attempt to palpate the thyroid gland for enlargement from both in front and in back of the person, even though the gland is generally not easily palpated. If the gland is enlarged, it must be determined whether the gland is diffusely enlarged (goiter) or exhibits discrete nodularity. Sometimes a bruit may be heard over vascular thyroid lesions, and occasionally a thrill is felt. Thyroid disease in older adults is notorious for subtle presentation. For example, hypothyrodism may manifest solely as depression or mental deterioration. The symptoms of hypothyroidism are easily misinterpreted by the older adult or the physician and include dry skin, constipation, sleepiness, lethargy, cold intolerance, and fatigue. Periodic evaluation of serum thyroid-stimulating hormone levels has been suggested in order to detect impending hypothyroidism.[51,52]

Hyperthyroidism or thyrotoxicosis may present without the signs and symptoms usually found in younger persons, such as exophthalmos, restlessness, hyperactivity, and tachycardia. Atrial fibrillation occurs in half of older hyperthyroid persons, but in only 10% of younger persons, whereas ocular changes are less common in older adults who are hyperthyroid. The term "apathetic thyrotoxicosis" has been used to refer to hyperthyroidism in older persons with nonspecific signs and symptoms. Constipation, weight loss, and anorexia of hyperthyroidism may resemble a gastrointestinal carcinoma. The hyperthyroid state may precipitate heart failure as the presenting illness.

## Heart and Lungs

The heart and lungs may be examined next while the client is still seated. Cardiovascular disease is common in older adults.[53] In older persons, angina pectoris may very well present as dyspnea, palpitations, or syncope on exertion, rather than as pain.[54] Patients presenting with transient ischemic attack, stroke, or an episode of confusion should have myocardial infarction considered in the differential diagnosis. Even when the pain is typical, an older person may ascribe it to other causes so that jaw pain is attributed to arthritis and epigastric pain to hiatal hernia or ulcer.[53] Heart disease may be associated with nonspecific fatigue or weakness.

The palm of the examiner's hand is placed over the apex of the patient's heart to palpate the apex pulsation. Normally the apex pulsation covers an area the size of a half-dollar. If the apex pulsation is not easily palpated, the person may be asked to lean forward or to move into a left lateral decubitus position. Cardiac hypertrophy as a result of hypertension, for example, produces a small vigorous apical beat. Dilated ventricles, as from mitral regurgitation, cause the apex beat to be lateral to the midclavicular line. The heart size generally remains unchanged in healthy older persons.[55]

In auscultating the heart, the examiner should start at the apex using the diaphragm, inch across to the left lower sternal border, and then to the left second intercostal space, then cross to the right and down the right sternal border. The first and second heart sounds are listened to first. Simultaneous palpation of the carotid pulse may help identify which sound is the first heart sound. Because the first heart sound is produced by the closure of the mitral and tricuspid valves, it sounds louder than the second heart sound over the mitral and tricuspid areas (the apex of the heart and the right lower sternal border, respectively).

The sequence of auscultation is repeated to listen for murmurs and for silence in systole and diastole. High-pitched clicks and many murmurs will best be heard using the diaphragm of the stethoscope. Lower-pitched sounds such as gallops and diastolic rumbles arising from the mitral and tricuspid valves will best be heard with the bell of the stethoscope. Diastolic murmurs are always significant and may be caused by mitral stenosis. Aortic or pulmonic regurgitation may also be associated with diastolic murmurs. Mitral stenosis may be silent in older adults. Atrial fibrillation, particularly when accompanied by mitral stenosis or an enlarged left atrium, is a significant risk factor for stroke.

Systolic murmurs are very common in persons over the age of 65 years. Functional flow murmurs from a dilated aortic annulus are short, early systolic murmurs heard at the cardiac base. The second heart sound is normally split, and the carotid upstrokes are normal. The murmur of aortic stenosis is a systolic ejection (diamond-shaped murmur) at the base classically with diminished carotid upstrokes, sustained apical impulse, and a fourth heart sound. These findings may not be present in the older person. Mitral regurgitation in older persons is commonly due to ischemic heart disease and results in a holosystolic murmur.[53] Because systolic murmurs are so common in older adults, distinguishing benign murmurs from significant murmurs in asymptomatic patients can be difficult.

Abnormalities of the heart rhythm may be poorly tolerated by older adults who generally have less reserve capacity than younger persons. Atrial fibrillation, for example, may not be tolerated because early diastolic filling in the older heart is considerably diminished. The contribution of the atrial "kick" to ventricular filling, lost in atrial fibrillation, becomes critical to appropriate cardiac output.

Arrhythmias are apparently quite prevalent in otherwise healthy older persons, with prognosis and significance depending on the presence of overt or unrecognized coronary artery disease.[56–60] In one study of 106 older adults studied with 24-hour electrocardiographic monitoring, one fourth had multifocal premature ventricular contractions, and four had ventricular tachycardia. After 18 months of follow-up, recordings showed no difference among the 13 persons who died compared with the group as a whole.[60] In another study, supraventricular tachycardia was present in 28% of 50 persons over the age of 80 years who were studied with 24-hour ambulatory electrocardiographic monitoring. Every person exhibited supraventricular ectopic beats, and 65% had more than 20 ectopic beats per hour. Premature ventricular contractions were also quite common, occurring in 32% of the persons at a rate of greater than 10 premature beats per hour. In 18% of the persons, the premature contractions were multifocal.[61]

After the cardiac examination, the lungs are examined by auscultation and percussion. Assessment of respiration begins when the person came into the examining room. The rate and depth of breathing, as well as any use of accessory muscles of respiration, were observed. The aged lung has less elasticity because of a loss of elastin and because of collagen crosslinking. While listening over the chest and asking the person to take a few deep breaths, the physician must be alert for signs of hyperventilation, such as dizziness, especially in the older person, to avoid inducing syncope. Normally, only so-called vesicular breath sounds are heard over the chest. Bronchial or tubular breath sounds can be heard over the trachea. If one hears such sounds over the peripheral lung fields, consolidation is suggested.

Rales are sounds produced by the movement of fluid or exudate in the airways. Small amounts of fluid may be detected as posttussive rales. For posttussive rales to be heard, the person must expire fully and cough. When he or she inspires with the next breath, fine crackles can be heard. The cough collapses some wet alveoli, which are then heard opening in inspiration. Moist rales or rhonchi are gurgling sounds arising from larger bronchi. Moist breath sounds at the bases in older adults often do not represent congestive heart failure. Such marginal or atelectatic rales are heard most frequently in aged, debilitated, or bedridden patients or in habitual shallow breathers. These sounds should disappear after the person takes a few deep breaths. Other adventitious sounds heard in the lungs are friction rubs and wheezes.

The lung fields are percussed for areas of dullness or hyperresonance as further maneuvers to detect any abnormality. An underlying consolidation or effusion will yield dullness or flatness on percussion. In chronic obstructive pulmonary disease, the lungs are often hyperresonant (i.e., the pitch on percussion is higher than that over the normal lung). A check is then made for tactile fremitus: after the ulnar surfaces of both the examiner's hands are applied to either side of the person's chest, the patient is asked to speak ("say 99"). Differences in vibration from one side to another may be significant. Consolidation as in pneumonia increases fremitus. Sometimes it is helpful to auscultate the lung fields and simultaneously tap the sternum. Increased transmission of the sound through areas of consolidation is sometimes identified more readily when using this technique rather than simple percussion. The clinician listens over the lung fields and asks the person to say "E." The "E" will frequently sound like "A" over a pleural effusion (egophony).

## Musculoskeletal System

At the time the lungs are auscultated, any kyphosis or scoliosis is noted. Severe kyphosis can interfere with breathing and cardiovascular function. Tenderness over the spinous processes may portend a vertebral fracture. The joints are inspected next, particularly the joints of the hands. Osteoarthritis is common and especially affects the distal interphalangeal joints of the hands as well as the knees. Bony overgrowths at the distal interphalangeal joint are called Heberden's nodes. Limitation of external rotation of the hip can be an early sign of osteoarthritic involvement. Indeed, the range of motion of all the joints should be assessed.

Rheumatoid arthritis in the hands tends to affect the proximal interphalangeal joints. Joint swelling seen in rheumatoid joints is not bone, but rather synovia and soft tissue swelling that can be felt along the dorsal surface of the involved interphalangeal joint. Progression of the disease produces ulnar deviation in the hands at the metacarpophalangeal joints, as well as a tendency for joints to sublux. Morning pain and stiffness may last several hours for the person with rheumatoid arthritis, whereas the person with osteoarthritis is relieved from pain after a short period of limbering up the affected joints.

Clubbing of the fingers may indicate an underlying chronic disorder resulting in hypoxia. A normal nail, when viewed from the side, forms an angle with the skin of the nail bed. Clubbing results when the angle is greater than normal, and the finger has a "rounded" appearance. Clubbing is seen in chronic lung disorders, carcinoma of the lung, and other disorders associated with chronic hypoxia. The feet may be examined for changes in the joints and for clubbing as well. Frequently, the examination of the foot reveals evidence of diabetes, neglect, or peripheral vascular disease. The examination of the lower extremities may be deferred until the abdominal examination when the person will be supine.

## Abdomen

The patient is placed supine so that the abdomen, breasts, peripheral pulses, genitalia, and the rectum may be examined. It is important to make the older person as comfortable as possible for this part of the examination. A pillow can be used or the head of the examining table elevated slightly to support the head and upper back; a perfectly flat position is uncomfortable for some older adults.

Examination of the abdomen begins with inspection, noting any distention or scars from previous surgery. The examiner should listen to the abdomen before proceeding with palpation to avoid inducing peristaltic activity. Partial bowel obstruction produces rushing sounds, and when obstruction is complete, the sounds may become tinkling or very high pitched. Ileus produced by obstruction or from other causes, such as pneumonia or appendicitis, may result in absence of bowel sounds. Abdominal wall rigidity is not as common a sign of peritoneal irritation among the older as among younger persons.

Constipation may produce a mass of feces that can easily be palpated and mistaken for a tumor. Conversely, a silent abdominal mass may be the only sign of a gastrointestinal carcinoma. Tortuosity or aneurysm of the abdominal aorta may be felt as a pulsatile mass in the abdomen. An abdominal aortic aneurysm may have lateral as well as anteroposterior pulsation, which distinguishes it from a mass in front of the aorta, which merely transmits the pulsations to the examining hand. In thin persons, the aortic pulsation may be felt normally and may be quite alarming to the unsuspecting examiner. An abdominal ultrasound is a noninvasive way to evaluate the person for the possibility of an aneurysm. Leaking aneurysm or mesenteric ischemia should be considered in the differential diagnosis of abdominal pain in older adults.

In addition to palpating and percussing the liver to estimate its size, the midlower abdomen is palpated to check for bladder distention. Such a finding may be important in the evaluation of incontinence or as a sign of urinary retention from prostatic hypertrophy. Urinary retention may be the cause of otherwise unexplainable confusion. With the patient still supine, the peripheral pulses in the feet are checked. The femoral arteries may be palpated in the groin and auscultated for bruits. Bruits heard in the femoral arteries are evidence of diffuse artherosclerotic disease. While examining the area of the groin, the physician can check for lymph node swelling. The feet and lower legs can be examined for skin changes and skin breakdown. Diabetics are at increased risk for foot ulcers and infection. Decubiti and heel sores are common, particularly in those persons who are bedfast. The legs are examined for evidence of arterial insufficiency: namely, laterally placed ulcers, loss of the skin appendages, and delayed capillary refill when the toenails are pressed and released. Venous insufficiency may be manifest by pigmented, medially placed ulcers.

## Breasts

Palpation and examination of the breasts should not be neglected. Ideally, this examination is done both while the patient is sitting and again while the patient is supine during the abdominal examination. A search is made for nipple retraction, skin changes, and masses, which because of loss of connective tissue and adipose are often more easily appreciated in the older woman. Retraction of the nipple secondary to age-related changes can be everted with gentle pressure around the nipple. Retraction caused by an underlying growth, however, cannot be everted by such gentle pressure. The nipples are palpated so as to express any discharge present. All four quadrants of both breasts are examined, including the axillary tail, and a careful inspection made for any asymmetry. The skin under large, pendulous breasts is examined for maceration due to perspiration. The male breasts are not exempt from disease and should also be examined.

Gynecomastia (breast enlargement) in an older male can result from a variety of causes, including bronchiogenic carcinoma, thyroid disease, testicular tumors, drugs (such as spironolactone), liver cirrhosis, and other types of cancer.

## Genitourinary System

The genitalia in both men and women may be conveniently examined in conjunction with the rectal examination. This part of the examination may be deferred but never neglected. The male genitalia should be examined for sores, discharge, and testicular masses. The glans of the penis in an uncircumcised man is checked by retracting the foreskin. The prostate is palpated during the rectal examination. The prostate is frequently enlarged in older men but should normally feel soft and nonnodular. The two lobes of the prostate can usually be distinguished by the median furrow between them. Because lobes of the prostate not palpable by the examining finger may enlarge centrally and cause obstruction, a normal-sized gland on physical examination does not rule out urinary obstruction from prostatic enlargement. Do not neglect the evaluation of the prostate in the work-up of back pain.

The female genitalia should at a minimum be inspected for lesions of the skin, although a bimanual and speculum pelvic examination, which is often neglected, is mandatory if urinary incontinence is a problem or if the woman is due for a Papanicolaou smear. Note is made of any cystocele, rectocele, or uterine prolapse that may occur as the pelvic musculature becomes lax with age. After menopause, the estrogen-responsive tissues of the genitalia and the lower urinary tract atrophy. This leads to dryness of the vagina, shrinkage of the vagina and its surrounding structures, altered bacterial resistance, and weakened uterine ligaments. Urinary incontinence and infections may result. Postmenopausal changes in the vagina cause itching, burning, and dyspareunia (painful intercourse), which are symptoms that most older women are reluctant to volunteer spontaneously. The context of the pelvic examination, however, is a natural one in which to broach such subjects in a straightforward and supportive manner. Vaginal atrophy may also be associated with bleeding, but it should be emphasized that all postmenopausal bleeding must be suspect for uterine carcinoma until proved otherwise. Additionally, palpable ovaries are never normal in an older woman.

Rectal examination may be performed after the patient is helped into the lateral decubitus position (alternatively, the patient may be asked to bend over the examination table). The examiner should tell the patient what to expect and when. The anus is inspected for tears, irritation, and external hemorrhoids, and the tone of the anal sphincter, which may diminish with age, is noted. A gloved finger is used to make a sweep of the entire rectum, being sure to take in its entire circumference. The patient is asked to strain, as at stool, to bring down any lesions just outside the reach of the examining finger. A stool sample to test for occult blood is obtained.

Older adults may not want to bring urinary incontinence to the attention of their doctor, preferring instead to make adjustments on their own, such as decreasing fluid intake and using absorbent napkins. In addition to a neurologic examination that includes testing for perineal sensation and sacral reflexes, and a pelvic examination in women and prostate examination in men, examine the abdomen for a grossly distended bladder and look for leaking of urine in the supine and standing position.[62] Fecal incontinence is a serious problem among institutionalized older adults and is a significant risk factor for formation of decubiti.[63] Guidelines for the evaluation and treatment of urinary incontinence provide detailed information on the office assessment.[64]

## SEXUAL HEALTH ASSESSMENT

The sexual health of older adults is an important component of the overall health assessment. Unfortunately, this area may inadvertently be omitted because of stereotypic beliefs regarding aging and sexuality. There is clear evidence that although certain physiologic functions related to sexuality change with aging, healthy sex lives among older adults are the norm. In the 1940s and 1950s, with the groundbreaking work of Kinsey and colleagues,[65,66] we began to understand sexuality in later life. While those early studies documented sexual functioning and capacity in older adults, they also documented changes in sexual capacity with aging. A recent study on sexual activity and satisfaction among 1,216 older adults (mean age 77.3) found that almost 30% engaged in sexual activity in the past month, with 67% noting satisfaction with their sexual activities. That study noted that men were more likely to be sexually active but less apt than women to be satisfied with their sexual activity.[67,68] It is also true, however, that sexual activity is affected by declining health and selected medications. Libido and sexual response are inhibited when individuals are ill or on medications that may blunt sexual arousal response. In conducting a sexual health history, it is important to review systematically the individual's regular patterns of sex, expectations related to sex, and any changes in capacity or enjoyment, as well as to elicit the client's goals for a healthy sex life. Once the clinician understands these goals, he or she can recommend appropriate treatment and/or actions such as counseling, adjunct therapy, or physical aides to increase sexual capacity.[69]

It is key that the clinician understand that sexuality in late life is a normal and positive experience of aging. Clinicians need to assess their own level of comfort in eliciting a sexual history from the older adult, in that any discomfort on their part is likely to inhibit the older adult's ability to discuss his or her sexual life frankly. Key components of a sexual history should include an understanding of what the older adult's normal sexual patterns and interests have been over the course of his or her life and whether any changes have transpired that now affect sexual capacity and performance. Biologic factors, illness, and medication (Table 12–1) should all be reviewed. Medications are often contributors to sexual dysfunction. (In fact, individuals over age 65 years take 25% of all prescription drugs and account for over half of all adverse drug reactions.)[70] Certain biologic factors that affect sexual interests and behaviors relate to normal aging. For men, the duration and intensity of sexual response changes with aging. Older men may

**Table 12–1** Drugs That Can Diminish Sexual Function in Women

| *Type of Agent* | *Example* |
| --- | --- |
| Hypnotic agents | Alcohol, barbiturates |
| Tranquilizers | Chlordiazepoxide, diazepam |
| Narcotics | Heroin, methadone |
| Antipsychotic agents | Phenothiazines, butyrophenones |
| Antidepressants | Tricyclic agents, monoamine oxidase inhibitors |
| Stimulants | Cocaine, amphetamines |
| Anorectic agents | Fenfluramine |
| Hallucinogens | THC, LSD, PCP, mescaline |
| Hormones | Progestins, oral contraceptives |
| Antihypertensive agents | Reserpine, propranolol, methyldopa |
| Anticholinergic agents | Propantheline bromide |
| Diuretics | Acetazolamide |

*Note:* THC, tetrahydrocannabinol; LSD, lysergic acid diethylamide; and PCP, phenylcyclohexylpiperidine

*Source:* Reprinted with permission from AE Reading and JR Bragonier, Human Sexuality and Sexual Assault. In NF Hacker and JG Moore, Eds., *Essentials of Obstetrics and Gynecology*, 3rd ed. pp. 534–536, W.B. Saunders Company.

take longer to achieve an excitement phase and experience a shortened, less forceful orgasm phase (Exhibit 12–3). Their resolution phase is more rapid with an increased refractory period between erections. In older women, the time needed to experience a sexual cycle (excitement, orgasm, and resolution) is increased with decreased vaginal expansion and lubrication. In some cases, uterine atrophy can cause painful intercourse.[69] Sexual desire is thought to be controlled by a dopamine-sensitive excitatory center along with serotonin-sensitive inhibitory centers.[71] True sexual dysfunction is described as the absence of one or more phases of the sexual response cycle: desire, excitement, orgasm, and/or resolution. Clinically, dysfunction could be further subdivided into (1) primary sexual dysfunction, which is defined as realistic sexual expectations that have never been met under any circumstances; (2) secondary dysfunction, all phases have functioned in the past, but are no longer doing so; or (3) situational dysfunction, defined as the response cycle functions under some circumstances, but not others (Table 12–2).[71]

The clinician should elicit any sexual concerns or chief complaints during the course of the overall health assessment. At this juncture, there is the opportunity to educate the client about myths related to

**Exhibit 12–3** Sexual Problems That Occur in Older Patients

---

**Women**
*Arousal*
- Foreshortening of the vagina
- Slower and decreased vaginal lubrication
- Delayed and reduced vaginal expansion

*Orgasm*
- Fewer contractions
- Occasional painful uterine spasms
- Greater need for direct clitoral stimulation

*Postorgasm*
- No dilation of external cervical orifice
- Vaginal irritation and clitoral pain as a result of the thinner and more atrophic vaginal epithelium, which is more susceptible to mechanical trouble

**Men**
*Arousal*
- Delayed and less firm erection
- Longer interval to ejaculation
- Impaired sense of timing of orgasm

*Orgasm*
- Shorter ejaculation event
- Fewer expulsion contractions
- Less forceful expulsion of semen
- Reduced volume of seminal fluid

*Postorgasm*
- Rapid loss of erection
- Longer refractory period

*Source:* Reprinted with permission from A.E. Reading and J.R. Bragonier, Human Sexuality and Sexual Assault, in N.F. Hacker and J.G. Moore, Eds., *Essentials of Obstetrics and Gynecology,* 3rd ed., pp. 534–536, W.B. Saunders Company.

---

sexuality in aging: specifically, the myth that sexual behavior is aberrant in older individuals and that there is no longer an opportunity for a healthy sex life in aging. Most important, the clinician must determine whether the individual's sexual activities are meeting his or her expectations and whether that person perceives there to be any sexual difficulties. In some cases, it might be useful to interview the older adult's partner, as his or her responses may be different. The clinician can then recommend counseling for couples who have different expectations. After a problem is identified, it should be fully documented with regard to perception, duration, precipitating events, and change. After the nature of the problem has been discerned, the provider can reassure and educate the client as well as institute counseling and referral. The provider may be able to treat

**Table 12–2** Classification of Sexual Dysfunction*

| Category | Characteristics | Etiology |
|---|---|---|
| Primary | Sexual expectations have never been met | Usually psychogenic |
| Secondary | All phases functioned in the past, but one or more no longer do so | May be organic or pharmacologic |
| Situational | Response cycle functions under some circumstances, but not others | May be psychogenic or relationship-related |

*Any of the dysfunctions may involve desire, excitement, or orgasm.

*Source:* Reprinted with permission from A.E. Reading and J.R. Bragonier, Human Sexuality and Sexual Assault, in N.F. Hacker and J.G. Moore, Eds., *Essentials of Obstetrics and Gynecology,* 3rd ed., pp. 534–536, W.B. Saunders Company.

certain conditions such as vaginismus, which is pain with penile penetration, or lack of desire, which may be due to psychologic distress or biologic conditions.

In summary, the clinician needs to understand whether the older adult perceives there to be any sexual dysfunction, what his or her expectations are of normal sexuality in later life, and any existing diseases or medications that may affect sexual function. The clinician then needs to develop strategies for resolving sexual concerns that are noted during the sexual assessment. Sexual options for older adults are as varied as they are for younger adults. Finally, homosexuality, unsafe intercourse resulting in venereal disease, including HIV infection, sexual trauma from rape, and other types of sexual assault are all issues that should not be overlooked because of stereotypes held about older people.

## Nervous System

The neurologic examination is performed after bringing the person to a sitting position. The neurologic examination is composed of six components: intellectual function, the cranial nerves, motor examination, sensory examination, reflexes, and cerebellar examination. The mental status examination was discussed at length in Chapter 7. The importance of the mental status examination should be emphasized again. Unless in an advanced stage, patients with Alzheimer's disease have a normal neurologic examination to an examiner who neglects to specifically test cognitive functioning.

Age-related changes in the nervous system include decreased vibratory sensation (especially in the legs), less brisk deep tendon reflexes, and decreased ability for upward gaze.[72] The Achilles tendon reflex is frequently unobtainable. The so-called pathologic reflexes such as the grasp, palmomental, glabellar, and snout reflexes are characteristic of release of cortical inhibition but are fairly common in normal older persons. Concomitant presence of these release signs may signal arteriosclerotic changes in the brain or dementia.[73] Demented persons with pathologic reflexes may have more functional impairment and poorer prognosis, but the release signs may also be present in persons with dementia.[74,75]

Sensation may be tested by evaluation of the person's ability to feel a soft cotton-tipped applicator, sharp pinprick, and vibrating tuning fork. Such examination is often quite subjective, and sometimes deficits are not reproducible. Impaired mental status or aphasia may make sensory examination more difficult, prone to error, or even impossible. More complex sensory integration is examined by asking the patient to identify common objects placed in his or her hands, such as a coin, comb, or paper clip (stereognosis). Position sense (proprioception) is examined by asking the patient to identify the direction in which the toes or fingers are displaced by the examiner. Older persons asked to stand with their feet together and eyes closed (Romberg test) may have some difficulty, because of impaired proprioception, decreased strength, and slowed reaction time.

Motor tone is frequently increased in older persons. Passive movement of the person's limb by the examiner may commonly demonstrate gegenhalten, or involuntary rigidity, which should not be mistaken for lack of cooperation. Strength is decreased as is muscle mass, especially in the small muscles of the hands. Coarse senile tremors may involve the head as well as the hands, may improve after alcohol use, and may worsen with stress or fatigue.

## Gait and Balance

Falling is an example of a geriatric problem with multiple contributing causes and serious consequences requiring careful delineation of the circumstances of the fall and thorough search for underlying physical illness. The risk of falling increases with advancing age, and simple diagnostic evaluation may identify persons at increased risk.[76–79] The patient can be observed as he or she is requested to sit and rise from a chair, walk and turn around, and bend down to pick up an object off the floor.[80] Does the individual rise from a chair in a single movement? Is he or she steady in walking and turning without grasping for support while using smooth continuous movement? Does the person seem sure of himself or herself when bending? Observe if possible the patient climbing and descending a flight of stairs.[81] A relatively quick screen is the 8-foot up-and-go test. The patient is seated and instructed to stand, walk 8 feet forward (a spot on the floor may be indicated), turn, return to the chair, and sit. The patient is asked to do this as quickly as safety allows. This task assesses speed, agility, and dynamic balance.[82] Testing balance and gait in a standard way (Exhibit 12–4) would be indicated

---

**Exhibit 12–4** Tinetti Balance and Gait Evaluation

BALANCE
*Instructions:* Seat the subject in a hard armless chair. Test the following maneuvers. Select one number that best describes the subject's performance in each text, and add up the scores at the end.

1. Sitting balance
   Leans or slides in chair $\qquad$ = 0
   Steady, safe $\qquad$ = 1 ____

2. Arising
   Unstable without help = 0
   Able but uses arms to help = 1
   Able without use of arms = 2 ____

3. Attempt to arise
   Unable without help = 0
   Able but requires more than one attempt = 1
   Able to arise with one attempt = 2 ____

4. Immediate standing balance (first 5 seconds)
   Unsteady (staggers, moves feet, marked trunk sway) = 0
   Steady but uses walker or cane or grabs other objects = 1
   for support
   Steady without walker, cane, or other support = 2 ____

5. Standing balance
   Unsteady = 0
   Steady but wide stance (medial heels more than 4 inches = 1
   apart) or uses cane, walker, or other support
   Narrow stance without support = 2 ____

*continues*

**Exhibit 12–4** continued

6. Nudging (With subject's feet as close together as possible,
   push lightly on the sternum with palm of hand three times.)
   Begins to fall                                    = 0
   Staggers and grabs, but catches self              = 1
   Steady                                            = 2 ____

7. Eyes closed (at same position as in No. 6)
   Unsteady                                          = 0
   Steady                                            = 1 ____

8. Turning 360 degrees
   Discontinuous steps                               = 0
   Continuous steps                                  = 1 ____
   Unsteady (grabs and staggers)                     = 0
   Steady                                            = 1 ____

9. Sitting down
   Unsafe (misjudges distance, falls into chair)     = 0
   Uses arms or lacks smooth motion                  = 1
   Safe, smooth motion                               = 2 ____

GAIT
*Instructions:* The subject stands with the examiner, and then walks down
hallway or across room, first at the usual pace and then back at a rapid but safe
pace, using a cane or walker if accustomed to one.

10. Initiation of gait (immediately after being told to go)
    Any hesitancy or several attempts to start       = 0
    No hesitancy                                      = 1 ____

11. Step length and height
    Right swing foot:
        Fails to pass left stance foot with step      = 0
        Passes left stance foot                       = 1 ____
        Fails to clear floor completely with step     = 0
        Completely clears floor                       = 1 ____
    Left swing foot:
        Fails to pass right stance foot with step     = 0
        Passes right stance foot                      = 1 ____
        Fails to clear floor completely with step     = 0
        Completely clears floor                       = 1 ____

12. Step symmetry
    Right and left step length unequal               = 0
    Right and left step equal                        = 1 ____

13. Step continuity
    Stopping or discontinuity between steps                              = 0
    Steps appear continuous                                             = 1 ____

14. Path (Observe excursion of either left or right foot over
    about 10 feet of the course.)
    Marked deviation                                                    = 0
    Mild to moderate deviation or uses walking aid                      = 1
    Walks straight without aid                                          = 2 ____

15. Trunk
    Marked sway or uses walking aid                                     = 0
    No sway but flexion of knees or back or spreads arms out
    while walking                                                       = 1
    No sway, flexion, use of arms, or use of walking aid                = 2 ____

16. Walking stance
    Heels apart                                                         = 0
    Heels almost touch while walking                                    = 1 ____

Balance score: ____ /16                                    Gait score: ____ /12
                        Total score: ____ /28

*Source:* Adapted with permission from M Tinetti, Performance-Oriented Assessment of Mobility Problems in Elderly Patients, *Journal of the American Geriatric Society*, Vol. 34, pp. 119–126, © 1986, Lippincott Williams & Wilkins.

for persons with neurologic disorders as well as to assess the effect of medications that might interfere with balance.

## CONCLUSION

The observation of mobility and strength during the exam, or more formal evaluation by the 8-foot up-and-go test or Tinetti Balance and Gait Evaluation, may suggest mobility deficits and an increased risk of falling. A multifaceted intervention may reduce this risk, including assistive devices (cane, quad-cane, or walker), gait training and strengthening (physical therapy), improving vision (cataract evaluation), discontinuing sedating medications, and evaluating the home for areas of risk.

Another important function of the physical exam in the older patient is to evaluate for possible abuse or neglect by caregivers. In situations where there is abuse or neglect, it is often not described in the history, and thus, the examiner must keep these issues in mind during the physical evaluation of the patient. In a retrospective emergency department study of protective service records of old people known to be victims of physical older person abuse, physicians rarely asked patients about abuse or made the diagnosis, even when the clinical presentation suggested a substantial possibility of mistreatment.[83] A diagnosis of abuse should be considered whenever there are multiple injuries in different stages of evolution or when injuries are unexplained or the explanations provided are implausible. The possibility of significant neglect should be considered whenever a dependent patient presents with malnutrition, dehydration, or gross inattention to hygiene.[84]

After abuse is suspected, a thorough examination is required. The general appearance of patients and the nature of their interactions with their alleged abusers may be revealing. A full examination of the entire body is performed, with particular attention to the skin, hair, and orthopedic injuries. The size, location, and number of any skin lesions must be documented. As cognitive impairment is a risk factor for abuse, mental status screening suggesting dementia should increase vigilance for abuse and neglect. Also, addressing competency and decision-making capacity is necessary before many protective interventions that require the victim's consent.[85] Careful documentation of findings is essential, as the medical record often becomes part of a legal record.[86] Verbatim transcription of described events and drawings or photographs of injuries can be very helpful. Whole-body x-rays for healing fractures, and computed tomography scanning of the head should be considered when history and exam suggest abnormalities.

Also, additional history from the patient without the caregiver present, as well as from the caregiver, concerning the injuries or neglect is important. However, care must be exercised to not alienate the caregiver, who will generally continue to have responsibility for the patient. Such alienation may lead to abandonment of the clinical relationship and further harm to the patient. Early consultation with social work and involvement of clinicians with expertise in older person abuse and neglect may be valuable, as well as legally prudent.[84]

The physical examination of the older person is not markedly different than the physical examination of any adult. The focus on contributing factors to functional loss, the frequent barriers to communication present in older adults (such as impaired special senses), and the difficulty of many older adults in obtaining adequate access to medical care (because of their values or inadequate transportation) distinguish the examination of the older adult from examination of younger persons. In addition, the increased morbidity incurred as a person ages cannot be neglected. The physical examination is complementary to functional, social, economic, and values assessment. For the older adult, evaluation of these other domains is often the key to the solution of the multifaceted problems of living presented by older adults to the primary care practitioner and others who care for older persons.

**REFERENCES**

1. Galazka S. Preoperative evaluation of the elderly surgical patient. *J Fam Pract.* 1988;27:622–632.

2. Goldman L. Cardiac risks and complications of noncardiac surgery. *Ann Intern Med.* 1983;98:504–513.

3. Keeler E, Solomon D, Beck J. Effect of patient age on duration of medical encounters with physicians. *Med Care.* 1982;20:1101–1108.

4. Frankl VE. *Man's Search for Meaning.* Boston: Beacon Press; 1959.

5. Frankl VE. *The Doctor and the Soul.* New York: AA Knopf; 1995.

6. Yalom ID. *Existential Psychotherapy.* New York: Basic Books; 1980.

7. Sulmasy DP. *The Healer's Calling.* Mahwah, NJ: Paulist Press; 1997.

8. Matthews DA, McCullough ME, Larson DB. Religious commitment and health status. *Arch Fam Med.* 1998;7:118–124.

9. King DE, Bushwick B. Beliefs and attitudes of hospital inpatients about faith healing and prayer. *J Fam Pract.* 1994;39:349–352.

10. Cadieux R, Kales J, Zimmerman L. Comprehensive assessment of the elderly patient. *Am Fam Phys.* 1985;31:105–111.

11. Ham RJ. *Geriatrics I: American Academy of Family Physicians Home Study Self-Assessment.* Kansas City, MO: American Academy of Family Physicians; 1986. Monograph 89.

12. Besdine RW. The educational utility of comprehensive functional assessment in the elderly. *J Am Geriatr Soc.* 1983;31:651–656.

13. Williams TF. Assessment of the geriatric patient in relation to needs for services and facilities. In: Reichel W, ed. *Clinical Aspects of Aging,* 2nd ed. Baltimore: Williams & Wilkins; 1983:543–548.

14. Williams T. Comprehensive functional assessment: An overview. *J Am Geriatr Soc.* 1983;31:637–641.

15. Mader S. Aging and postural hypotension: An update. *J Am Geriatr Soc.* 1989;37:129–137.

16. Caird F, Andrews G, Kennedy R. Effect of posture on blood pressure in the elderly. *Br Heart J.* 1973;35(5):527–530.

17. Mader S, Josephson K, Rubenstein L. Low prevalence of postural hypotension among community-dwelling elderly. *JAMA.* 1987;258:1511–1514.

18. Shannon R, Wei J, Rosa R. The effect of age and sodium depletion on cardiovascular response to orthostatis. *Hypertension.* 1986;5:438–443.

19. Messerli F, Ventura H, Amodeo C. Osler's maneuver and pseudohypertension. *N Engl J Med.* 1985;312:1548–1551.

20. Hansen A, Jensen H, Laugesen L. Withdrawal of antihypertensive drugs in the elderly. *Acta Med Scand.* 1983;676:178–185.

21. Amery A, Birkenhager WH, Brixko P, et al. Mortality and morbidity results from the European Working Party on high blood pressure in the elderly trial. *Lancet.* 1985;1:1349–1354.

22. National Heart Foundation of Australia. Treatment of mild hypertension in the elderly: Report by the management committee. *Med J Aust.* 1981;2:398–402.

23. Dahlof B, Lindholm L, Hansson L. Morbidity and mortality in the Swedish trial in old persons with hypertension (STOP-hypertension). *Lancet.* 1991;338:1281–1285.

24. MRC Working Party. Medical Research Council trial of treatment of hypertension in older adults. *Br Med J.* 1992;304:405–412.

25. Hulley S, Feigal D, Irelan C. Systolic Hypertension in the Elderly Program (SHEP): The first three months. *J Am Geriatr Soc.* 1986;34:101–105.

26. Gifford R. Isolated systolic hypertension in the elderly. *JAMA.* 1982;247:781–785.

27. Hypertension Detection and Follow-Up Program Cooperative Group. Five-year findings of the Hypertension Detection and Follow-Up Program: II: Mortality by race, sex, and age. *JAMA.* 1979;242:2572–2577.

28. Hypertension Detection and Follow-Up Program Cooperative Group. Five-year findings of the Hypertension Detection and Follow-Up Program: I: Reduction in mortality of persons with high blood pressure, including mild hypertension. *JAMA.* 1979;242:2562–2571.

29. Kannel W. Implications of Framingham Study data for treatment of hypertension: Impact of other risk factors. In: Laragh JH, Buhler FR, Seldin DW, eds. *Frontiers in Hypertension Research.* New York: Springer-Verlag; 1981:17–21.

30. Applegate WB, Rutan GH. Advances in the management of hypertension in older persons. *J Am Geriatr Soc.* 1992;40:1164–1174.

31. SHEP Cooperative Research Group. Prevention of stroke by antihypertensive drug treatment for older persons with isolated systolic hypertension. *JAMA.* 1991;265:3255–3264.

32. Meyer JS, Judd BW, Tawakina T, et al. Improved cognition after control of risk factors for multi-infarct dementia. *JAMA.* 1986;256:2203–2209.

33. Morley J, Solomon D. Major issues in geriatrics over the last five years. *J Am Geriatr Soc.* 1994;42:218–225.

34. The Nutrition Screening Initiative. *Report of Nutrition Screening: Toward a Common View.* Washington, DC: Nutritional Screening Initiative; 1991.

35. Haboubi N, Hudson P, Pathy M. Measurement of height in the elderly. *J Am Geriatr Soc.* 1990;38:1008–1010.

36. National Heart Lung and Blood Institute and the National Institute of Diabetes and Digestion and Kidney Diseases. *Clinical Guidelines on the Identification, Evaluation, and Treatment of Overweight and Obesity in Adults.* Bethesda, MD: National Institutes of Health; 1998.

37. Dwyer J, Gallo J, Reichel W. Assessing nutritional status in elderly patients. *Am Fam Phys.* 1993;47:613–620.

38. Detsky A, Smalley P, Chang J. Is this patient malnourished? *JAMA.* 1994;271:54–58.

39. O'Malley TA, Everitt DE, O'Malley HC, et al. Identifying and preventing family-mediated abuse and neglect of elderly persons. *Ann Intern Med.* 1983;98:998–1005.

40. Council on Scientific Affairs of the American Medical Association. Elder abuse and neglect. *JAMA.* 1987;257:966–971.

41. Taler G, Ansello E. Elder abuse. *Am Fam Phys.* 1985;32:107–114.

42. Rathbone-McCuan E, Goodstein RK. Elder abuse: Clinical considerations. *Psychiatr Ann.* 1985;15:331–339.

43. Allman R. Pressure ulcers among the elderly. *N Engl J Med.* 1989;320:850–853.

44. Brandeis G, Morris J, Nash D, Lipsitz L. The epidemiology and natural history of pressure ulcers in elderly nursing home residents. *JAMA.* 1990;264:2905–2909.

45. Clinical Practice Guidelines. *Pressure Ulcers in Adults.* Rockville, MD: US Department of Health and Human Services, Public Health Service, Agency for Health Care Policy and Research; 1992.

46. Steffes R, Thralow J. Visual field limitation in the patient with dementia of the Alzheimer's type. *J Am Geriatr Soc.* 1987;35:198–204.

47. Mader S. Hearing impairment in elderly persons. *J Am Geriatr Soc.* 1984;32:548–553.

48. Gordon S, Jahnigen D. Oral assessment of the edentulous elderly patient. *J Am Geriatr Soc.* 1983;31:797–801.

49. Gordon S, Jahnigen D. Oral assessment of the edentulous elderly patient. *J Am Geriatr Soc.* 1986;34:276–281.

50. Sauve JS, Laupacis A, Ostbye T, Feagan B, Sackett DL. Does this patient have a clinically important carotid bruit? *JAMA.* 1993;270:2843–2845.

51. Livingston EH, Hershman JM, Sawin CT, et al. Prevalence of thyroid disease and abnormal thyroid tests in older hospitalized and ambulatory persons. *J Am Geriatr Soc.* 1987;35:109–114.

52. Cooper DS. Subclinical hypothyroidism. *JAMA.* 1987;258:246–247.

53. Wei J, Gersh B. Heart disease in the elderly. *Curr Probl Cardiol.* 1987;12:1–65.

54. Agency for Health Care Policy and Research. *Heart Failure: Evaluation and Care of Patients with Left Ventricular Failure.* Rockville, MD: US Department of Health and Human Services, Public Health Service, Agency for Health Care Policy and Research; 1994.

55. Potter J, Elahi D, Tobin J, et al. The effect of age on the cardiothoracic ratio of man. *J Am Geriatr Soc.* 1982;30:404–409.

56. Martin A, Benbow L, Butrous G, et al. Five-year follow-up of 101 elderly subjects by means of long-term ambulatory cardiac monitoring. *Eur Heart J.* 1984;5:592–596.

57. Heger J. Cardiac arrhythmias in the elderly. *Cardiovasc Clin.* 1981;12:145–159.

58. Fleg J, Kennedy H. Cardiac arrhythmias in a healthy elderly population: Detection by 24-hour ambulatory electrocardiography. *Chest.* 1982;81:302–307.

59. Dreifus L. Cardiac arrhythmias in the elderly: Clinical aspects. *Cardiol Clin.* 1986;4:273–283.

60. Camm A, Evans K, Ward D, et al. The rhythm of the heart in active elderly subjects. *Am Heart J.* 1980;99:598–603.

61. Kantelip J, Sage E, Duchene-Marullaz P. Findings on ambulatory electrocardiographic monitoring in subjects older than 80 years. *Am J Cardiol.* 1986;57:398–401.

62. Vernon M. Urinary incontinence in the elderly. *Primary Care.* 1989;16:515–528.

63. Madoff R, Williams J, Caushaj P. Fecal incontinence. *N Engl J Med.* 1992;326: 1002–1007.

64. Urinary Incontinence Guideline Panel. *Urinary Incontinence in Adults.* Rockville, MD: US Department of Health and Human Services, Public Health Service, Agency for Health Care Policy and Research; 1992.

65. Kinsey AC, Pomeroy WB, Martin CE. *Sexual Behavior in the Human Male.* Philadelphia: WB Saunders; 1948.

66. Staff of the Institute for Sex Research, Indiana University. *Sexual Behavior in the Human Female.* Philadelphia: WB Saunders; 1953.

67. Matthias RE, Lubben JE, Atchison KA, Schweitzer SO. Sexual activity and satisfaction among very old adults: Results from a community-dwelling Medicare population survey. *Gerontologist.* 1997;37:6–14.

68. Helgason AR, Adolfsson J, Dickman P, et al. Sexual desire, erection, orgasm and ejaculatory functions and their importance to elderly Swedish men: A population-based study. *Age Aging.* 1996;25:285–291.

69. Levy JA. Sexuality and aging. In: Hazzard WR, Bierman EL, Blass JP, Ettinger WH, Halter JB, Reubin A, eds. *Principles of Geriatric Medicine,* 3rd ed. New York: McGraw-Hill; 1994:115–123.

70. Besdine RW, Beers MH, Bootman JL. *When Medicine Hurts Instead of Helps: Preventing Medication Problems in Older People* (Congressional Briefing). Washington, DC: Alliance for Aging Research; 1998.

71. Reading AE, Bragonier JR. Human sexuality and sexual assault. In: Hacker NF, Moore JG, Gambone JC, eds. *Essentials of Obstetrics and Gynecology,* 3rd ed. Philadelphia: WB Saunders; 1998:532–542.

72. Katzman R, Terry R. *The Neurology of Aging.* Philadelphia: FA Davis Co; 1983.

73. Thomas R. Blinking and the releasing reflexes: Are they clinically useful? *J Am Geriatr Soc.* 1994;42:609–613.

74. Molloy D, Clarnette R, McIlroy W, et al. Clinical significance of primitive reflexes in Alzheimer's disease. *J Am Geriatr Soc.* 1991;39:1160–1163.

75. Hodges J. Neurological aspects of dementia and normal aging. In: Huppert F, Brayne C, O'Connor D, eds. *Dementia and Normal Aging.* Cambridge: Cambridge University Press; 1994:118–129.

76. Nevitt M, Cummings S, Kidd S, Black D. Risk factors for recurrent nonsyncopal falls: A prospective study. *JAMA.* 1989;261:2663–2668.

77. Tinetti M, Speechley M, Ginter S. Risk factors for falls among elderly persons living in the community. *N Engl J Med.* 1987;319:1701–1705.

78. Studenski S, Duncan P, Chandler J, et al. Predicting falls: The role of mobility and nonphysical factors. *J Am Geriatr Soc.* 1994;42:297–302.

79. Rogers ME, Rogers NL, Takeshima N, et al. Methods to assess and improve the physical parameters associated with fall risk in older adults. *Prev Med.* 2003;36: 255–264.

80. Tinetti M, Speechley M. Prevention of falls among the elderly. *N Engl J Med.* 1989;320:1055–1059.

81. Tinetti M. Performance-oriented assessment of mobility problems in elderly patients. *J Am Geriatr Soc.* 1986;34:119–126.

82. Rikili R, Jones CS. Development and validation of a functional fitness test for community-residing older adults. *J Aging Phys Act.* 1999;7:129–161.

83. Lachs MS, Williams CS, O'Brien S, et al. Emergency department utilization by older victims of family violence. *Ann Emerg Med.* 1997;30:448–454.

84. Lachs MS, Pillemer K. Elder abuse. *Lancet.* 2004;364:1263–1272.

85. Butler RN. Warning signs of elder abuse. *Geriatrics.* 1999;54:3.

86. Lachs MS, Pillemer K. Abuse and neglect of elderly persons. *N Engl J Med.* 1995; 332:437–443.

# 13

# *Pain Assessment*

James P. Richardson

## CASE VIGNETTE

*Mrs. H, a 78-year-old widow, sees you for the first time because "no one has been able to help me with my pain." She has hypertension and diet-controlled diabetes, but her principal concern is chronic pain. She says that the pain is "all over" and has been present for weeks. After a cursory exam (limited by time), which reveals nothing alarming or emergent, you ask Mrs. H to keep a pain diary (discussed later). Although skeptical at first, she eventually agrees.*

*Two weeks later she is back in your office. Her pain diary, although not thorough, reveals that she has difficulty moving in the morning and completing her morning activities of daily living, but this improves somewhat later in the day. The pain is primarily in her upper arms, back, and neck. An over-the-counter nonsteroid had some effect, but did not eliminate the pain. She also notes some "feverishness." Armed with this new information, you direct your exam to the appropriate areas, finding limited active and passive range of motion of the shoulders, but no findings of frank arthritis. Temporal arteries are normal to palpation. The erythrocyte sedimentation rate is 95, and Mrs. H's symptoms improve*

> *dramatically with low-dose prednisone within a few days, con-*
> *firming the diagnosis of polymyalgia rheumatica.*

Acute and chronic non–cancer-related pains are among the most common complaints of older adults. Acute pain may be caused by exacerbation of a chronic problem (e.g., a vertebral fracture in a person with osteoporosis) or a new injury from a recent fall. Chronic pain may result from osteoarthritis, rheumatoid arthritis, chronic back pain, myalgias, other rheumatologic conditions, or cancer. This chapter reviews acute and chronic pain assessment in older adults. For a comprehensive review of pain therapy, the reader is referred to the recently revised clinical practice guidelines published by the American Geriatrics Society on the management of persistent pain in older persons and to other sources.[1–3]

Although definitions of chronic pain vary, a common and useful operating definition is persistent pain that does not respond to usual treatments within the expected time frame. Chronic pain in older adults is common. For example, a recent telephone survey found that one fifth of older adults surveyed took analgesic medications regularly. Patients who are taking analgesics regularly tend to see multiple physicians, usually primary care doctors.[4] Chronic pain also is common in nursing home residents.[5]

Multiple patient and physician barriers might interfere with the assessment and successful treatment of chronic pain in older adults (Exhibit 13–1). Some older individuals will deny having pain but will admit to experiencing discomfort, aching, or pressure. In addition, older adults may not receive adequate treatment because they and their doctors fear addiction.

---

**Exhibit 13–1** Patient/Physician Beliefs and Barriers to Effective Pain Assessment/ Treatment in Older Adults

*Patient*
- Pain is a normal part of aging
- Stoicism
- Complaining of pain represents a moral failing
- Fear of the cause of the pain (e.g., cancer)

*Physician*
- Inadequate time for assessment
- Lack of interest in assessment and treatment
- Lack of expertise

## HISTORICAL ASSESSMENT OF PAIN

Assessment of pain in the older adult can be problematic and provoke anxiety in the examiner. However, keeping in mind some general principles of pain assessment will help (Exhibit 13–2). Although it has long been postulated that older adults do not experience pain with the same intensity as younger adults because of age-related changes in the nervous system, it is doubtful that these changes are clinically significant. In particular, it is important to stress that there is no evidence that pain perception is decreased in older adults compared with younger adults.[3,6] It is now understood that only the patient truly knows the severity of the pain that he or she is experiencing. "Accurate pain assessment begins when the physician believes patients and takes their complaints of pain seriously" (p. 682).[5] Therefore, physicians should focus on quantifying the individual's subjective experience of pain.

---

**Exhibit 13–2** Special Considerations in Geriatric Pain Assessment

1. General considerations
   A. Recognize that age itself does not reduce pain sensitivity.
   B. Recognize that there is no evidence that age, *per se,* influences qualitative properties of pain.
   C. Recognize the importance of encouraging the patient to discuss the pain.
2. Co-morbidity: Illness and symptom presentation in the elderly, particularly the frail and the "old-old," is often characterized by multiplicity, duplicity, and chronicity.
3. Mental status: Assess for cognitive impairment—dementia of the Alzheimer's type, pseudodementia secondary to depression, multiinfarct dementia—and refer if necessary.
4. Depression: Pain is likely a major source of depression in the elderly.
5. Activities of daily living: Differentiate between limitations caused by non–pain-related dysfunction and limitations in activities due to the fact that their performance is painful. Pain-related dysfunctions and limitation in activities of daily living are likely a significant source of depression in the old.
6. Medications: Assess all current and recent medications (look in the "brown bag of pills"). Start low and go slow, but remember 1-A and 1-B above.
7. Family and social support systems: Maintain these systems in the physically or mentally impaired elderly.

Reprinted from Harkins SW, Scott RB. Pain and presbyalgos. In: Birren J, ed. *Encyclopedia of gerontology.* San Diego: Academic Press, 1996:247–260, with permission.

## Unidimensional Pain Scales

Numerous means are available for recording pain. Unidimensional scales record the intensity of the pain but do not address other pain characteristics, such as affective components. An example is a verbal descriptor scale, in which persons are asked to choose from five words that reflect increasing severity of pain: mild, discomforting, distressing, horrible, and excruciating.[7] The disadvantages of a verbal descriptor scale are the limited words to choose from and that individuals tend to choose moderate words rather than those expressing the extremes.[7]

In common use today in most care settings is the numeric rating scale (NRS). When an NRS is used, persons are asked to rate the pain from 0 to 10, with 0 representing absolutely no pain and 10 the worst possible pain the person can imagine. A visual analog scale (VAS) is similar to an NRS in that persons rate pain from 0 to 10,[7] but do so by marking a 10-cm line that is labeled on one end as "no pain" and on the other as "worst imaginable pain." VASs appear to be valid and reliable indicators of chronic pain in older patients attending a chronic pain clinic, but have not been extensively tested in the general population of older persons who are suffering pain.[8] NRSs and VASs are widely used in acute care settings such as hospitals because of their simplicity and because they are easily understood by patients. In addition, these scales can reflect small changes in pain that can be helpful in monitoring the response to therapy. However, NRSs and VASs do not reflect changes in psychologic distress or physical function caused by pain.

## Multidimensional Pain Scales

Multidimensional pain scales are useful because they assess more than just the intensity of pain; they are affective for other components of pain. The best known and most studied of these is the McGill Pain Questionnaire (MPQ).[3,9] The MPQ assesses pain along three dimensions: sensory, affective, and evaluative. The three components of pain are derived from the gate-control theory of pain.[10] Each of the three components is subdivided into 20 subclasses. A person is asked to classify his or her pain by picking words in each subclass that are closest to the person's experience of pain. Each category is scored, and a total score is calculated.

Although the MPQ has been used in a variety of clinical settings, its complexity (it is not self-administered and may take 20 minutes to complete) makes it most suitable for use in chronic pain clinics or as a research tool. As is true for many pain-assessment or quality-of-life instruments, some controversy attends the use of the MPQ as well.[10]

## Other Historical Data

The quality of the pain can guide the practitioner as to the type of pain; the type of pain may then be helpful in deciding treatment options.[1] *Nociceptive pain* is either visceral (caused by mechanical deformation mediated by stretch receptors) or somatic (caused by tissue injury mediated by pain receptors). Examples include pain from a bowel obstruction or joint pain caused by osteoarthritis. Most often, the degree of pain is proportional to the degree of tissue injury. All tissue types may cause nociceptive pain except the central nervous system. Nociceptive pain usually responds to traditional treatments for pain.

*Neuropathic pain* involves disease or injury to either the central or peripheral nervous system. Neuropathic pain is often described as "burning," "aching," or "deep" in quality. Examples include post-stroke pain, phantom limb pain, or painful extremities from diabetic neuropathy. The pain may continue without ongoing tissue damage. This type of pain may not respond to the usual analgesic therapies but may respond to treatment with tricyclic antidepressants, anticonvulsants, or antiarrhythmic drugs.[1] So-called *central pain* is a special case of neuropathic pain that is caused by damage to pain transmission pathways, such as the spinothalamic tract or the thalamus itself. Allodynia (i.e., a painful response to a nonpainful stimulus) or hyperesthesia (i.e., increased sensitivity to a stimulus) may present because of neuropathic pain.[7]

*Mixed pain,* such as recurrent headaches or vasculitic pain, appears to be caused by unknown mechanisms. Treatment is often difficult and usually requires a combination of therapies. *Psychogenic pain,* the final category of pain, is said to be present when psychologic influences (e.g., somatization or conversion disorder) are a major factor in the etiology or persistence of the pain symptoms. In these cases, the usual pain treatments are not advised, and psychiatric intervention is necessary.[1]

After the intensity and the quality of the pain have been evaluated and quantified, the other usual descriptors of pain should be elicited: location and radiation, duration, frequency or pattern, and precipitating and ameliorating factors. The person can describe or mark the location of the pain on a body diagram. Persons who cover a large part of a body diagram, especially when previous evaluation has shown involvement limited to one or two nerve roots, are more focused on their pain and may be more disturbed.[11] An attempt should be made to determine whether the pain is localized or referred from another site and whether it is superficial or visceral. Examples of referred pain include shoulder pain resulting from diaphragmatic irritation and back pain from kidney or prostate disease. Pain that is superficial is easily localized, whereas visceral pain is diffuse. A pain diary helps to clarify relationships between ameliorating and precipitating factors, pain duration, and frequency. Completion of a pain diary also helps to assess the relationship between pain and activity.[1] For example, persons who identify particular activities as pain producing rather than certain movements may be having their pain behaviors reinforced by activity avoidance.[11] On the other hand, when pain-relieving factors are limited to medications, activity avoidance, or massage by family members, these persons may be having their pain behavior reinforced.[11] In the pain diary, pain intensity can be recorded according to an NRS (from 0 to 10) during various activities. Other helpful information may be recorded, such as the effect of medicines or other therapies or emotional state and interactions with family members.[7]

Additional history taking should focus on the sequence of events that led to the chronic pain, as well as the treatments, especially over-the-counter and prescription medicines, along with the person's assessment of the results of treatments. This type of information becomes especially important when evaluating persons with psychogenic pain. Persons with psychogenic pain will benefit from a full psychologic evaluation that includes an assessment of the impact of the pain on the person's life, his or her premorbid personality, and a consideration of the financial aspects.[11] Assessment of activities of daily living and instrumental activities of daily living is very helpful in delineating the impact of the person's pain on function (see Chapter 10).

## PHYSICAL ASSESSMENT OF PAIN

The evaluation of the older person with pain, as with all medical evaluations, should include a comprehensive physical examination. The physical assessment may not always be completed on the first visit because persons with pain often present as urgent visits and because more time is usually necessary to evaluate older adults. Although the goal is a "complete" examination, the neurologic and musculoskeletal systems will require more attention and time when considering the person with pain. Because a physical examination of the older adult is explored in detail in Chapter 12, in this chapter, only topics that are pertinent in assessing pain syndromes are highlighted.

General observations are important and may begin with the person's entrance to the waiting area. Does the patient walk in unassisted, or is he or she using a wheelchair or other assistive device? Can the patient stand up from a sitting position without assistance or pain? Is the patient's gait normal or antalgic? Is the patient anxious or in obvious pain? Is the patient accompanied by a family member? What is the interaction between the patient and caregiver? Further general observations can occur in the exam room during history taking.[12] The patient's dress and body language are observed. Poor grooming and personal hygiene suggest depression and/or dementia. The patient's posture and side-to-side symmetry can be assessed.[12] Kyphosis or scoliosis could indicate osteoporosis with compression fractures. Odors suggestive of poor hygiene, recreational substance use, or metabolic abnormalities should be noted. The patient should be observed while she or he is undressing to see whether an extremity is favored due to pain.[7] Although a person in acute pain may manifest elevated pulse rate and blood pressure, these may not be present in someone with chronic pain because of physiologic adaptation.[12]

## Skin

In addition to the usual observations, surgical scars should be noted that may indicate procedures that patients do not recall during history taking. Other scars may indicate trauma or infections. Lesions that may indicate a systemic condition (e.g., neurofibromatosis) should be noted.[12] Excoriations may be a sign of dysesthesias or pruritus. Color changes over the extremities may mean arterial or venous insufficiency (discussed later). Signs of trauma could be evidence of older person abuse. Pressure sores may mean abnormal posture or poor mobility. Evidence of trophic skin and nail changes should be sought.

## Head, Eyes, Ears, Nose, Throat, and Neck

Evidence of head trauma, systemic disease that affects the sclera or iris, and the results of ophthalmoscopy should all be noted. Examination of the ears may reveal cerumen, impaction, or otitis. The condition of the teeth may reveal caries or other painful dental conditions. Foul breath may result from periodontal disease or sinusitis. The carotid arteries should be palpated and auscultated. Enlarged or tender lymph nodes (cervical, submandibular, supraclavicular) should be noted. The thyroid should be examined as well.

## Chest, Abdomen, Genitalia, Pelvis, and Extremities

Breasts and axillae should be examined for tenderness, masses, or discharge. The sternum and the sternocostal, costoclavicular, and costochondral joints should be palpated for swelling or tenderness. The heart, lungs, and abdomen are examined in the usual fashion. If urinary pathology is suspected, be sure to percuss the flanks. The bladder should be palpated for the possibility of urinary retention. Lower abdominal or back pain complaints may require examination of the genitalia. Women should have a careful pelvic examination, including bimanual examination for masses or tenderness. Men should have inspection and palpation of the scrotum and a prostate examination. Both men and women should have rectal examinations to check for masses and tenderness and, if applicable, to check stool for occult blood. Tenderness of the ischia and coccyx might be noted during rectal exam. The bones of the pelvis should be palpated for tenderness. Pulses should be palpated. Notation should be made of skin changes suggestive of ischemia (e.g., pallor, coolness, or ulcers) or venous insufficiency (e.g., edema, hyperpigmentation, or ulcers) or thrombophlebitis (e.g., swelling or pain).

## Musculoskeletal System

Along with the neurologic exam, the musculoskeletal exam deserves the most emphasis in persons with chronic pain. In addition to the points raised in Chapter 12, a thorough musculoskeletal exam in older persons with pain should include palpation of muscles, looking for spasm and referred pain.[12] Trigger points may be identified. Active range of motion of symptomatic joints should be checked. If limited, then the person is gently assisted to determine passive range of motion. Joint disease limits both active and passive motion, whereas greater passive than active range of motion suggests disease of the muscle or tendon. If contraction of the muscles of the affected joint against sufficient resistance to prevent movement is painful, this may also indicate muscular or supporting structure pathology. Joints should be examined for swelling, erythema, sponginess (suggestive of synovitis), and bony enlargement.[13] The areas surrounding joints should be examined for soft tissue pathology that may produce pain, such as ganglion cysts, bursitis, or tenosynovitis.[13] The spine deserves special emphasis. The person is asked to stand for this exam, and the spine is viewed from behind for symmetry and symmetric muscle bulk of the paraspinal and shoulder muscles. The iliac crests should be level. Forward flexion and extension, as well as lateral flexion and rotation, test range of motion. Pain on percussion of the spinous processes may indicate vertebral fractures or ligamentous pathology or may represent referred tenderness.[12]

A few special maneuvers deserve mention.[11] Pain in the cervical spine with Valsalva's maneuver suggests increased intrathecal pressure caused by a space-occupying lesion in the spinal canal. If pain occurs on the concave side with lateral flexion of the thoracic spine, intercostal nerve root compression is likely; if the pain is on the convex side, pleural pathology with fixation to the chest wall is more likely. Straight leg raising tests for sciatic nerve irritation. An observation of the person's gait should be included (see Chapter 12).

## Neurologic System

A careful neurologic examination is necessary in many individuals with chronic pain, especially if neuropathic pain is suspected. The usual neurologic examination is reviewed in Chapter 12. Parts of the neurologic examination that are particularly important in the older adult with pain will be emphasized. Pain in an area of hypoesthesia, allodynia, and hyperpathia (i.e., increased response to a repetitive, nonpainful stimulus) are indicative of neural pathology. Peripheral lesions may be distinguished from central lesions if typical radicular findings of motor weakness, reflex changes, and hypoesthesia are present. The reader is referred to standard medical or neurologic texts for detailed information on nerve root lesions and the expected motor, reflex, and dermatome patterns.

Evidence of autonomic dysfunction may be alteration in skin temperature or color or decreased or increased sweating. Abnormal hair or nail growth may occur. If these signs are present in a painful extremity, complex regional pain syndrome (formerly reflex sympathetic dystrophy) may be present.[12] Mental status testing is important because persons with dementia may complain of pain or other somatic symptoms (see Chapter 7). It is difficult to complete a precise examination of persons with pain and advanced dementia because so much of the exam requires the person's cooperation. Examiners may need to rely on nonverbal expressions of pain, such as grimacing, agitation, or withdrawal, discussed in more detail later.

## PAIN ASSESSMENT IN COGNITIVELY IMPAIRED OLDER ADULTS

As noted earlier, pain is common in nursing home residents, the majority of whom are cognitively impaired.[14] Although nursing home residents are difficult to evaluate for pain, there is no evidence that cognitive impairment "masks" the pain. However, impaired cognition may be associated with reduced pain complaints, even after adjustment for co-morbidities and altered function.[14] Reports of current pain in demented persons are usually valid and reliable.[5,14] Recall of past episodes of pain may be less reliable. Chronic pain complaints may be attributed to depression because depression is so common in nursing home residents. However, psychogenic pain is rare in long-term care residents.

When older persons have cognitive impairment or language barriers, the report of the caregiver or family should be sought.[5] Examples of information that caregivers may provide include changes in function, such as altered gait or falls, agitation, and moaning or crying. Functional decline may be the most noticeable change in a nursing home resident with pain.

## CONCLUSION

Increased recognition of the problem of pain in older adults brings with it the need for new assessment techniques and knowledge. Although much more research needs to be done for a more complete understanding of pain and its treatment, the geriatric practitioner can improve skills in this area by keeping in mind the principles of assessment discussed in this chapter. For more in-depth discussion, readers are referred to other sources.[1,3,7,10] Improving pain assessment and treatment in the hospital, nursing home, hospice, and ambulatory care settings is a worthwhile effort with the potential for a considerable effect on the quality of life of older persons.

**REFERENCES**

1. American Geriatrics Society Panel on Persistent Pain in Older Persons. The management of persistent pain in older persons. *J Am Geriatr Soc.* 2002;50:S205–S224.

2. Ferrell BR, Ferrell BA, eds. *Pain in the Elderly.* Seattle, WA: IASP Press; 1996.

3. Harkins SW. Aging and Pain. In: Loeser JD, Butler SH, Chapman CR, Turk DC, eds. *Bonica's Management of Pain,* 3rd ed. Philadelphia: Lippincott Williams & Wilkins; 2001:813–823.

4. Cooner E, Amorosi S. *The Study of Pain and Older Americans.* New York: Louis Harris and Associates; 1997.

5. Ferrell BA. Pain evaluation and management in the nursing home. *Ann Intern Med.* 1995;123:681–687.

6. Harkins SW. Geriatric pain: Pain perceptions in the old. *Clin Geriatr Med.* 1996;12:435–459.

7. LeBel AA. Assessment of pain. In: Ballantyne J, Fishman SM, Abdi S, eds. *The Massachusetts General Handbook of Pain Management,* 2nd ed. Boston: Little, Brown, and Company; 2002:58–75.

8. Harkins SW, Price DD, Bush FM, Small RE. Geriatric pain. In: Wall PD, Melzack R, eds. *Textbook of Pain,* 3rd ed. New York: Churchill Livingstone; 1994.

9. Melzack R. The McGill Pain Questionnaire: Major properties and scoring methods. *Pain.* 1975;1:277–299.

10. Valley MA. Pain measurement. In: Raj PP, ed. *Pain Medicine: A Comprehensive Review.* St. Louis: Mosby; 1996:36–46.

11. Doleys DM, Murray JB, Klapow JC, Coleton MI. Psychologic assessment. In: Ashburn MA, Rice LJ, eds. *The Management of Pain.* New York: Churchill Livingstone; 1998;27–49.

12. Weinstein SM. Physical examination. In: Ashburn MA, Rice LJ, eds. *The Management of Pain.* New York: Churchill Livingstone; 1998:17–25.

13. Cash JM. History and physical examination. In: Klippel JH, ed. *Primer on the Rheumatic Diseases,* 11th ed. Atlanta, GA: Arthritis Foundation; 1997:89–94.

14. Parmelee PA. Pain in cognitively impaired older persons. *Clin Geriatr Med.* 1996; 12:473–487.

# 14

# *Health Promotion*

Meredith Wallace, Joyce Shea, and Carrie Guttman

Clinicians who care for older adults are often under the impression that older persons are immune to the effects of health promotion. Many believe that so much physiologic damage is done before the first 6 or 7 decades of life that changes in lifestyle are ineffective later in life. For example, the lungs may already have sustained damage from smoking, and the person may even already be battling chronic obstructive lung disease. Years of obesity may already have resulted in the onset of Type II diabetes mellitus and pathologic changes to the bones. Failure to get a yearly influenza vaccine may have already resulted in a 5-day hospitalization, and a mass in the breast may have already metastasized more significantly because the older adult did not undergo yearly mammograms. However, while these scenarios are possible they are not inevitable. In fact, older adults are not too old to benefit from health promotion activities even in the 7th, 8th, or 9th decades of life. Padula and McNatt[1] reported that although interest in the health promotion of older adults is increasing, caution must be paid to the unique needs of this population.

The ability of older adults to benefit from health promotion activities has been underscored by the development and implementation of *Healthy People 2010: National Health Promotion and Disease-Prevention*

*Objectives*. These objectives, which largely focus on older adults (see Exhibit 14–1), consist of increasing the access and involvement of the US population in health-promotion programs. In promoting the health of older adults, evidence based studies have shown that it is possible that the damage caused to the pulmonary system from years

---

**Exhibit 14–1** Selected National Health-Promotion and Disease-Prevention Objectives for the Older Adult

| | |
|---|---|
| 1–4 | Increase the proportion of persons who have a specific source of ongoing care. |
| 1–9 | Reduce hospitalization rates for three ambulatory-care-sensitive conditions—pediatric asthma, uncontrolled diabetes, and immunization-preventable pneumonia and influenza in older adults. |
| 2–9 | Reduce the overall number of cases of osteoporosis. |
| 2–10 | Reduce the proportion of adults who are hospitalized for vertebral fractures associated with osteoporosis. |
| 3–12 | Increase the proportion of adults who receive a colorectal cancer screening examination. |
| 4–1 | Reduce the rate of new cases of end-stage renal disease. |
| 4–5 | Increase the proportion of dialysis patients registered on the waiting list for transplantation. |
| 4–6 | Increase the proportion of patients with treated chronic kidney failure who receive a transplant within 3 years of registration on the waiting list. |
| 4–7 | Reduce kidney failure due to diabetes. |
| 5–1 | Increase the proportion of persons with diabetes who receive formal diabetes education. |
| 5–2 | Prevent diabetes. |
| 5–3 | Reduce the overall rate of diabetes that is clinically diagnosed. |
| 5–4 | Increase the proportion of adults with diabetes whose condition has been diagnosed. |

5–5        Reduce the diabetes death rate.

5–6        Reduce diabetes-related deaths among persons with diabetes.

5–7        Reduce deaths from cardiovascular disease in persons with diabetes.

5–10       Reduce the rate of lower extremity amputations in persons with diabetes.

5–12       Increase the proportion of adults with diabetes who have a glycosylated hemoglobin measurement at least once a year.

5–13       Increase the proportion of adults with diabetes who have an annual dilated eye examination.

5–14       Increase the proportion of adults with diabetes who have at least an annual foot examination.

5–15       Increase the proportion of persons with diabetes who have at least an annual dental examination.

5–16       Increase the proportion of adults with diabetes who take aspirin at least 15 times per month.

5–17       Increase the proportion of adults with diabetes who perform self-blood glucose monitoring at least once daily.

6–3        Reduce the proportion of adults with disabilities who report feelings such as sadness, unhappiness, or depression that prevent them from being active.

6–4        Increase the proportion of adults with disabilities who participate in social activities.

6–5        Increase the proportion of adults with disabilities reporting sufficient emotional support.

6–6        Increase the proportion of adults with disabilities reporting satisfaction with life.

6–7        Reduce the number of people with disabilities in congregate care facilities, consistent with permanency planning principles.

6–8        Eliminate disparities in employment rates between working-aged adults with and without disabilities.

*continues*

**Exhibit 14–1** continued

| | |
|---|---|
| 7–12 | Increase the proportion of older adults who have participated during the preceding year in at least one organized health promotion activity. |
| 8–22 | Increase the proportion of persons living in pre-1950s housing that have tested for the presence of lead-based paint. |
| 10–1 | Reduce infections caused by key food borne pathogens. |
| 12–6 | Reduce hospitalizations of older adults with heart failure as the principal diagnosis. |
| 14–5 | Reduce invasive pneumococcal infections. |
| 14–28 | Increase hepatitis B vaccine coverage among high-risk groups. |
| 14–29 | Increase the proportion of adults who are vaccinated annually against influenza and ever vaccinated against pneumococcal disease. |
| 15–1 | Reduce hospitalization for nonfatal head injuries. |
| 15–15 | Reduce deaths caused by motor vehicle crashes. |
| 15–16 | Reduce pedestrian deaths on public roads. |
| 15–25 | Reduce residential fire deaths. |
| 15–27 | Reduce deaths from falls. |
| 15–28 | Reduce hip fractures among older adults. |
| 17–3 | (Developmental) Increase the proportion of primary care providers, pharmacists, and other health care professionals who routinely review with their patients aged 65 years and older and patients with chronic illnesses or disabilities all new prescribed and over-the-counter medicines. |
| 18–14 | Increase the number of states, territories, and the District of Columbia with an operational mental health plan that addresses mental health crisis interventions, ongoing screening, and treatment services for older persons. |
| 19–1 | Increase the proportion of adults who are at a healthy weight. |
| 19–2 | Reduce the proportion of adults who are obese. |

19–5    Increase the proportion of persons aged 2 years and older who consume at least two daily servings of fruit.

19–6    Increase the proportion of persons aged 2 years and older who consume at least three daily servings of vegetables, with at least one third being dark green or deep yellow vegetables.

19–7    Increase the proportion of persons aged 2 years and older who consume at least six daily servings of grain products, with at least three being whole grains.

19–8    Increase the proportion of persons aged 2 years and older who consume less than 10 percent of calories from saturated fat.

19–9    Increase the proportion of persons aged 2 years and older who consume no more than 30% of calories from fat.

19–11   Increase the proportion of persons aged 2 years and older who meet dietary recommendations for calcium.

19–17   Increase the proportion of physician office visits made by patients with a diagnosis of cardiovascular disease, diabetes, or hyperlipidemia that include counseling or education related to diet and nutrition.

19–18   Increase food security among US households and in so doing reduce hunger.

21–4    Reduce the proportion of older adults who have had all their natural teeth extracted.

21–10   Increase the proportion of children and adults who use the oral health care system each year.

22–1    Reduce the proportion of adults who engage in no leisure-time physical activity.

22–2    Increase the proportion of adults who engage regularly, preferably daily, in moderate physical activity for at least 30 minutes per day.

22–3    Increase the proportion of adults who engage in vigorous physical activity that promotes the development and maintenance of cardiorespiratory fitness 3 or more days per week for 20 or more minutes per occasion.

*continues*

**Exhibit 14–1** continued

| | |
|---|---|
| 22–4 | Increase the proportion of adults who perform physical activities that enhance and maintain muscular strength and endurance. |
| 22–5 | Increase the proportion of adults who perform physical activities that enhance and maintain flexibility. |
| 24–1 | Reduce asthma deaths. |
| 24–2 | Reduce hospitalizations for asthma. |
| 24–3 | Reduce hospital emergency department visits for asthma. |
| 24–9 | Reduce the proportion of adults whose activity is limited due to chronic lung and breathing problems. |
| 24–10 | Reduce deaths from chronic obstructive pulmonary disease among adults. |
| 27–10 | Reduce the proportion of nonsmokers exposed to environmental tobacco smoke. |

From http://www/health.gov/healthypeople

of smoking may be reversed,[2] obese older adults may lose weight and eliminate the need for daily insulin injections or arthritis medications,[3] unnecessary cases of viral influenza and pneumonia[4] will be avoided, and malignancies detected at an earlier and more treatable stage.[5] Moreover, because the Centers for Disease Control and Prevention (CDC) reported that chronic conditions such as arthritis, chronic obstructive pulmonary disease, and non–insulin-dependent diabetes mellitus substantially limit daily activity for 39% of persons over 65 years of age, health promotion among the older adult population is particularly important. The implementation of health promotion activities in the older adult population has already played a significant role in increasing the percentage of older adults from approximately 12% of the population in 1990 to an estimated 18% by the year 2030. With these figures in mind, it is exciting to imagine the impact of enhanced health promotion on expanding the opportunities for healthy living more appreciably in the future.

One framework within which to categorize health promotion is levels of prevention. There are three levels of prevention that focus interventions for promoting the health of the population, especially older adults. The first level of prevention is called *primary prevention*. This level includes interventions to prevent illness or disease from occurring. Examples of interventions within the primary prevention level include smoking cessation, immunizations, proper nutrition, and regular exercise.[6] The next level of prevention is called *secondary prevention* and includes interventions focused on detecting the presence of disease as early as possible, increasing the effectiveness of available treatments. Examples of interventions in this level include routine mammograms, hypertension screening, and prostate-specific antigen blood tests. The third level of prevention is *tertiary prevention*. Interventions within this category are aimed at treatment of disease after the disease has already been diagnosed in order to prevent the impact of disease on functional decline of older adults. As the tertiary level of prevention involves effective disease management among older adults, it is beyond the scope of discussion in this chapter. This chapter explores the primary and secondary levels of prevention among older adults. The incidence and prevalence of harmful health behaviors, best assessment practices, and interventions to reduce these behaviors are discussed in this chapter. Current research supporting the effectiveness of interventions will be reported and recommendations provided.

## PRIMARY HEALTH PROMOTION AND DISEASE PREVENTION

Primary health promotion interventions are designed to prevent the occurrence of a disease. Interventions at the primary prevention level afford the patient and care provider opportunities to promote health and prevent both morbidity and mortality. For example, primary prevention is used to prevent obesity and the related complications such as arthritis, diabetes, and heart disease; cardiovascular diseases, cancer, and other disorders; and promote overall health and well-being. In so doing, both quality of life and function will be maximized. The following section summarizes key interventions and activities in the primary prevention category of health promotion.

### Nutrition

Older adults' lives in the past did not have the benefit of the science base that currently guides nutrition. Older adults ate the foods that were available and the effects of different foods was unknown. The high fat content of meat and eggs was both unknown and unavoidable. The risk factors inherent in high-carbohydrate diets were previously unidentified and consequently not considered when making food choices. The end result was that older adults sustained considerable physiologic damage from poor diets.[5] Furthermore, many older adults are still unfamiliar with healthier dietary guidelines.

Older adults are fully capable of experiencing the health effects from dietary changes late in life. There is sufficient clinical evidence that weight loss reduces arthritis-related pain and dependence on insulin and oral hypoglycemic medication, as well as reducing the risk of heart disease. A recent study revealed that 4 of the 10 leading causes of death are related to poor diet.[3] Improved nutrition greatly impacts the health and quality of life of older adults.

Padula and McNatt[1] reported that diet is among the most important health behaviors and activities ranked by older adult couples in promoting their health. However, many barriers to good nutrition exist among older adults. Normal age-related changes in digestion of nutrients as well as reduction in smell, vision, and taste sensations put older adults at an increased risk of malnutrition. The prevalence of dental conditions and ill-fitting dentures among the older populations also contributes to the inability to meet recommended daily allowances.

Appropriate nutritional interventions may be most successfully implemented after a comprehensive nutritional assessment. The *Nutritional Screening Initiative Checklist*[7] is an instrument that has been effectively used for both initial and successive assessment of nutrition in older adults. The Nutritional Screening Initiative Checklist is a 14-item instrument that may be given to the older adult for self-assessment or may be administered in an interview format. The instrument collects nutritional information on the effect of illness on nutrition, as well as effects of dietary consumption. Among older adults, it is also important to consider financial, logistical, and emotional capacity to select, purchase, prepare, and consume food, as well as the environment in which food is eaten. Often, older adults cannot afford the foods that will provide them with appropriate nutrients, do not have transportation for food shopping, or are unable to prepare food. Moreover, the presence of depression and loneliness may precipitate malnutrition among older adults.[8]

Older adults, even in later decades of life, are amenable to dietary changes to improve their nutrition. A recent study revealed that dietary counseling was an effective intervention for producing small to moderate dietary changes in a primary care population.[9] This supports the deployment of health care professionals to teach and coun-sel older adults about appropriate dietary choices in all care settings. The Food Guide Pyramid is a helpful tool for providing this educa-tion. Older adults should be assessed for the ability to obtain, afford, and prepare food.

## Sleep

The relationship between healthful sleep and morbidity in older adults is strong, and the positive effects of a good night's sleep are abundant.[8] Sleep results in improved energy, motivation to work, and participation in both activities of daily living and instrumental activi-ties of daily living.[10] Furthermore, adequate sleep contributes to the enjoyment of a high quality of life. The impact of sleep disorders on the health of older adults is profound. Failure to get a "good night's sleep" is a prevalent concern among older adults[11] and results from both the inability to fall asleep and the ability to sleep throughout the night. One study ($n = 1,118$) reported that approximately 25% of older adults stated that they had difficulty falling asleep, and 52% had difficulty remaining asleep.[10] Moreover, 28% of this sample reported early awakening, and 12% reported daytime sleepiness.

The numerous sleep complaints reported by older adults are a prod-uct of several normal aging changes in circadian rhythms. These changes result in nocturnal awakenings, decreased periods of sleep, and a reduction in slow wave activity. Montgomery[12] reported that al-though the issue has been hotly debated, it is unclear whether or not older adults actually require less sleep than their younger counterparts.

Montgomery[12] reported that despite the numerous sleep concerns among older adults, little research is available to improve the assess-ment and management of this frequently occurring problem. Several reasons account for the lack of sleep assessment and intervention by health professionals. These reasons include lack of time for assess-ment and lack of knowledge regarding supported interventions. Older adults may view sleep problems as part of the normal aging process and do not report them to their health care providers. However, given the impact of poor sleep on health and functioning, sleep assessment must be given priority by health professionals caring for older adults. Moreover, evidence-based sleep interventions must be implemented and evaluated regularly for effectiveness.

The first step in helping older adults improve sleep is to administer a standardized sleep assessment instrument. The Pittsburgh Sleep Quality Index[13] is an instrument that has been used effectively for both initial and follow-up evaluation of sleep quality among older adults. The Pittsburgh Sleep Quality Index quantifies seven areas of sleep, including subjective sleep quality, sleep latency, sleep duration, habitual sleep efficiency, sleep disturbances, use of sleeping medication, and daytime dysfunction over a period of 1 month. The instrument may be given to older adults to complete or may be administered in an interview format. The instrument is very thorough; however, scoring requires the assistance of a health professional.

Interventions to enhance the sleep quality of older adults begin with teaching about the normal changes in circadian rhythms and their effect on nighttime sleep. Montgomery[12] reported that other interventions include bright-light therapy, exercise, and passive body heating, but all interventions lack clear scientific support. Wallace[14] reported that improving pain control in the nighttime may help those older adults who are awakened by pain to obtain better rest at night. In addition, modifications in noise and lighting may assist older residents of long-term care facilities to improve sleep.

The pharmacologic treatment of sleep disorders is common in older adults and may be effective for short alterations in sleep quality. Newer medications with low side-effect profiles are recommended for a 2-week or as-needed period. Benzodiazepines should be used carefully because of the possibility of rebound and morning insomnia, as well as hangover effect, delirium, and daytime sedation among older adults.[11]

## Smoking

There is no greater modifiable risk factor for developing preventable diseases than smoking. Among older adults, the long-term effects of smoking have been linked with the development of bladder, cervical, esophageal, kidney, laryngeal, lung, oral, pancreatic, and stomach cancers as well as leukemia and abdominal aortic aneurysm, atherosclerosis, cataracts, cerebrovascular disease, coronary heart disease, chronic obstructive pulmonary disease, hip fractures, low bone density, peptic ulcer disease, and pneumonia (Table 14–1). The death toll from smoking-related diseases is estimated to be 440,000 each year.[15] The year 2004 marked the 40th anniversary of the Surgeon General's warning about the dangers of smoking. Although there has been increased legislation regarding the reduction of this known risk factor over the past 40 years, the prevalence of smoking among older adults continues to remain among the most substantial, modifiable risk factors for the development of disease.

It is often believed that the substantial amount of time in which older adults have smoked places them beyond intervention and help.

---

**Table 14–1** Primary and Secondary Prevention Strategies for Older Adults

| *Interventions Considered and Recommended for the Periodic Health Examination* | |
|---|---|
| | *Leading Causes of Death* |
| | Heart disease |
| | Malignant neoplasm (lung, colorectal, breast) |
| | Cerebrovascular disease |
| | Chronic obstructive pulmonary disease |
| | Pneumonia and influenza |

*Interventions for the General Population*

**SCREENING**
Blood pressure
Height and weight
Fecal occult blood test[1] and/or
   sigmoidoscopy
Mammogram ± clinical breast exam[2]
   (women ≤69 yr)
Papanicolaou (Pap) test (women)[3]
Vision screening
Assess for hearing impairment
Assess for problem drinking

**COUNSELING**
*Substance Use*
Tobacco cessation
Avoid alcohol/drug use while driving,
   swimming, boating, etc.*

*Diet and Exercise*
Limit fat and cholesterol; maintain caloric
   balance; emphasize grains, fruits,
   vegetables
Adequate calcium intake (women)
Regular physical activity*

*Injury Prevention*
Lap/shoulder belts
Motorcycle and bicycle helmets*
Fall prevention*
Safe storage/removal of firearms*
Smoke detector*
Set hot water heater to <120–130° F*
CPR training for household members

*Dental Health*
Regular visits to dental care provider*
Floss, brush with fluoride toothpaste daily*

*Sexual Behavior*
STD prevention: avoid high-risk sexual
   behavior;* use condoms*

**IMMUNIZATIONS**
Pneumococcal vaccine
Influenza[1]
Tetanus-diphtheria (Td) boosters

**CHEMOPROPHYLAXIS**
Discuss hormone prophylaxis
   (women)

*continues*

---

**Table 14–1** Continued

---

*Interventions for High-Risk Populations*

---

| POPULATION | POTENTIAL INTERVENTIONS<br>(see detailed high-risk definitions) |
|---|---|
| Institutionalized persons | PPD (HR1); hepatitis A vaccine (HR2); amantadine/rimantadine (HR4) |
| Chronic medical conditions; TB contacts; low income; immigrants; alcoholics | PPD (HR1) |
| Persons ≥75 yr; or ≥70 yr with risk factors for falls | Fall prevention intervention (HR5) |
| Cardiovascular disease risk factors | Consider cholesterol screening (HR6) |
| Family h/o skin cancer; nevi; fair skin, eyes, hair | Avoid excess/midday sun, use protective clothing* (HR7) |
| Native Americans/Alaska Natives | PPD (HR1); hepatitis A vaccine (HR2) |
| Travelers to developing countries | Hepatitis A vaccine (HR2); hepatitis B vaccine (HR8) |
| Blood product recipients | HIV screen (HR3); hepatitis B vaccine (HR8) |
| High-risk sexual behavior | Hepatitis A vaccine (HR2); HIV screen (HR3); hepatitis B vaccine (HR8); RPR/VDRL (HR9) |
| Injection or street drug use | PPD (HR1); hepatitis A vaccine (HR2); HIV screen (HR3); hepatitis B vaccine (HR8); RPR/VDRL (HR9); advice to reduce infection risk (HR10) |
| Health care/lab workers | PPD (HR1); hepatitis A vaccine (HR2); amantadine/rimantadine (HR4); hepatitis B vaccine (HR8) |
| Persons susceptible to varicella | Varicella vaccine (HR11) |

---

[1]Annually .[2]Mammogram q1–2 yr, or mammogram q1–2 yr with annual clinical breast exam. [3]All women who are or have been sexually active and who have a cervix: q<3 yr. Consider discontinuation of testing after age 56 yr if previous regular screening with continuously normal results.

*The ability of clinician counseling to influence this behavior is unproven.

Adapted from http://odphp.osophs.dhhs.gov/pubs/guidecps/PDF/Frontmtr.PDF

---

In other words, since so much damage has been done, why expend resources to stop after 40 or 50 years of smoking? However, the fact remains that older adults may still experience positive results from smoking cessation even after decades of smoking. Moreover, it is believed that older adults may be more highly motivated to quit smoking because the effects of smoking on various organ systems, such as the eyes or lungs, are more profoundly notable than among younger adults. For most people, smoking cessation will be perceived as a cure for these health problems. Because of these reasons, the report of the Surgeon General on the health effects of smoking stated that the health risks of smoking may be reduced among all age groups and recommended that "geriatricians should counsel their patients who smoke, even the oldest, to quit."[15]

Despite the great impetus to stop smoking and the projected positive effects of success in this area, smoking cessation is one of the greatest challenges to both smokers and health care providers working with older smokers.[2] The long-standing use of tobacco in older adults' lives may place them in a position to forget what it was like not to smoke. Consequently, smoking cessation in older adults takes time, and it is not unusual for multiple setbacks to occur. Appel and Aldrich[2] encourage health care providers who work with older smokers to maximize every opportunity to help them quit. In working with older adults who are considering smoking cessation, it is important to discuss this with them and reassure them that setbacks do not mean that health care providers will stop working with them.

The first step in helping older adults to quit smoking is to assess their readiness and motivation, as well as the resources available to them. Mackey[16] suggested making statements such as "I feel that your smoking poses a significant health risk" to define the problem and begin the dialogue with the patient. It is important to determine what factors inspired the decision to quit and what position they are in to do so. The Centers for Disease Control[17] recommended five steps to quit smoking: (1) *Get ready.* This requires determining a start date in which the older adult will wake up cigarette-free. The older adult should be counseled to dispose of all cigarettes from their environments, including the home, work, car, and frequently traveled places. (2) *Get support.* The health care professional should encourage the older adult to announce plans to quit smoking to family and friends and ask for their assistance by not smoking around them. Support may also include visits to a counselor, physician, or support group to assist the older adult with quitting. (3) *Learn new skills and behaviors.* The older adult should be encouraged to avoid habits that are associated with smoking, such as drinking coffee or alcohol, and to substitute these unhealthy habits with healthy ones, such as drinking water or exercise. (4) *Get medication and use it correctly.* The use of nicotine products, such as nicotine gum, patches, inhalers, or nasal spray, are very helpful in the physical withdrawal from nicotine experienced during smoking cessation. Moreover, the adjunct use of the antidepressant therapy Bupropion SR among older adults has also been shown to assist in smoking cessation.[2] (5) *Be prepared for relapse or difficult situations.* Quitting smoking is one of the most difficult tasks to accomplish, as relapses are extremely common in all age groups. Older adults try several times before they successfully quit smoking for good. If older adults experience relapses, they should be encouraged to try again, as soon as they are able.

## Alcohol Abuse Among Older Persons

It is often thought that alcohol problems that are prevalent in younger adult populations cease by the time people enter older age. However, this notion is among the many myths of aging and is perpetuated by the difficulty in identifying alcohol problems among older adults. Levin and Kruger[18] referred to alcoholism as an "invisible epidemic" among older adults. The percentage of alcohol abuse among the older population ranges from 2% to 20%, underscoring the variation in detection efficacy among clinical settings.[19] Moreover, The Robert Wood Johnson Foundation[20] reported that the number of substance dependent and abusing adults over the age of 50 years is projected to increase from 1.7 million to 4.4 million by 2020.

The deleterious health effects of alcoholism among older adults are widespread. Mokdad et al.[21] reported approximately 85,000 deaths in older adults related to excessive or risky alcohol usage in the United States, making alcohol the third leading actual cause of death. Alcohol results in motor vehicle accidents and other violent and unintentional injuries among older adults. In addition, alcohol use has been associated with increased risk of sexually transmitted diseases, hepatitis C and chronic liver disease, as well as oral–pharyngeal, esophageal, prostate, liver, and breast cancer.[22] For older adults, changes in organ systems, including hepatic and nephritic changes, often alter the ability to metabolize and excrete alcohol, effectively resulting in greater concentrations and sensitivity to the substance.[23] Hall et al.[24] reported that alcohol consumption is an essential warning sign for suicide among older adults.

Drinking more than seven drinks each week or more than three drinks per day during an occasion is considered at risk for alcohol abuse according to the National Institute on Alcohol and Alcoholism.[25] However, assessing the use of alcohol among older adults is extremely challenging and presents a large barrier to successful treatment in this population. One of the great challenges lies in the confusion of alcohol-induced symptoms with those of delirium, depression, and dementia.[18] For example, an individual under the influence of alcohol may be unable to articulate his or her thoughts or feelings, which is also symptomatic of more commonly occurring cognitive disorders among older adults. Mersey[26] stated that caution should be paid to several "red-flag" symptoms of alcohol abuse, such as missing appointments, history of accidents, depression, labile hypertension, vague gastrointestinal symptoms, and sexual and sleep disorders. Moreover, Mersey reports that gamma-glutamyl transpeptidase, mean corpuscular volume, and carbohydrate-deficient transferring are helpful laboratory tests in making the diagnosis[26].

One of the most widely used assessment instruments to detect alcohol use among older adults is the CAGE. CAGE is an easily used, four-question instrument that focuses the interview on aspects of drinking indicative of problems. The questions include the following: (1) Have you ever tried to cut down on your drinking? (2) Do you become annoyed when others ask you about drinking? (3) Do you ever feel guilty about your drinking? (4) Do you ever use alcohol in the morning, as an eye opener? Although the instrument is not diagnostic of alcoholism, affirmative responses to any of the four questions should lead the health care provider to refer the patient for further assessment of alcohol-related problems and treatment.

Research shows that older adults with alcohol problems who received treatment specific to their needs can achieve positive health outcomes.[27] As with any long-standing habit, eliminating alcohol from older adults' lives is often complex and challenging. Alcohol rehabilitation requires psychoeducational, personal, and family counseling, support, and cognitive behavioral therapy, as well as physiologic support. These are best provided through skilled alcohol rehabilitation specialists in either an inpatient or outpatient setting.

## Adult Immunization

The United States has substantially increased the amount of children who currently receive childhood vaccinations. This was accomplished in great part by implementing mandatory childhood vaccination as a requirement to enter public and most private schools. However, no such requirement is present for older adults. It is not necessary to be up to date on vaccinations in order to receive Medicare, participate in most work or volunteer activities or to attend a senior center. In fact, without the presence of external motivators to enhance immunization among older adults, personal motivation in the form of health promotion and illness prevention, as well as health care provider influence remain the key factors in promoting vaccination in this population.

As with children, it is essential that older adults remain immunized against all vaccine-preventable illnesses, including diphtheria, tetanus, and pertussis. The recommended vaccination schedule for older adults is contained in Table 14–2. In addition, influenza and pneumococcal are two vaccine-preventable diseases that result in great morbidity and mortality among older adults.[28] In spite of the improvement among the number immunized against these two diseases witnessed in the past 2 decades, and recent Medicare payment for vaccination, influenza vaccination rates among older adults in senior housing remains between 30% and 60% of older residents. This occurs amidst great expense and public relations efforts to promote vaccination among the public. Telford and Rogers[4] reported that older adults' distrust of modern medicine and prior bad experiences with the flu vaccine (i.e., perceptions that they received the flu from the vaccine) were among reasons cited for avoiding it.

Vaccination to prevent influenza can substantially decrease the rate of illness, hospitalizations, and death from the disease.[29] The influenza vaccine is composed of inactivated whole virus or virus subunits and is grown in chick embryo cells. Because of its inactive composition, older adults must be reassured that the influenza vaccination cannot give them the flu. It must be administered annually to all older adults, especially those with chronic conditions such as chronic obstructive pulmonary disease or heart disease. Vaccination is contraindicated only among older adults who have experienced a reaction to the vaccine in the past, and caution should be exercised in administering the vaccine to older adults who have allergies to eggs. Older adults in long-term care facilities must also be vaccinated, despite their medical history, because of the great risk of disease spread in these areas. The percentage of institutionalized older persons who are immunized against influenza is approximately 80%.[29]

Although health care providers are obviously concerned with the individual health of patients, influenza is a public health threat. Yet, every year, there are problems with accessing adequate flu vaccinations. The year 2004 witnessed a rationing of the flu vaccine to only the oldest and sickest citizens. Although younger, healthier people probably will not die from the flu, they can very easily spread it to older, unvaccinated, and immunocompromised persons. It is important for health care providers to advocate for universal vaccination among health care priorities in order to decrease

# Table 14–2 CDC Recommendations for Adult Immunizations

## Recommended Adult Immunization Schedule, United States, 2004–2005

### By Age Group

| Age group (yrs)► Vaccine ▼ | 19–49 | 50–64 | ≥65 |
|---|---|---|---|
| Tetanus Diphtheria (Td)* | 1 dose booster every 10 years[1] | | |
| Influenza | 1 dose annually[2] | 1 dose annually[2] | |
| Pneumococcal (polysaccharide) | 1 dose[3,4] | | 1 dose[3,4] |
| Hepatitis B* | 3 doses (0, 1, 2, 4-6 months)[5] | | |
| Hepatitis A* | 2 doses (0, 6-12 months)[6] | | |
| Measles, Mumps, Rubella (MMR)* | 1 of 2 doses[7] | | |
| Varicella* | 2 doses (0, 4-8 weeks)[8] | | |
| Meningococcal (polysaccharide) | 1 dose[9] | | |

\* Covered by the Vaccine Injury Compensation Program.

See Footnotes for Recommended Adult Immunization Schedule on back cover.

| For all persons in this group | For persons lacking documentation of vaccination or evidence of disease | For persons at risk (i.e., with medical/exposure indications) |
|---|---|---|

This schedule indicates the recommended age groups for routine administration of currently licensed vaccines for persons aged ≥19 years. Licensed combination vaccines may be used whenever any components of the combination are indicated and when the vaccine's other components are not contraindicated. Providers should consult manufacturers' package inserts for detailed recommendations.

Report all clinically significant postvaccination reactions to the Vaccine Adverse Event Reporting System (VAERS). Reporting forms and instructions on filing a VAERS report are available by telephone, 800-822-7967, or from the VAERS website at http://www.vaers.org.

Information on how to file a Vaccine Injury Compensation Program claim is available at http://www.hrsa.gov/osp/vicp or by telephone, 800-338-2382. To file a claim for vaccine injury, contact the U.S. Court of Federal Claims, 717 Madison Place, N.W., Washington, DC 20005, telephone 202-219-9657.

Additional information about the vaccines listed above and contraindications for immunization is available at http://www.cdc.gov/nip or 800-CDC-INFO [800-232-4636] (English or Spanish).

The Recommended Adult Immunization Schedule is Approved by the Advisory Committee on Immunization Practices (ACIP), the American College of Obstetricians and Gynecologists (ACOG), and the American Academy of Family Physicians (AAFP).

### By Medical Condition

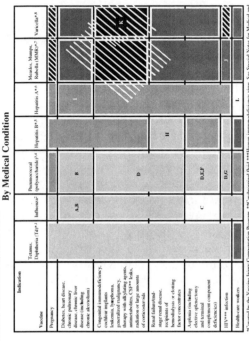

| Indication Vaccine | Tetanus, Diphtheria (Td)*[1] | Influenza[2] | Pneumococcal (polysaccharide)[2,3] | Hepatitis B*[5] | Hepatitis A*[6] | Measles, Mumps, Rubella (MMR)*[7] | Varicella*[8] |
|---|---|---|---|---|---|---|---|
| Pregnancy | | | | | | | |
| Diabetes, heart disease, chronic pulmonary disease, chronic liver disease (including chronic alcoholism) | | A,B | B | | I | | |
| Congenital immunodeficiency, cochlear implants leukemia, lymphoma, generalized malignancy, therapy with alkylating agents, antimetabolites, CSF** leaks, radiation or large amounts of corticosteroids | | | D | | | K | |
| Renal failure/end-stage renal disease, recipients of hemodialysis or clotting factor concentrates | | | | H | | | |
| Asplenia (including elective splenectomy and terminal complement component deficiencies) | | C | D,E,F | | | | |
| HIV*** infection | | | D,G | H | | J | |
| Healthcare workers | | | | | L | | |

\*Covered by the Vaccine Injury Compensation Program. \*\*Cerebrospinal fluid. \*\*\*Human immunodeficiency virus. See Footnotes for Recommended Adult Immunization Schedule on back cover.

Other Indications below. Also see Footnotes for Recommended Adult Immunization Schedule.

| For all persons in this group | For persons lacking documentation of vaccination or evidence of disease | For persons at risk (i.e., with medical/exposure indications) | Contraindicated |
|---|---|---|---|

## Special Notes for Medical and Other Indications

A. Although chronic liver disease and alcoholism are not indications for influenza vaccination, administer 1 dose annually if the patient is aged ≥50 years, has other indications for influenza vaccine, or requests vaccination.

B. Asthma is an indication for influenza vaccination but not for pneumococcal vaccination.

C. No data exist specifically on the risk for severe or complicated influenza vaccination.

D. For persons aged <65 years, revaccinate once after ≥5 years have elapsed since initial vaccination.

E. Administer meningococcal vaccine and consider Haemophilus influenzae type b vaccine.

F. For persons undergoing elective splenectomy, vaccinate ≥2 weeks before surgery.

G. Vaccinate as soon after diagnosis as possible.

H. For hemodialysis patients, use special formulation of vaccine (40 µg/ml) or two 20 µg/ml doses administered at one body site. Vaccinate early in the course of renal disease. Assess antibody titers to hepatitis B surface antigen (anti-HBs) levels annually. Administer additional doses if anti-HBs levels decline to <10 mIU/mL.

I. For all persons with chronic liver disease.

J. Withhold MMR or other measles-containing vaccines from HIV-infected persons with evidence of severe immunosuppression (see MMWR 1998;47 [No. RR-8];21-2 and MMWR 2002;51[No. RR-2];22-4).

K. Persons with impaired humoral immunity but intact cellular immunity may be vaccinated (see MMWR 1999;48[No. RR-6]).

L. No data to support a recommendation.

the great amount of morbidity and mortality related to this preventable disease.

Pneumococcal pneumonia is a respiratory disease that presents with high fever, cough, and chest pain among older adults. Along with influenza, it is one of the most common causes of preventable morbidity and mortality among the older population. In fact, the Centers for Disease Control and Prevention reported that this disease results in more deaths in the United States each year than all other vaccine-preventable diseases combined.[30] Pneumococcal vaccination is recommended in all older adults aged 65 years and over, especially those with chronic respiratory and immunodeficiency illnesses. Moreover, the Centers for Disease Control recommends that Alaskan Natives and those from specific Native American populations are at higher risk.[30] The pneumococcal polysaccharide vaccine provides protection against the 23 most common types of pneumococcal bacteria. Vaccination once in a lifetime is usually sufficient. However, a second dose is necessary if the first dose was received under the age of 65 years or if certain chronic medical conditions place the older adult at high risk for respiratory infection. The vaccination is very safe, with minor side effects appearing in less than 1% of the population and adverse reactions reported rarely.

## Exercise

Researchers have shown that exercise has substantial impacts on the overall health of older persons. Exercise is an integral component to health maintenance and improvement in the older population. Resnick and Spellbring[6] reported that exercise has many obvious and supported benefits, including improving strength, preventing disease, decreasing falls, improving sleep, enhancing mood, and reducing physical disabilities. Moreover, exercise is an important component in fighting depression.

Research has clearly supported the benefits of exercise as key to health promotion in the older population. However, only a fraction of people over 65 years old participate in exercise programs on a regular basis or have a personal exercise regimen. Resnick and Spellbring[6] reported that in the United States 40% of persons aged 65 years and older do not exercise, and less than 10% exercise vigorously. One of the many reasons for lack of exercise among older adults lies in the fact that older adults did not grow up during a period in history when society valued exercise for its health benefits, social fun, and pleasure.

The first step in helping older adults to begin an exercise program is to assess their readiness and motivation to start. Many factors precipitate inactivity in older adults that must be assessed, including lack of motivation, social issues and cultural expectations, environmental factors, co-morbidity, fear of falling, impaired health, unpleasant sensations associated with exercise, and lack of knowledge about benefits. Furthermore, an even greater challenge is convincing older adults to maintain an exercise regimen. Resnick and Spellbring[6] found that half of sedentary adults who begin a program stop exercising after 6 months. As stated earlier in discussing smoking cessation with older adults, Mackey[16] suggested making statements such as "I feel that your lack of exercise poses a significant health risk" to define the problem and begin the dialogue with the patient.

Health care providers are ideally suited to act as coaches in order to assist older adults to begin and maintain a program of exercise in their lives. Coaching should begin with a discussion of the benefits of exercise, followed by assistance with the selection of exercises that older adults find fun and exciting. The health care providers should recommend that older adults find exercise partners, as this is a key ingredient to maintaining an exercise program. Exercise programs should be designed to include strength training, flexibility, and balance. One of the well-accepted exercises among older adults is walking. Walking is an exercise that requires only a good pair of shoes and can take place anywhere at any time. Older adults also enjoy weight-bearing and aquatic exercises that reduce muscle wasting, support and maintain functional mobility, promote independence, and prevent falls. Aquatic exercises are also a pain-free method of promoting health and increasing functional ability for older adults with arthritis and osteoporosis.

Resnick and Spellbring[6] recommended several interventions that may improve adherence to exercise programs, including teaching about the benefits of exercise, establishing appropriate exercise goals for individual participants, and increasing pleasant sensations associated with exercise. Moreover, exercise regimens must be individualized because of the heterogeneous nature of older adults with varying needs and influencing factors. Motivation is a key factor in convincing older people to exercise. Health care providers must focus on the integrity and individuality of each client and work creatively in partnership with the person to find what motivates them to a higher level of physical activity. Grove and Elliott[31] found that continuity, simplicity, cognitive motivational techniques, and consistent leadership are hallmarks of successful exercise programs whose participants adhere to a regular exercise regime.

## SECONDARY PREVENTION

Because primary health promotion activities are not always able to prevent the occurrence of a disease, secondary prevention efforts become crucial in detecting the disease at the earliest possible stage. Early detection affords the patient and care provider maximum choice and maximum effect in terms of response to the identified disease. In particular, secondary prevention is practiced in order to decrease the risks associated with certain medical conditions (such as diabetes, hypertension, coronary heart disease, osteoporosis, and cancer) that have been linked to significant loss of functioning in older adults.[32] In addition, researchers have cited the benefit of secondary prevention to "reduce the potential years of life lost in premature mortality and ensure better quality of remaining life".[33] A discussion of secondary prevention efforts with older clients is clearly warranted, given the conflicting data on the usefulness of certain screening mechanisms, especially with those over 85 years of age.[34] Geriatric health care providers need to develop a *consensus* on best practices to incorporate with their patients. The discussion is also necessary in order to understand the factors that specifically influence the likelihood that older adults will participate in secondary health-promoting activities.[32] Such a focus would allow care providers to recognize the *barriers* to secondary prevention measures that need to be reduced. Table 14–3 includes the recommended secondary screening tests for older adults. The following will provide an overview of key areas amenable to secondary prevention efforts.

### Cardiovascular Disease

This constellation of disorders presents a major focus of concern for older persons because approximately 84% of deaths related to cardiovascular disease (CVD) in the United States occur in people age 65 years and older.[35] In 2001, over 4 million individuals in this age group were discharged from acute care facilities with a primary diagnosis of CVD. Williams et al.[36] noted that, on autopsy, obstructive coronary artery disease was found in approximately 50% of older women and 70% to 80% of older men. Even with proper diagnosis and management, patients face increased morbidity and mortality risks. Earlier identification of CVD could conceivably reduce the progression of the disease and the occurrence of adverse coronary events.[37] Secondary prevention efforts would, therefore, focus on screening for the risk factors of

**Table 14–3** Diseases and Other Adverse Health Effects for Which Smoking Is Identified as a Cause in the Current Surgeon General's Report

| Disease | Highest Level Conclusion from Previous Surgeon General's Reports (Year) | Conclusion from the 2004 Surgeon General's Report |
| --- | --- | --- |
| **Cancer** | | |
| Bladder cancer | "Smoking is a cause of bladder cancer; cessation reduces risk by about 50 percent after only a few years, in comparison with continued smoking." (1990, p. 10) | "The evidence is sufficient to infer a causal relationship between smoking and . . . bladder cancer." |
| Cervical cancer | "Smoking has been consistently associated with an increased risk for cervical cancer." (2001, p. 224) | "The evidence is sufficient to infer a causal relationship between smoking and cervical cancer." |
| Esophageal cancer | "Cigarette smoking is a major cause of esophageal cancer in the United States." (1982, p. 7) | "The evidence is sufficient to infer a causal relationship between smoking and cancers of the esophagus." |
| Kidney cancer | "Cigarette smoking is a contributory factor in the development of kidney cancer in the United States. The term 'contributory factor' by no means excludes the possibility of a causal role for smoking in cancers of this site." (1982, p. 7) | "The evidence is sufficient to infer a causal relationship between smoking and renal cell, [and] renal pelvis . . . cancers." |
| Laryngeal cancer | "Cigarette smoking is causally associated with cancer of the lung, larynx, oral cavity, and esophagus in women as well as in men. . . ." (1980, p. 126) | "The evidence is sufficient to infer a causal relationship between smoking and cancer of the larynx." |
| Leukemia | "Leukemia has recently been implicated as a smoking-related disease . . . but this observation has not been consistent." (1990, p. 176) | "The evidence is sufficient to infer a causal relationship between smoking and acute myeloid leukemia." |

*continues*

**Table 14–3**   continued

| Disease | Highest Level Conclusion from Previous Surgeon General's Reports (Year) | Conclusion from the 2004 Surgeon General's Report |
|---|---|---|
| Lung cancer | "Additional epidemiological, pathological, and experimental data not only confirm the conclusion of the Surgeon General's 1964 Report regarding lung cancer in men but strengthen the causal relationship of smoking to lung cancer in women." (1967, p. 36) | "The evidence is sufficient to infer a causal relationship between smoking and lung cancer." |
| Oral cancer | "Cigarette smoking is a major cause of cancers of the oral cavity in the United States." (1982, p. 6) | "The evidence is sufficient to infer a causal relationship between smoking and cancers of the oral cavity and pharynx." |
| Pancreatic cancer | "Smoking cessation reduces the risk of pancreatic cancer, compared with continued smoking, although this reduction in risk may only be measurable after 10 years of abstinence." (1990, p. 10) | "The evidence is sufficient to infer a causal relationship between smoking and pancreatic cancer." |
| Stomach cancer | "Data on smoking and cancer of the stomach . . . are unclear." (2001, p. 231) | "The evidence is sufficient to infer a causal relationship between smoking and gastric cancers." |
| **Cardiovascular diseases** | | |
| Abdominal aortic aneurysm | "Death from rupture of an atherosclerotic abdominal aneurysm is more common in cigarette smokers than in nonsmokers." (1983, p. 195) | "The evidence is sufficient to infer a causal relationship between smoking and abdominal aortic aneurysm." |
| Atherosclerosis | "Cigarette smoking is the most powerful risk factor predisposing to atherosclerotic peripheral vascular disease." (1983, p. 8) | "The evidence is sufficient to infer a causal relationship between smoking and subclinical atherosclerosis." |

| Disease | *Highest Level Conclusion from Previous Surgeon General's Reports (Year)* | *Conclusion from the 2004 Surgeon General's Report* |
|---|---|---|
| **Cardiovascular diseases** | | |
| Cerebrovascular disease | "Cigarette smoking is a major cause of cerebrovascular disease (stroke), the third leading cause of death in the United States." (1989, p. 12) | "The evidence is sufficient to infer a causal relationship between smoking and stroke." |
| Coronary heart disease | "In summary, for the purposes of preventive medicine, it can be concluded that smoking is causally related to coronary heart disease for both men and women in the United States." (1979, p. 1–15) | "The evidence is sufficient to infer a causal relationship between smoking and coronary heart disease." |
| **Respiratory diseases** | | |
| Chronic obstructive pulmonary disease | "Cigarette smoking is the most important of the causes of chronic bronchitis in the United States, and increases the risk of dying from chronic bronchitis." (1964, p. 302) | "The evidence is sufficient to infer a causal relationship between active smoking and chronic obstructive pulmonary disease morbidity and mortality." |
| Pneumonia | "Smoking cessation reduces rates of respiratory symptoms such as cough, sputum production, and wheezing, and respiratory infections such as bronchitis and pneumonia, compared with continued smoking." (1990, p. 11) | "The evidence is sufficient to infer a causal relationship between smoking and acute respiratory illnesses, including pneumonia, in persons without underlying smoking-related chronic obstructive lung disease." |
| **Other effects** | | |
| Cataract | "Women who smoke have an increased risk for cataract." (2001, p. 331) | "The evidence is sufficient to infer a causal relationship between smoking and nuclear cataract." |

*continues*

**Table 14–3**    continued

| Disease | Highest Level Conclusion from Previous Surgeon General's Reports (Year) | Conclusion from the 2004 Surgeon General's Report |
|---|---|---|
| Diminished health status/morbidity | "Relationships between smoking and cough or phlegm are strong and consistent; they have been amply documented and are judged to be causal. . . ." (1984, p. 47) | "The evidence is sufficient to infer a causal relationship between smoking and diminished health status that may be manifest as increased absenteeism from work and increased use of medical care services." |
| | "Consideration of evidence from many different studies has led to the conclusion that cigarette smoking is the overwhelmingly most important cause of cough, sputum, chronic bronchitis, and mucus hypersecretion." (1984, p. 48) | "The evidence is sufficient to infer a causal relationship between smoking and increased risks for adverse surgical outcomes related to wound healing and respiratory complications." |
| Hip fractures | "Women who currently smoke have an increased risk for hip fracture compared with women who do not smoke." (2001, p. 321) | "The evidence is sufficient to infer a causal relationship between smoking and hip fractures." |
| Low bone density | "Postmenopausal women who currently smoke have lower bone density than do women who do not smoke." (2001, p. 321) | "In postmenopausal women, the evidence is sufficient to infer a causal relationship between smoking and low bone density." |
| Peptic ulcer disease | "The relationship between cigarette smoking and death rates from peptic ulcer, especially gastric ulcer, is confirmed. In addition, morbidity data suggest a similar relationship exists with the prevalence of reported disease from this cause." (1967, p. 40) | "The evidence is sufficient to infer a causal relationship between smoking and peptic ulcer disease in persons who are *Helicobacter pylori* positive." |

Sources: U.S. Department of Health, Education, and Welfare 1964, 1967, 1979; U.S. Department of Health and Human Services 1980, 1982, 1983, 1984, 1989, 1990, 1994, 2001.

Adapted from http://www.cdc.gov/tobacco/sgr/sgr_2004/pdf/executivesummary.pdf

hypertension (HTN) and cholesterol levels in order to reduce the morbidity and mortality rates associated with diseases such as coronary heart disease (CHD) and the occurrence of myocardial infarction (MI) and stroke. The incidence of CHD is significant for those aged 65 to 74 years (approximately 10 to 14 of 1,000 for women and 22 of 1,000 for men), and rates rise sharply (particularly for non-black women) in those aged 75 years and older (approximately 25 to 28 of 1,000 for women and 31 to 35 of 1,000 for men).[35] Women are noted to have MIs at older ages than men do, explaining in part their greater likelihood to die from the MI within a few weeks.[35]

Stroke is the other major vascular event and is noted to be a "leading cause of serious, long-term disability" in the United States.[35] The majority of deaths from stroke occur in people age 65 years and older, and more than 25% of the people from this age group who experience a stroke die within a year of the event.[35] HTN has been defined by the Joint National Committee (JNC)-VII criteria as systolic pressure of 140 mm Hg or higher or diastolic pressure of 90 mm Hg or higher or taking antihypertensive medications. HTN is considered to be a major risk factor for CHD, peripheral artery disease, and cerebrovascular disease.[36] Uncontrolled HTN can often lead to heart failure and/or chronic renal failure. It is common among older men and especially older women. The National Health and Nutrition Examination Survey IV (NHANES IV) found increasing rates of HTN in each of the three oldest age groups, reporting that 43% of men and 58% of women in the 55 to 64 years age group, 55% of men and 65% of women in the 65 to 74 years age group, and 59% of men and 71% of women in the 75 years and older age group were found to have HTN.

Studies have shown that patients 60 to 80 years old clearly benefit from antihypertensive treatment, including prevention of strokes and heart failure and reduced mortality rates.[38] There have been fewer studies involving patients older than 80 years from which to draw conclusions, but one meta-analysis by Gueyffier et al.[39] provided support for the benefits of active antihypertensive treatment to reduce the risks of stroke, major cardiovascular events, and heart failure in this age group. Guidelines issued by the World Health Organization[40] also identify the clear link between control of HTN and reduction in morbidity and mortality related to stroke, CHD, heart failure, and chronic renal failure. The US Preventive Services Task Force[41] recommended screening at least every 2 years for adults, with more frequent screening if the blood pressure readings are borderline.

The American Heart Association considers adults whose total cholesterol level (TCL) is 240 mg/dL or higher to be at high risk for both

CHD and adverse coronary events.[35] TCLs between 200 and 239 mg/dL are believed to place the individual in the borderline high-risk range. Low-density lipoprotein cholesterol levels of 130 mg/dL or higher are also believed to place the individual at higher risk of CHD, as do high-density lipoprotein cholesterol levels of less than 40 mg/dL.[42] An alarming number of older people in the United States fall into these high-risk categories. Over 60% of men and over 76% of women aged 65 to 74 years have TCLs greater than or equal to 200 mg/dL; for those age 75 years and older, the percentages fall slightly to approximately 42% of men and 66% of women.[42] Those individuals at greatest risk (i.e., with TCLs greater than or equal to 240 mg/dL) include roughly 19% of men and 37% of women aged 65 to 74 years and 10% of men and 27% of women aged 75 years and older.[42]

Racial and ethnic factors appear to interact with gender in influencing prevalence rates as well. In general, by the age of 45 years, there is a greater percentage of women than men who have TCLs of 200 mg/dL or higher. Among women, whites have the highest percentage (54%), followed by blacks (46%), Mexican Americans (45%), and Native Americans (38%). The ranking for men by racial and ethnic background falls out slightly differently, with Mexican American men ranking highest (54%), followed by whites (51%), Japanese Americans (42%), Native Americans (38%), and then blacks (37%).[42] Age, gender, and racial and ethnic backgrounds all need to be considered in assessing an individual's risk for developing CHD.

Screening for cholesterol and lipid levels in older persons has been influenced by the debate on the value of lipid-lowering treatment in older individuals.[36] Several studies have documented the fact that high cholesterol levels in older persons who are at risk for a cardiovascular event are both underdiagnosed and undertreated.[43,44] Older individuals without CHD have generally not been included in studies exploring the value of cholesterol-lowering therapy as primary prevention.[37] However, because the cholesterol level needed to produce significant atherosclerotic plaque burden decreases with age,[45] even older individuals with currently "normal" cholesterol levels are faced with a certain disease risk that warrants ongoing monitoring and/or consideration of pharmacotherapy. Older patients are also considered to face a greater absolute risk for CHD and cardiovascular events, leading some researchers to draw the conclusion that treatment with lipid-lowering agents produces therefore a greater absolute benefit for older individuals.[36] Finally, although there are few actual data available to guide practice with patients who are 75 years and older, there is also no evidence of decreased effect with age. However, as cautioned by Williams et al.,[36] "The clinician should not overlook quality of life issues, concomitant illness, and remaining life expectancy in these patients" (p. 1742). In terms of scheduled screening, the US Preventive Services Task Force[46] recommended having cholesterol measured every 5 years after the age of 45 years, with more frequent measurements if the levels are abnormal or if the patient is at high risk for CHD.

In summary, CHD is the leading cause of morbidity and mortality in older persons.[47] Lowering blood pressure and cholesterol levels lowers the risk for CHD.[42] Studies have found alarming prevalence rates of HTN (43% to 71%) (NHANES IV) and hypercholesterolemia (42% to 76%)[42] among older persons in the United States. Care providers have a responsibility to meet their clients' needs, maintain their safety, and maximize the quality of their lives; screening for cholesterol and blood pressure levels can achieve all of these objectives.

## Diabetes

Diabetes mellitus (DM) is a group of diseases that affect multiple body systems and is considered to be a specific risk factor for the development of CHD and the occurrence of adverse coronary events in older persons.[48] There is an increase in the prevalence of both insulin resistance and DM with age.[36] Estimates have indicated that up to 20% of the US population will have developed Type II DM by the age of 75 years.[49] In people between the ages of 60 and 74 years, approximately 12% of men and 13% of women have physician-diagnosed diabetes. Prevalence rises slightly in men aged 75 years and older (14%) and remains unchanged in women of this age group. Rates are higher for Japanese-American men (ages 71 to 93 years) who have been found to have a 17% prevalence rate of diagnosed diabetes, with another 19% having unrecognized diabetes and 32% having prediabetes (based on impaired glucose tolerance testing).[35] A total of 8.6 million people aged 60 years and older (18% of all people in this age group) have recognized diabetes. This compares with a 6.3% prevalence rate in the general population.[50]

Long-term complications associated with DM include CHD and stroke, HTN, blindness, kidney disease, neuropathies, and amputations.[50] Having diabetes increases susceptibility to other illnesses, which in turn have worse prognoses in people with DM. In 2000, diabetes was the sixth leading cause of death in the United States, and the risk of death for people with diabetes is about twice that of people without diabetes.[50] Given these statistics, it is even more imperative to develop effective methods of screening to reduce both morbidity and mortality in individuals with DM. Screening for Type II DM can be accomplished when the disease is still asymptomatic.[49]

Effective screening, in part, means the identification of susceptible populations. In addition to age, race and ethnicity have been shown to be significant factors in identifying the most at-risk individuals.[50] Native Americans and Alaska Natives have a 14.5% prevalence rate of diabetes and are more than twice as likely to have diabetes as non-Hispanic whites. Non-Hispanic blacks have the next highest prevalence rate at 11.4% and are more than 1.5 times more likely than non-Hispanic whites to have diabetes. Both Mexican Americans and residents of Puerto Rico are approximately twice as likely to have diagnosed diabetes as non-Hispanic whites, who have a prevalence rate of 8.4%.[50]

Screening efforts need to be able to identify both prediabetes and diabetes in at-risk patients. Prediabetes is usually determined by impaired fasting glucose levels of between 100 and 125 mg/dL and/or impaired glucose tolerance where blood sugar is between 140 and 199 mg/dL after a 2-hour glucose tolerance test.[50] Patients so identified could begin programs to decrease weight and increase physical activity with the goal of preventing or at least delaying the onset of DM. Health care providers need to be aware that patients with prediabetes are already at increased risk for CHD and stroke.[50]

Although there are no preventive measures for Type I DM, patients who are identified with Type II DM can also be assisted in making lifestyle changes (e.g., alterations in diet and activity level) and consideration of oral medications to control, and in some cases reverse, the progression of DM.[50] It is especially important to detect and manage DM in older CHD patients in order to decrease the risk for an adverse cardiovascular event. Older women with a history of both CHD and DM are three times more likely to develop heart failure.[51]

In summary, older patients in general are at greater risk for developing DM. Individuals with CHD are also at high risk to develop DM, and as already noted, older persons are at high risk for CHD. Early detection and management of Type II DM follows the American Diabetes Association (ADA) 2001 recommendations and guidelines[49] and allows the care provider the chance to work with the patient in avoiding or minimizing complications, reducing associated morbidity and mortality, and improving the patient's overall quality of life. The ADA recommends that women over 45 years of age have their blood glucose level checked every 3 years, with greater frequency indicated if the individual is at higher risk or is reporting signs and symptoms of diabetes.[52]

## Cancer

Although cancer can happen to anyone at any age, studies have shown that the occurrence of cancer increases with age. Approximately three fourths of all cancers are diagnosed in patients age 55 years and older.[53] In the 2002 National Health Interview Survey,[54] approximately 20% of people aged 65 to 74 years were found to have cancer, and approximately 24% of those aged 75 years old and older were found to have cancer. Individuals aged 65 years and older were found to account for 56% of all cases of breast cancer and 80% of all prostate cancer in 2002.[54] Cancer is second only to heart disease as a leading cause of death in the United States, being responsible for one of every four deaths.[53] The rates of cancer diagnosis and mortality are further influenced by factors such as race and socioeconomic status.[53] Evidence clearly supports screening efforts focused on high-risk populations because early detection increases the likelihood of successful treatment. However, some researchers have questioned the usefulness of cancer screening efforts in older persons, raising issues of benefits versus risks in light of decreased life expectancy and the impact of additional diagnostic and treatment procedures on the quality of life of older individuals. The following discussion focuses on some common forms of cancer found in older persons (including breast, cervical/uterine, prostate, and colorectal), information on incidence, prevalence, survival and mortality rates, currently available screening mechanisms and their rates of use, and recommended guidelines for practice. Some barriers to effective screening are also discussed.

In 2004, officials expected that over 200,000 new cases of *breast cancer* would be diagnosed in the United States, making it the most frequent nonskin cancer in women.[53] The risk of developing breast cancer increases with age. Between 1986 and 2000, women aged 50 years old and older were the only group to experience an increased incidence of breast cancer.[53] Lung cancer is the only form of cancer that caused more deaths in women. Fortunately, earlier detection and improved treatment combined in the 1990s to cause a 23% reduction in the mortality rates, although this mostly affected younger women. Early detection has meant a greater chance of survival for localized breast cancer, which now has a 5-year survival rate of 97%. The survival rate for cancer that has spread regionally is 79%, and cancer with metastases has only a 23% survival rate.[53]

Mammography is considered the most effective screening tool to detect breast cancer, although American Cancer Society (ACS) guidelines also recommend an annual clinical breast exam for women 40 years and older. The US Preventive Services Task Force likewise recommends both a clinical breast exam and a mammography every 1 to 2 years beginning at age 40.[52] The percentage of women age 40 years and older who reported having had a mammogram within the previous 2 years increased from 29% in 1987 to 70% in 2000.[5] By 2008, the ACS hopes to increase this number to 90%. The benefits of mammography screening for women 65 years and older has been a point of controversy among researchers and clinicians alike; Johs-Artisensi and McGill[55] argued that the data do in fact support the efficacy and effectiveness of mammography screening programs for women up to 80 years old and even beyond that if the woman is otherwise in good health. Mandelblatt et al.[56] also supported the notion of the cost-effectiveness of mammograms for women over age 65 years but recommended conducting the screening every 2 years. Finally, in a review of a clinical case, Stegbauer et al.[57] also pointed out the importance of teaching women to conduct monthly self-breast exams, as "women discover 80% of breast lumps by themselves" (p. 52). Bogner and Wittink pointed out how depression can interfere with older women obtaining mammography.[58]

*Cervical cancer* is far less common than breast cancer. An estimated 10,500 cases were diagnosed in 2004. Screening via the Pap smear method has become increasingly popular and has directly contributed to the marked decrease in mortality rates over the past several decades.[53] Although the Pap smear is not perfect, it has allowed health care providers to detect early changes in cervical cells before the cancer has become invasive. Consequently, survival rates for persons with preinvasive lesions are now 100%. Invasive cervical cancer also has high success rates with early detection and treatment, with a 5-year survival rate of 92% for localized cancers. However, African Americans are far less likely than whites to be diagnosed at this early stage, with less than half of their cervical cancers diagnosed at the localized stage.[53] Guidelines suggested by the ACS recommend that women begin to have Pap smears no later than the age of 21 years and continue to be screened every year until about the age of 30 years. At that point, if the women has had normal Pap smears 3 years in a row, she may then arrange to be screened every 2 to 3 years. By the time a woman reaches the age of 70 years, the ACS suggests that if she has had three consecutive normal Pap tests in the past 10 years then she may choose to stop screening.[5] Sirovich et al.[59] questioned the continued rather large volume of Pap testing on women over 65 years old in the United States, citing the rarity of cervical cancer deaths and the "unknown benefits of screening in this age group" (p. 189).

*Prostate cancer* poses a major threat to older men, with approximately 230,000 new cases occurring in the United States in 2004.[53] It is the second leading cause of cancer death in men. Both incidence and death rates are significantly higher in African American men than white men, and more than 70% of all cases of prostate cancer are diagnosed in men over the age of 65 years.[53] Incidence rates rose dramatically in the early 1990s with the advent of prostate-specific antigen (PSA) testing but have since then begun to level off. The early detection afforded by the PSA test resulted in 86% of prostate cancers being discovered in either the localized or regional stages, with a 100% 5-year survival rate.[53] In spite of this success, there remains a lack of consensus among groups of experts about use of the prostate cancer screening mechanisms. The PSA is a marker for both benign and malignant prostate activity. There are age-specific PSA ranges, with a PSA cutoff value of 4.0 ng/ml providing the best specificity and sensitivity for prostate cancer.[60] Because prostate tumors grow slowly and the PSA test is able to detect them before they become clinically significant, some clinicians feel that this leads to the initiation of treatment at a time when it may not yet be clinically necessary. At this point, the ACS recommends that the PSA test and digital rectal examination should be offered to men starting at the age of 50 years, assuming that they have a life expectancy of at least 10 years.[5] Men who are at high risk (e.g., African-American men) should begin screening at the age of 45 years. The guidelines also specify, however, that the individual patient should be informed about the benefits and limitations of the tests in order to make an informed decision.[5] In a review of data from the 2000 National Health Interview Survey, Lu-Yao et al.[61] found that 32.5% of men aged 75 years and older underwent PSA screening on the advice of their care providers. The authors considered this rate high in light of questions about the efficacy of PSA screening and the long natural history of untreated prostate cancer and recommended that men aged 75 years and older not be screened. In spite of this controversy, the ACS has set, for one of their 2015 nationwide objectives, the goal of increasing to 90% the men age 50 years and older who follow their prostate cancer detection guidelines.[53]

Estimates of 147,000 cases of *colorectal cancer* to occur in 2004 bring to light another significant threat to both older men and women. Colorectal cancer is the third most common cancer in both men and women.[53] More than 90% of the cases are diagnosed in people age 50 years and above. Survival rates are less impressive than with other cancers, with 1- and 5-year survival rates of 83% and 62%, respectively. If the cancer is found at an early, localized stage, the 5-year survival rate is 90% (slightly more than one third of colorectal cancers are caught at this stage). If the cancer has spread regionally, the 5-year survival rate drops to 66%; if it has reached a stage of metastases, the rate is a grim 9%.[5] There are five possible colorectal cancer screening tests that the ACS offers in its guidelines for men and women age 50 years and beyond: a fecal occult blood test (FOBT) every year, a flexible sigmoidoscopy (FSIG) every 5 years, annual FOBT, *and* FSIG every 5 years, a double contrast barium enema every 5 years, and a colonoscopy every 10 years.[53] Positive results from noncolonoscopy tests should be followed up by colonoscopy. This is useful for detecting some cancers, preventing others, and removing polyps. Screening rates for all of these mechanisms are noted to be very low (e.g., 41% of those 50 years old and older having completed either the FOBT within the past year or the FSIG within the past 5 years)[62] and were found to be lowest among those with no health insurance, those with less than a high school education, among Hispanics and Asian Americans, and among recent immigrants.[5] In general, individuals aged 65 years and older were more likely to have had a colorectal cancer screening test than those 50 to 64 years old. The ACS has another 2015 nationwide objective to increase to 75% the proportion of people aged 50 years and older who follow their guidelines for colorectal screening.[5]

In summary, older persons face greater risks of developing cancer than younger age groups. There continues to be controversy about what screening mechanisms are useful and effective in this population, and what the longer term consequences are of their use. Keeping in mind that people will generally follow their care provider's recommendations,[5] clinicians should develop a framework to use in guiding them and their patients in making decisions regarding screening. Walter and Covinsky[34] offered just such a framework that incorporated estimates of life expectancy, risks of cancer death, and outcomes of screening mechanisms to determine the potential benefits of screening.

## Osteoporosis

Osteoporosis affects primarily postmenopausal white women, although it can also be seen in men and women of other ethnic backgrounds. It causes bone fragility secondary to low bone density and deterioration of bone tissue, which in turn increases the risk for fractures, especially in the areas of the hips, wrists, and spine.[63] As much as 70% of fractures that occur in people aged 45 years and older can be seen as related to the osteoporosis process.[64] Decreases in bone mineral density can be seen in both men and women by midlife, and estrogen deficiency as well as family history of osteoporosis increases an individual's risk for the disease.[63] Wrist fractures can often be seen in individuals from their late 50s to early 70s; the more serious hip and vertebral fractures tend to happen when the individuals get to their late 70s to 80s. Mortality risks are significant, in that one in five patients who fractures his or her hip dies within a year of the fracture.[63] In spite of the serious consequences, universal screening is not recommended; the National Osteoporosis Foundation recommends bone density screening by dual-energy x-ray absorptiometry for women identified as high risk, including women age 65 years and older, postmenopausal women under the age of 65 years who have specific risk factors for osteoporosis (estrogen deficiency, white race, low body mass index, family history, etc.), postmenopausal women who present with fractures, and women who have been on prolonged hormone replacement therapy.[63]

## Thyroid Dysfunction

The prevalence of thyroid disease increases with age; individuals over 60 years old have a prevalence of hyperthyroidism that ranges from 0.5% to 2.3%, and a prevalence of hypothyroidism that ranges from 2% to 7.4%.[65] The American Thyroid Association has reported that one of every five women is at risk for developing thyroid problems at some point in their lives.[64] Their clinical presentation is also often different from younger patients, and diagnosis is difficult, particularly if they are manifesting symptoms of a subclinical abnormality. Although the structure of the thyroid gland changes, results of thyroid function tests are often normal in patients.[65] There is no consensus as to when and how often screening should occur. Both the American Thyroid Association and the American Association of Clinical Endocrinologists have recommended that everyone over 35 years old be screened every 5 years using the thyroid stimulating hormone (TSH) test.[64] Other experts have recommended withholding the screening unless and until the patient shows actual symptoms of thyroid problems. The rationale for this position is based on the fact that there is little in the way of data demonstrating positive outcomes from treating early asymptomatic disease and that the patient faces some potential adverse effects of therapy.[65]

## SUMMARY AND CONCLUSION

Despite the many myths of aging that fuel public and health care providers' opinions of health promotion among older adults, it is clear that the older population may experience great benefits from health promotion. Although much damage may have been done through years of smoking, alcohol use, and obesity, lifestyle changes and early disease detection may result in great improvements in health, functional status, and quality of life. Older adults are never too old to benefit from health promotion activities. The implementation of health promotion activities in the older adult population has played a substantial role in expanding the life span of older adults already; it is exciting to envision the impact of greater health promotion implementation on future population projects.

This chapter presented health promotion assessment and intervention strategies within two levels of prevention. Primary prevention included interventions to prevent an illness or disease from occurring, such as smoking cessation, immunizations, proper nutrition, and regular exercise. Secondary prevention strategies included interventions focused on early disease detection through the use of interventions such as routine mammograms, hypertension screening, and PSA blood tests. Through the exploration of these primary and secondary levels of prevention among older adults, it is hoped that the incidence and prevalence of harmful health behaviors will be reduced through the implementation of best assessment practices and interventions.

## REFERENCES

1. Padula CA, McNatt M. Older married couples and health promotion. *J Gerontol Nurs.* 2004;30:38–46.

2. Appel DW, Aldrich TK. Smoking cessation in the elderly. *Clin Geriatr Med.* 2003;19:77–100.

3. Ammerman AA, Lindquist CH, Lohr KN, Hersey J. The efficacy of behavioral interventions to modify dietary fat and fruit and vegetable intake: A review of the evidence, *Prev Med.* 2002;35:25–41.

4. Telford R, Rogers A. What influences elderly people's decisions about whether to accept the influenza vaccination? A qualitative study. *Health Educ Res.* 2003;18:743–753.

5. American Cancer Society. *Cancer Prevention and Early Detection: Facts and Figures.* Atlanta, GA: Author; 2004.

6. Resnick B, Spellbring A. Understanding what motivates older adults to exercise. *J Gerontol Nurs.* 2000;26:34–42.

7. Dwyer JT. *Screening Older Americans' Nutritional Health: Current Practices and Future Responsibilities.* Washington, DC: Nutritional Screening Institute; 1991.

8. Robertson RG, Mantagnini M. Geriatric Failure to Thrive. *Am Fam Phys.* 2004;70(2): 343–351.

9. US Preventive Services Task Force. Behavioral counseling in primary care to promote a healthy diet: Recommendations and rationale. *Am J Nurs.* 2003;103: 81–91.

10. Zizi F, Jean-Louis G, Magai C, Greenidge KC, Wolintz AH, Heath-Phillip O. Sleep complaints and visual impairment among older Americans: A community-based study. *J Gerontol.* 2002;57A:10m691–m694.

11. Ramesh M, Roberts G. Use of night-time benzodiazepines in an elderly inpatient population. *J Clin Pharm Ther.* 2002;27:93–97.

12. Montgomery P. Treatments for sleep problems in elderly people. *BMJ.* 2002;325: 1049.

13. Buysse DJ, Reynolds III CF, Monk TH, Berman SR, Kupfer DJ. The Pittsburgh Sleep Quality Index: A new instrument for psychiatric practice and research. *J Psychiatr Res.* 1989;28:193–213.

14. Wallace M. Pain in older adults. *Ann Long Term Care.* 2001;9:50–58.

15. US Department of Health and Human Services. *The Health Consequences of Smoking. Executive Summary;* 2004. Available from http://www.cdc.gov/tobacco/sgr/sgr_2004/pdf/executivesummary.pdf

16. Mackey SL. Therapeutic lifestyle change. *Clin Rev.* 2004;14:56–62.

17. Centers for Disease Control and Prevention. *You can quit smoking consumer guide;* 2004. Available from http://www.cdc.gov/tobacco/quit/canquit.htm

18. Levin SM, Kruger J, eds. *Substance Abuse Among Older Adults: A Guide for Social Service Providers.* Rockville, MD: Substance Abuse and Mental Health Services Administration; 2000.

19. Menninger JA. Assessment and treatment of alcoholism and substance related disorders in the elderly. *Bull Menninger Clin.* 2002;66:166–184.

20. Robert Wood Johnson Foundation. *Substance Abuse: The Nation's Number One Health Problem.* Prepared by the Schneider Institute for Health Policy, Brandeis University; 2001. Available from http://www.rwjfliterature.org/chartbook/chartbook.htm. Princeton, NJ: Author.

21. Mokdad A, Marks J, Stroup D, Gerberding J. Actual cause of death in the United States. *JAMA.* 2004;291:1238–1245.

22. Centers for Disease Control and Prevention. *Measures of Alcohol Consumption and Alcohol-Related Health Effects from Excessive Consumption;* 2004. http://www.cdc.gov/alcohol/factsheets/general_information.htm

23. Ondus KA, Hujer ME, Mann AE, Mion LC. Substance abuse and the hospitalized elderly. *Orthoped Nurs.* 1999;18:27–36.

24. Hall RCW, Hall RCW, Chapman MJ. Identifying geriatric patients at risk for suicide and depression. *Clin Geriatr.* 2003;11:36–38, 40–44.

25. National Institutes of Health. The physicians' guide to helping patients with alcohol problems. US Department of Health and Human Services, Public Health Service. NIH Pub. No. 95-3769; 1995.

26. Mersey DJ. Recognition of alcohol and substance abuse. *Am Fam Physician.* 2003;67:1529–1532.

27. Blow FC, Walton MA, Chermack ST, Mudd SA, Brower KJ. Older adult treatment outcome following elder-specific inpatient alcoholism treatment. *J Substance Abuse Treat.* 2000;19:67–75.

28. Centers for Disease Control and Prevention. *Immunizations;* 2004. http://www.cdc.gov/programs/immun.htm

29. Centers for Disease Control and Prevention. *Key Facts About the Flu;* 2004. Available from http://www.cdc.gov/flu/keyfacts.htm

30. Centers for Disease Control and Prevention. *Pneumococcal Polysaccharide Vaccine: What You Need to Know;* 2004. Available from http://www.cdc.gov/nip/publications/vis-ppv.pdf

31. Grove N, Elliott B. Motivating the well elderly to exercise. *J Community Health Nurs.* 1999;16:179–190.

32. Wang L, van Belle G, Kukull WB, Larson EB. Predictors of functional change: A longitudinal study of nondemented people aged 65 and older. *J Am Geriatr Soc.* 2002;50:1525–1534.

33. Resnick B. Promoting health in older adults: A four-year analysis. *J Am Acad Nurse Pract.* 2001;13:23–33.

34. Walter LC, Covinsky KE. Cancer screening in elderly patients: A framework for individualized decision making. *JAMA.* 2001;285:2750–2756.

35. American Heart Association. *Older Americans and Cardiovascular Diseases: Statistics;* 2004. Available from http://www.americanheart.org/ (Accessed October 3, 2004).

36. Williams MA, Fleg JL, Ades PA, et al. Secondary prevention of coronary heart disease in the elderly (with emphasis on patients ≥75 years of age). *Circulation.* 2002;105:1735–1743.

37. LaRosa JC. Prevention and treatment of coronary heart disease: Who benefits? *Circulation.* 2001;104:1688–1692.

38. MacMahon S, Rodger A. The effects of blood pressure reduction in older patients: An overview of five randomized controlled trials in elderly hypertensives. *J Clin Exp Hyperten.* 1993;15:967–978.

39. Gueyffier F, Bulpit C, Boissel JP, et al. Antihypertensive drugs in very old people: A sub-group meta-analysis of randomized controlled trials. *Lancet.* 1999;353:793–796.

40. World Health Organization Society of Hypertension. Guidelines for the management of hypertension. *J Hypertens.* 1999;17:151–183.

41. US Preventive Services Task Force. *Screening for High Blood Pressure: Recommendations and Rationale.* Rockville, MD: Agency for Healthcare Research and Quality; 2003. Available from http://www.ahrq.gov/ (Accessed October 17, 2004).

42. AHA Cholesterol Statistics. *American Heart Association;* 2004. Available from http://www.americanheart.org (Accessed October 3, 2004).

43. Aronow WS. Underutilization of lipid-lowering drugs in older persons with prior MI and a serum low-density lipoprotein cholesterol >125 mg/dL. *Am J Cardiol.* 1998;82:668–669, A6, A8.

44. Clinical Quality Improvement Network Investigators. Low incidence of assessment and modification of risk factors in acute care patients at high risk for cardiovascular events, particularly among females and the elderly. *Am J Cardiol.* 1995;76: 570–573.

45. Grundy SM, Cleeman JI, Rifkind BM, Kuller LH, Coordinating Committee of the National Cholesterol Education Program. Cholesterol lowering in the elderly population. *Arch Intern Med.* 1999;159:1670–1678.

46. US Preventive Services Task Force. *Screening for Lipid Disorders: Recommendations and Rationale.* Rockville, MD: Agency for Healthcare Research and Quality; 2003. Available from http://www.ahrq.gov/ (Accessed October 17, 2004).

47. LaRosa JC. From bench to bedside. Prevention and treatment of coronary heart disease. Who benefits? *Circulation.* 2001;104(14):1688–1692.

48. Vokonas PS, Kannel WB. Diabetes mellitus and CHD in the elderly. *Clin Geriatr Med.* 1996;2:69–78.

49. Jones ED, Kennedy-Malone L, Wideman L. Early detection of type 2 diabetes among older African Americans. *Geriatr Nurs.* 2004;25(1):24–28.

50. Centers for Disease Control and Prevention. *National Diabetes Fact Sheet: General Information and National Estimates on Diabetes in the U.S., 2002.* Atlanta, GA: US Department of Health and Human Services, Centers for Disease Control and Prevention; 2003.

51. ADA—Diabetes News. Older women with heart disease, diabetes have triple the risk of heart failure. *In Diabetes Today;* 2004. Available from http://www.diabetes.org/ (Accessed October 3, 2004).

52. Women's Screening Tests. *Mayo Clinic;* 2004. Available from http://www.mayoclinic.com/ (Accessed October 17, 2004).

53. American Cancer Society. *Cancer Facts and Figures.* Atlanta, GA: Author; 2004.

54. Lethbridge-Cejku M, Schiller JS, Bernadel L. *Summary Health Statistics for U.S. Adults: National Health Interview Survey, 2002.* Washington, DC: National Center for Health Statistics; 2004.

55. Johs-Artisensi J, McGill J. Screening mammography for elderly women. *Cancer Pract.* 2001;9:128–133.

56. Mandelblatt J, Saha S, Teutsch S. The cost-effectiveness of screening mammography beyond age 65 years: A systematic review for the US Preventive Services Task Force. *Ann Intern Med.* 2003;139:835–842.

57. Stegbauer CC, Sandstrom-Wakeling SK, Nied L, Gambino K, Zak M, Duffy E. The importance of mammography screening in elderly women. *Nurse Pract.* 2003;28:50–53.

58. Bogner HR, Wittink MN. Depression as a risk factor for underuse of mammography. *J Womens Health.* 2004;13:739–742.

59. Sirovich BE, Gottlieb DJ, Fisher ES. The burden of prevention: Downstream consequences of Pap smear testing in the elderly. *J Med Screening.* 2003;10:189–195.

60. Caplan A, Kratz A. Prostate-specific antigen and early diagnosis of prostate cancer. *Am J Clin Pathol.* 2002;117(Suppl):S104–S108.

61. Lu-Yao G, Stukel TA, Yao S. Prostate-specific antigen screening in elderly men. *J Nat Cancer Inst.* 2003;95:1792–1797.

62. Burke W, Beeker C, Kraft JM, Pinsky L. Engaging women's interest in colorectal cancer screening: A public health strategy. *J Women's Health Gender-Based Med.* 2000;9: 363–371.

63. Crandall C. Osteoporosis: New guidelines for screening and diagnosis. *Consultant.* 2001;41:237–241.

64. Screening Tests for Adults. *Lab Tests Online;* 2004. Available from http://www. labtestsonline.org/ (Accessed October 14, 2004).

65. Mohandras R, Lal Gupta K. Managing thyroid dysfunction in the elderly. *Postgrad Med.* 2003;113:548–552.

# Section III
# Settings of Assessment

# 15

# Assessment of Older Adults in Their Home

Lucia C. Kim and Carmel B. Dyer

## CASE VIGNETTE

*After discharge from the hospital for pacemaker placement, a home health agency provided follow-up care to 82-year-old Mrs. S. The patient, however, began to decline their visits because she was fearful that the agency staff members were trying to harm her and that they were stealing from her. Her son called Adult Protective Services for help, and they determined that she suffered no theft or harm. In fact, Mrs. S. would often forget that she had paid a bill and often overpaid them. The agency referred Mrs. S. to the house call team to evaluate Mrs. S. in her home because she was fearful about coming to the clinic.*

*Mrs. S. was pleasant during the visit. The team learned that she had hypertension and diabetes that was treated with insulin. Further review of her medication list indicated that she also had congestive heart failure and Alzheimer's dementia. Mrs. S. admitted to visual hallucinations and paranoid ideation. Her physical examination showed a healing wound at the site of pacemaker placement, marked weight loss, and generalized weakness. It was difficult for Mrs. S. to get around in her own home because of a low chair and multiple throw rugs, furniture, and electrical cords. Her blood sugar was normal, as were other laboratory tests. The social worker on the team identified neighbors in the apartment building who were willing to help Mrs. S.*

The US Census 2000 data revealed that about 14 million adults who were 65 years of age or older had a disability. Of these, nearly 10 million had a physical disability, 3.5 million a mental disability, and 6.8 million a disability that prevented them from going outside of the home.[1] In the same year, however, only about 1.5 million adults who were 65 years of age or older were living in nursing homes.[2] Thus, the vast majority of older adults with disability are living in the community.

Although the American Medical Association's national survey in 1990 revealed that over 90% of primary care physicians agree on the importance of housecalls,[3] only 1.5 million home visits were made by physicians in 1994 to care for 3 million homebound Medicare patients.[4]

In general, older patients who need home visits tend to be frail and at high risk of hospitalization, medical and social complications, and institutionalization. Frail and disabled older patients need home visits for many reasons, including a decline in health or function, unexplained failure to thrive, suspicion for abuse or neglect, a patient's refusal to be seen in the office, unexplained failure of the care plan, and terminal illness.[4] Patients and family may also prefer to avoid hospitalization and request provision of care at home.[5] Goals of home visits by a medical practitioner include improving function, thereby preserving independent living, reducing hospitalizations, and preventing institutionalization.

## HOME VISIT VERSUS OUTPATIENT CLINIC VISIT

Seeing a patient in his or her home allows the medical practitioner to gather information that would not otherwise be apparent in any office or clinic setting. A home visit not only allows the medical practitioner to assess the patient in a more familiar setting to the patient but also to assess the patient's living condition and formal and informal support system. In addition, the medical practitioner can search for barriers to maintaining good health and to medical management in the patient's environment. Home assessment can also reveal potential safety risks for the patient. Furthermore, the clinician can better assess for caregiver issues, such as the caregiver's physical capability, in the patient's home. Thus, home visit assessment gives the clinician the bigger picture, and the information obtained during home visits can be useful in making critical decisions, such as safely discharging a patient from the hospital back to his or her home.

Limitations, however, do exist in the home setting. In the patient's home, the clinician does not have immediate support of nursing or ancillary staff. In addition, diagnostic facilities and consultants are not easily accessible. However, despite these limitations, the medical practitioner is able to obtain more accurate information about the patient in the patient's living environment.

## PRACTICAL TIPS ON MAKING HOME VISITS

Planning ahead and preparing for each home visit can help to improve efficiency and optimize the quality of care. This entails carrying the necessary items to assess the patient and knowing in advance what special issues need to be addressed on that visit. We recommend the following items in a designated home visit bag:

1.  A sphygmomanometer with at least two different cuff sizes (regular size and large size)
2.  An otoscope and funduscope
3.  A thermometer with disposable covers
4.  A plastic container with venipuncture supplies: tourniquets, needles, vacutainer, syringes, blood specimen tubes, alcohol pads, and gauze
5.  Sharps container
6.  Specimen bags
7.  Urine specimen containers
8.  Plenty of gloves
9.  A lubricant, stool guaiac cards, and developer
10. Wound dressing supplies (4 × 4 gauze, tape)
11. A glucometer
12. A pulsoximeter
13. Disposable ear curettes
14. A flashlight
15. Prescription forms
16. A note pad to write instructions for the patient and caregiver
17. Advance directive forms
18. A portable hearing amplification device

The patient's chart should be reviewed before the visit to determine specific issues to address on that visit and additional items (e.g., scale, vaccination supplies) may need to be added for that day.

## INITIAL/NEW PATIENT HOME VISIT

In-home comprehensive geriatric assessment (CGA) has been shown to delay the development of disability and reduce permanent nursing home admissions.[6] The CGA in the patient's home not only involves evaluation of medical, functional, mental, and social issues but also includes assessment of the patient's environment in which he or she lives and should be the crux of the initial visit to a patient's home. Although a complete history and physical exam are important in any initial assessment, emphasis should be placed on function, safety, nutrition, medications, cognitive function, and caregiver issues.

Functional impairment is the basic underlying problem that renders the patient homebound. Thus, assessing the patient's ability to perform basic activities of daily living and instrumental activities of daily living is a crucial part of the initial home visit. Information on the patient's function can be obtained by subjective report by the patient and/or caregiver or by direct observation by the practitioner during the examination. Vision and hearing often affect function and should also be assessed.

Cognitive impairment may be a major component of functional decline. Assessment tools such as the Folstein Mini-Mental State Examination[7] and the clock-drawing test[8] can easily be performed during the initial visit. In addition to allowing the medical professional to intervene with medications and safety measures if cognitive impairment is detected, knowing the older patient's cognitive status can also help determine the patient's ability to understand and implement a directed care plan. In certain situations, such as if there is a concern regarding the ability of the patient to care for his- or herself or if abuse or neglect is suspected, decision-making capacity assessment should be performed.

Safety is an important issue, especially for frail older patients with functional and/or cognitive impairment. Issues of safety such as fall risk and access to emergency services can best be accomplished by evaluating the patient's living environment. The following are some potential hazards to look for in the patient's home during the visit:

1. Loose rugs
2. Inadequate lighting

3. Lack of heating system during cold weather
4. Lack of cooling system during hot weather
5. Lack of grab bars in the bathroom
6. Inaccessible telephone
7. Cords in walkways
8. Obstruction in walkways
9. Lack of working smoke alarm

Sometimes safety issues pertain to people who live around or within the household of the patient. Elder abuse and neglect are prevalent in the community-dwelling older population. Older persons who are unable to care for themselves are more likely to suffer from abuse, and the majority of patients who are abused have mental impairment.[9] Thus, the medical professional should use the visit to assess for abuse and neglect.

Older patients, especially those with multiple chronic illnesses, are frequently on numerous medications. A thorough review of all medications, including over-the-counter medications, can help address compliance issues and prevent iatrogenic complications. In the patient's home, the medical practitioner can see how the medication bottles are organized or disorganized. The date and number of refills should be noted on each bottle. The patient's and the caregiver's understanding of the function and side effects should also be assessed.

Older patients who are disabled or have chronic illnesses are at high risk of malnutrition. Patients should be assessed for changes in body weight, eating habits, access to food and water, and ability to swallow.[10] It is often helpful to investigate the refrigerator and food storage area with permission from the patient or other members of the household. It is also important to determine the patient's ability to purchase and prepare food. An oral and dental exam should also be performed.

Substance abuse is often a hidden problem in the older population. Alcohol abuse, especially, is a significant problem that is often unrecognized in older persons because the symptoms are nonspecific, such as self-neglect, depression, falls, confusion, and malnutrition. The medical practitioner can better obtain clues of potential alcohol abuse in the older patient's home than in a clinic or office setting. Some clues include inebriation during the visit and presence of empty wine or liquor bottles and beer cans around the house. Risk factors that increase an older patient's propensity to begin drinking in his or her later years of life include loss of spouse, family or friends, depression or other psychiatric condition, and a family history of alcohol or substance dependence.[11]

Many homebound older persons depend on the help of caregivers to remain living in the community. Therefore, the assessment of the caregiver's ability to provide for the needs of the older patient is an essential part of the initial assessment. The following are some questions for the medical practitioner to ask regarding the caregiver:

1. Does the caregiver have the physical ability to care for the patient?
2. Does the caregiver understand and have knowledge about the older patient's medical, functional, social, and nutritional needs?
3. Does the caregiver have outside support (family or friends) in taking care of the older patient?

Furthermore, because caring for a frail older person can often be overwhelming, the medical practitioner should inquire about caregiver stress and depression during the visit.

Because homebound older patients are often frail and on the verge of institutionalization, an important question to ask at the end of the initial and subsequent visits pertains to whether the older patient is safe to remain at home. The answer to this question depends on all of the information obtained from the assessment discussed previously here. Information regarding function, cognition, nutrition, safety, medication, and caregiver help the medical practitioner determine the needs of the older patient. In some situations, resources may not be adequate or available to meet these needs for the older patient to remain safe in his or her home.

## FOLLOW-UP VISITS

Although the CGA does not need to be repeated on subsequent visits, many components of CGA must be addressed on each follow-up visit. Besides managing chronic diseases, the medical practitioner should remain cognizant of safety, nutrition, and caregiver stress. A thorough medication review should be part of each follow-up visit. The patient should also be assessed for any changes in cognition or function, which would in turn change the patient's needs.

## ACUTE VISITS

The majority of house calls are routinely made for the management of chronic medical conditions. However, acute problems may be noted during a routine visit, or the patient or the caregiver may contact the house call team if an acute problem is recognized. Acute illnesses can often be managed over the phone; however, an urgent medical assessment and intervention may be necessary in some cases.

Common acute conditions include infection, abdominal conditions, cardiac symptoms, and behavioral problems. The most common infections that occur in homebound patients are the same as those seen in nursing home patients, and they include urinary tract infections, pneumonia, and infection of ulcers.[12] Fever and/or delirium are common presenting signs of an acute infection. Patients, however, may develop an acute confusional state without elevated temperatures or other typical symptoms seen in younger patients. Family members often do not recognize confusion as a sign of illness or wait for the mental status to clear before seeking medical attention. It is important to advise family members that confusion is a common presenting sign of acute illness, especially infection, in both homebound and ambulatory geriatric patients. In other instances, patients, especially those with dementia, may simply experience a change in activity level.

Acute abdominal conditions often present insidiously. Common abdominal problems include fecal impaction both high and low in the colon, diarrheal disorders, or gastrointestinal bleeding.[13] Patients may present with obvious abdominal pain or discomfort; however, at times, the presentation of abdominal problems is obscured, and again, acute confusion may be the most common presenting sign. Alerting family members to take note of the patient's bowel habits and to report changes is an important way to detect abdominal disorders.

Caregivers frequently call because of behavioral problems such as hallucinations, irritability, agitation, or aggression, although family members who care for homebound patients often do not complain about the difficult work of caregiving. However, behavioral problems test the patience of even the most dedicated caregiver. These behavioral changes can be due to delirium caused by an acute medical problem or simply a worsening of dementing illness. A thorough history and physical examination can guide the clinician.

## TRIAGE OF ACUTE PROBLEMS

When the clinician or the nurse case manager receives a phone call from the patient or the caregiver about an acute problem, enough information must be obtained to decide on the following courses of action:[14]

1. Manage the problem over the phone
2. Give a referral to a home health agency for a nurse visit to assess the problem
3. Schedule an urgent visit by the home visit medical professional to assess the problem
4. Schedule an urgent clinic/office visit
5. Send the patient to the emergency department

At times, the nurse case manager or the clinician will receive a call from the caregiver or the patient about an acute problem that clearly needs to be treated in an inpatient setting. Changes that involve difficulty breathing or chest pain and place the patient or caregiver in imminent danger require triage to the emergency department. Caregivers should be advised to call 911 in these cases. If the problem is not immediately life threatening but the house call team is not staffed to make urgent house calls, it may also be appropriate to triage the patient to the emergency department.

If a home visit by the house call team can be done in a timely manner, the homebound patient can potentially avoid emergency room visit and hospitalization, as the hazards of hospitalization have been well documented.[14] Often, these patients experience long waits or may be seen by clinicians who are not familiar with geriatric syndromes or care of homebound patients. In many instances, patients or their caregivers request only interventions that can be administered at home and decline transport to the hospital.

Acute problems can often be managed over the phone, or if the medical professional can provide an urgent home visit, the patient can remain in the home setting. Tests such as blood chemistries, complete blood counts, and urinalysis can easily be performed by home health agencies or the medical professional during the home visit. Home management can be undertaken if the patient or the caregiver can carry out the therapy, the home health agency can follow the patient's progress, or if there is a neighbor or family member who can monitor the care and report any decline.

**AFTER THE VISIT**

Follow-up after a house call for a homebound patient is quite important and more labor intensive than the follow-up of ambulatory outpatients. Much of the responsibility falls to the members of the house call team along with the caregivers. In hospital or clinic settings, processes are in place for tracking laboratory results or monitoring progress; house call teams must establish similar processes to achieve quality care of homebound patients.

## PHONE CALLS

Often a myriad of phone calls is required after the house call. The home health agency may need to be notified about any necessary tests, treatment, or monitoring. Medical professionals may sometimes contact out-of-town family members or family members who were at work during the time of the visit if they are the ones who have primary responsibility for the homebound patient. The clinician may need to place a call to the pharmacy for prescriptions. If any abuse or neglect is seen, the medical professional may be required to call Adult Protective Services in accordance with state laws.

## INTERDISCIPLINARY TEAM MEETING

An effective practice for the management of complex homebound geriatric patients is to hold interdisciplinary team meetings.[15] House call teams are not dissimilar to other geriatric assessment teams. This is a time for all members of the house call team to provide the pieces of the history that they have obtained. The nurse case manager may provide information received through phone calls or reported by other agencies that go into the home. The social worker may comment on the caregiver's ability to carry out instructions or the economic means to achieve the team's goal at home. The clinicians who visited the patient in home can comment on the physical examination and the environment. With this multidimensional information the team members can fashion the joint care plan.

The workload associated with the joint care plan can be distributed to the various house call team members. Certain members take on the tasks that require follow-up. Dates are set for the next visit, along with the parameters for monitoring. It is here that the processes for long-term follow-up are developed and carried out. Documentation of the interdisciplinary meeting can help team members track their duties and provide a written description of the progress of the case to date. In academic settings, health profession students can present their cases and interact with and learn from the entire interdisciplinary team.

## CONCLUSION

Visiting an older patient in his or her home allows access to medical care for those who are disabled and homebound. The medical professional can obtain a more accurate and detailed information about the older patient through home visits. Assessment of the older patient in his or her home begins with a comprehensive geriatric assessment with emphasis on function, safety, nutrition, medications, cognitive function, and caregiver issues. Along with management of chronic illnesses, many of these issues are reviewed during the follow-up visits in the home.

When an acute illness or problem arises, the older patient may require a visit to the emergency department, or if possible, an urgent home visit may be made to prevent a hospital visit. In some cases, acute problems can be managed over the phone.

Interdisciplinary discussions are an important part of managing a homebound older patient because of the multiple issues that interplay in a frail homebound older patient. Medical, social, functional, cognitive, and care-taking issues must be addressed to keep the older patient safe in his or her home.

### REFERENCES

1. US Census Bureau. *Disability Status: 2000—Census 2000 Brief.* http://www.census.gov/hhes/www/disable/disabstat2k/table1.html/. Accessed October 4, 2004.

2. US Census Bureau. *Census 2000 Special Tabulation.* http://www.census.gov/prod/2001pubs/c2kbr01-10.pdf. Accessed October 4, 2004.

3. Keenan JM, Boling PA, Schwartzberg JG, et al. A national survey of the home visiting practice an attitudes of family physicians and internists. *Arch Intern Med.* 1992; 152:2025-2032.

4. American Medical Association. *Report 9 of the Council on Scientific Affairs (I-96).* http://www.ama-assn.org/ama/pub/article/2036-7135.html. Accessed October 4, 2004.

5. Fried TR, Wachtel TJ, Tinetti ME. When the patient cannot come to the doctor: A medical housecall program. *J Am Geriatr Soc.* 1998;46:226-231.

6. Stuck AE, Aronow HU, Steiner A, et al. A trial of annual in-home comprehensive geriatric assessments for elderly people living in the community. *N Engl J Med.* 1995; 333:1184-1189.

7. Folstein MF, Folstein SE, McHugh PE. "Mini-mental state": A practical method for grading the cognitive state of patients for the clinician. *J Psychiatr Res.* 1975;12:189-198.

8. Watson YI, Arfken CL, Birge SJ. Clock completion: An objective screening test for dementia. *J Am Geriatr Soc.* 1993;41:1235-1240.

9. The National Elder Abuse Incidence Study. http://www.aoa.gov/eldfam/Elder_Rights/Elder_Abuse/Abuse Report_full.pdf. Accessed October 4, 2004.

10. Omran ML, Salem P. Diagnosing undernutrition. *Clin Geriatr Med.* 2002;18: 719-736.

11. Sattar SP, Petty F, Burke WJ. Diagnosis and treatment of alcohol dependence in older alcoholics. *Clin Geriatr Med.* 2003;19:743–761.

12. Bentley DW, Bradley S, High K, Schoenbaum S, Taler G, Yoshikawa TT. Practice guideline for evaluation of fever and infection in long-term care facilities. *J Am Geriatr Soc.* 2001;49:210–222.

13. Dang C, Aguilera P, Dang A, Salem L. Acute abdominal pain: Four classifications can guide assessment and management. *Geriatrics.* 2002;57:30–32, 35–36, 41–42.

14. Creditor MC. Hazards of hospitalization of the elderly. *Ann Intern Med.* 1993;118: 219–223.

15. Dyer CB, Hyer K, Feldt K, et al. Frail older patient care by interdisciplinary teams: A primer for generalists. *Gerontol Geriatr Educ.* 2003;24:51–62.

# 16

# *Geriatric Assessment in Nursing Homes*

Miriam B. Rodin

This chapter discusses geriatric assessment in nursing homes. The topic is, on one hand, exceedingly straightforward because the assessments have been both standardized and mandated by Medicare for over a decade. On the other hand, a variety of well-validated instruments are described in other chapters in this book. Each discipline and specialty has its own preferred tools, such as the Functional Independence Measure (FIM) for physical therapy or the Braden Risk for nursing. These tools work very well in long-term care, and the reader is referred to those chapters. Therefore, here we focus attention on a discussion of a critical tool of geriatric assessment in the nursing home, the Minimum Data Set (MDS), its history, supplemental assessments, limitations, and applications.

In order to understand the form of the MDS, it is important to understand the why and when of the MDS. Briefly, the Medicare Act of 1965 for the first time provided federal dollars for skilled nursing care and rehabilitation outside of hospitals. The flood of dollars into small residential enterprises coincided with reforms in the mental health systems in a number of states. These reforms displaced chronic psychiatric and developmentally disabled patients from state hospitals to "community" facilities. Thus, the influx of money and patients stimulated a population explosion in nursing homes, as well as introducing a diversity of needs that had been previously unknown.

Before the enactment of Medicare, nursing homes provided relatively unregulated "invalid" care and supported living for older adults (e.g. the "old soldiers' home"). Hospital stays were unlimited, and the acuity of convalescents was therefore low. The introduction of prospective payment (PPS) to hospitals based on diagnostic-related groups (DRGs) changed the case mix for nursing homes. The incentive to discharge "quicker and sicker" led to an influx of sicker patients for which few nursing homes were prepared. Not surprisingly, the quality of care, the requirements for care, and the cost of care in nursing homes became a source of rising dissatisfaction among legislators, patients, families, and the general public.

In response, the Health Care Finance Agency (now the Center for Medicare and Medicaid Services [CMS]) sponsored the 1986 Institute of Medicine report, which determined that "providing high quality care requires careful assessment of each resident's functional, medical, mental, and psychosocial status upon admission, and reassessment periodically thereafter."[1] This was embodied in the Nursing Home Reform Act of 1986 and incorporated into the Omnibus Budget Reconciliation Act of 1987 (OBRA 87). OBRA 87 mandated the development of a standardized Resident Assessment Instrument to be used by all long-term care facilities licensed to receive payment from Medicare and subsequently from Medicaid as well. The resultant assessment tool is the MDS. It is required for all residents admitted to long-term care under Medicare or Medicaid. Assessments are due within 5 days of admission and then at 14, 30, 60, and 90 days. It also is required for long-stay residents quarterly or whenever a "significant change" in health or functional status occurs.

## MDS AND ITS IMPLICATIONS

The MDS began as an inventory of function, including physical capacities, self-care, mental and medical co-morbidity, and psychologic and social assets. Using expert opinion and extensive field testing, the result was a checklist that combined the observations of various nursing home personnel, patient self-reports, family proxies, and medical records. Each domain is scored by either summed or assigned points. Each item checked in a domain triggers the assessment specialist to complete a specific supplementary problem-focused Resident Assessment Protocol (RAP). The RAP directs the evaluator to consult with other disciplines, perform additional structured assessments, and obtain further medical examinations to determine individualized care plans. Each RAP is linked to a Key, essentially a differential diagnosis for the problem with suggestions for additional evaluations for reversible causes. Keys vary in the specificity of assessments and interventions that are required or suggested. Furthermore, reference tables guide the evaluator to "crosswalks," that is, additional RAPs that are likely to be related to the triggered RAP. Table 16–1 lists the domains of the MDS. Table 16–2 lists the RAPs, the problem-specific assessments triggered by a positive MDS finding.

The MDS is continually updated. The CMS website (http://www.cms.hhs.gov) provides a portal to updates of the MDS, RAPs, Keys, and scoring criteria. The site provides extensive case vignettes to describe how resident needs are to be documented, how "triggers" are to be identified, and how RAPs are to be completed. The realistic case vi-

---

**Table 16–1** Domains Assessed by the Minimum Data Set (MDS 2.0)

| | |
|---|---|
| 3.3 Section AA. Identification Information for MDS | 3-6 |
| SECTION AB. DEMOGRAPHIC INFORMATION | 3-12 |
| SECTION AC. CUSTOMARY ROUTINE | 3-22 |
| SECTION AD. FACE SHEET SIGNATURES | 3-27 |
| SECTION A. MDS IDENTIFICATION AND BACKGROUND INFORMATION | 3-28 |
| 3.4 Clinical Items for the MDS | 3-41 |
| SECTION B. COGNITIVE PATTERNS | 3-41 |
| SECTION C. COMMUNICATION/HEARING PATTERNS | 3-51 |
| SECTION D. VISION PATTERNS | 3-58 |
| SECTION E. MOOD AND BEHAVIOR PATTERNS | 3-60 |
| SECTION F. PSYCHOSOCIAL WELL-BEING | 3-71 |
| SECTION G. PHYSICAL FUNCTIONING AND STRUCTURAL PROBLEMS | 3-76 |
| SECTION H. CONTINENCE IN LAST 14 DAYS | 3-119 |
| SECTION I. DISEASE DIAGNOSES | 3-127 |
| SECTION J. HEALTH CONDITIONS | 3-138 |
| SECTION K. ORAL/NUTRITIONAL STATUS | 3-149 |
| SECTION L. ORAL/DENTAL STATUS | 3-158 |
| SECTION M. SKIN CONDITION | 3-159 |
| SECTION N. ACTIVITY PURSUIT PATTERNS | 3-169 |
| SECTION O. MEDICATIONS | 3-176 |
| SECTION P. SPECIAL TREATMENTS AND PROCEDURES | 3-182 |
| SECTION Q. DISCHARGE POTENTIAL AND OVERALL STATUS | 3-207 |
| SECTION R. ASSESSMENT INFORMATION | 3-210 |
| SECTION S. STATE-DEFINED SECTION | 3-214 |
| SECTION T. THERAPY SUPPLEMENT FOR MEDICARE PPS | 3-214 |
| SECTION U. MEDICATIONS | 3-223 |
| SECTION V. RESIDENT ASSESSMENT PROTOCOL SUMMARY | 3-237 |

---

**Table 16–2** Resident Assessment Protocols (RAP) Triggered by MDS 2.0

1. Delirium
2. Cognitive loss/dementia
3. Visual function
4. Communication
5. ADL function/rehabilitation
6. Urinary incontinence and indwelling catheter
7. Psychosocial well-being
8. Mood state
9. Behavior symptoms
10. Activities
11. Falls
12. Nutritional status
13. Feeding tubes
14. Dehydration/fluid maintenance
15. Dental care
16. Pressure ulcers
17. Psychotropic drug use
18. Physical restraints

---

gnettes demonstrate a recursive process of assessment, care planning, and evaluation. The MDS relies heavily on nursing staff documentation of their observations and impressions in detailed nursing notes. The MDS 2.0 is in use at this writing. Full text forms and instructional and interpretative guidelines are available on the CMS website using the search term MDS. There are working drafts of the MDS 3.0 as well.

The Budget Reform Act of 1999 extended the doctrine of PPSs to long-term care. Implementation was phased in state by state beginning in 2002. PPS defined resource utilization groups (RUGs), the long-term care equivalent of hospital DRGs. The RUGs are currently in Version III, available on the CMS website contained within the MDS documents or separately under the search term RUGs-III. There are 44 categories, grouped into seven major classifications of resource utilization intensity. The top 26 RUGs (in four classifications) qualify for Medicare payment under Parts A and B for skilled nursing and rehabilitation in a long-term care facility. Table 16–3 lists the seven major classes of RUG groups, and shows a definition or example of each RUG and the coding or billing group generated by the RUG.

MDS assessments are now universally entered on standardized software. The documents are electronically submitted to the states and then forwarded to CMS, where they are archived in the MDS repository, about which more will be said later. Private vendor and CMS

**Table 16–3** There Are Seven Major Resource Utilization Groups (RUG-III)

| Major RUG-III Group | Definition of RUG | Coding Groups |
|---|---|---|
| Rehabilitation | Resident receives physical, speech, and/or occupational therapy | RUA, RUB, RUC, RVA, RVB, RVC, HB, RHC, RMA, RMB, RMC, RLA, RLB |
| Extensive services | Complex clinical care or complex clinical needs, for example, IV, suctioning, tracheostomy care, ventilator, or other co-morbidities that exclude resident from other RUG | SE1, SE2, SE3 |
| Special care | Complex clinical care for serious diseases such as multiple sclerosis, quadriplegia, cerebral palsy, respiratory therapy, decubitus ulcers stages III and IV, radiation treatment, surgical wound care, tube feeding aphasia, fever with dehydration, pneumonia, vomiting, and weight loss | SSA, SSB, SSC |
| Clinically complex | Complex clinical care or conditions require skilled nursing (registered nurse) for burns, coma, sepsis, pneumonia, foot wounds, internal bleeding, dehydration, tube feeding, oxygen, transfusion, hemiplegia, chemotherapy, dialysis, or change of physician orders/physician visit | CA1, CA2, CB1, CB2, CC1, CC2 |
| Impaired cognition | Impairment in decision making, recall and short-term memory, MDS 2.0 cognitive performance scale $\geq 3$ | IA1, IA2, IB1, IB2 |
| Behavior problems | Wandering, verbally or physically abusive, socially inappropriate, hallucinations, or delusions | BA1, BA2, BB1, BB2 |
| Reduced physical functions | Needs are primarily ADL and general supervision (custodial) | PA1, PA2, PB1, PB2, PC1, PC2, PD1, PD2, PE1, PE2 |

software can score the MDS, trigger RAPs, compute the appropriate RUG, and then generate a care plan from menu-driven choices. Software can track individual and facility MDS scores over time.

The MDS was intended as a tool to promote patient-centered individualized care planning. To promote individualization of care, the MDS translates directly into RUGs. Effectively, there are financial incentives for the long-term care facility to identify the highest skilled nursing and highest intensity rehabilitation needs that can be justified by the MDS algorithms. In other words, the MDS is the documentation that supports billing claims. The recursive step in the process is outcomes evaluation, and the MDS documents do not specifically address evaluation in the same detail as the RAPs, Keys, and RUG coding. Outcomes must be easily measured and have an obvious relationship to care. The care given ought to be based on evidence of clinical efficacy. There must be a systematic approach to problem solving when appropriate care does not result in expected outcomes. This process is not addressed in the MDS source ware, although several items in MDS and the Keys do contain prognostic information, for example, recording of terminal diagnoses such as cancer or irreversible neurodegenerative diseases, including end-stage dementia. Certain MDS items have been designated as quality indicators regardless of the reliability of the record or clinical context in which the data were recorded. A recent Institute of Medicine report has cited the extreme variability in the quality of these data and of state survey data for fairly judging the quality of nursing home care.[2]

Nonetheless, in a general way, the reforms of OBRA 87 have improved care in US nursing homes, despite the trend for sicker, more complex patients. However, it is not entirely clear whether the quality of care is in any direct way related to the specifics of the MDS assessments or the specific items selected as quality indicators.[3] In other words, certain good outcomes are fairly straightforward, such as a resident who cannot walk at admission but can now walk without assistance at a standardized physical therapy 30-day reassessment. However, failure to achieve the obvious good outcome could reflect either poor care or the expected outcome for a resident with a poor prognosis. The rehabilitative disciplines—physical, occupational, speech, and language therapies—routinely provide prognostic evaluations with each assessment and tailor goals to what professional experience would suggest is attainable. However, failure to improve could represent the failure of standard but ineffective care or decline due to a problem unrelated to nursing home care, such as extreme old age with primary frailty.

Fourteen of the MDS assessments have been selected to provide a snapshot for comparing facilities across the nation. The 14 quality indicators and additional data about individual nursing homes have been collated by the On-line Survey, Certification, and Reporting (OSCAR) system since 2002. These data can be viewed for any nursing home in the country on www.medicare.gov/NHcompare. The OSCAR database for each facility is updated quarterly and contains results of state surveys over 15 months for every Medicaid nursing home in the country. These data include citations for deficiencies at state surveys. Table 16–4 lists the MDS items selected as quality indicators that are included in the on-line nursing home quality database referred to previously. Percentile rankings of facilities on each indicator are based on the percentage of residents triggering an assessment for that indicator in the most recent sample of MDS forms submitted from the facility. CMS spokesmen believe that this resource has been highly effective as an incentive for nursing homes to improve quality of care.[4] The adequacy of the quality indicator approach has been questioned by authorities in the field, but more meaningful measures have yet to be agreed on.[5,6]

Masses of MDS data in the MDS repository comprise a rich administrative database to be mined for a variety of research purposes, including quality monitoring. However, administrative data such as the MDS should be viewed with caution. Composition of the long-term care population varies markedly by region, facility type, and over

---

**Table 16–4** The MDS Enhanced Quality Indicators

For chronic care: The percentage of (long-stay) residents who
    Need for help with ADLs has increased
    Have moderate to severe pain
    Were physically restrained
    Spent most of their time in bed or in a chair
    Had their ability to move about in and around their room get worse
    Had a urinary tract infection
    Have become more depressed or anxious
    Are high risk and have pressure sores
    Are low risk and have pressure sores
    Are low risk and lose control of bowels or bladder
    Have/had a catheter inserted and left in their bladder
For postacute care: The percentage of short-stay residents who
    Had moderate to severe pain
    Had delirium
    Had pressure sores

---

time. Facility characteristics reflect local labor market forces, hospital factors, payer mix, size, and ownership. Examinations of MDS archives provide a way to think about standards of care, evaluate the effects of major shifts in national policy, or compare the impact of state programs on resident outcomes. The interpretation of large-scale data may not be relevant for quality assurance/quality improvement at the facility level. In other words, the grand pattern viewed from 42,000 feet may have little relevance to the bug's eye view on the ground. The MDS has come to serve a great many more purposes than comprehensive assessment of individual patients. Is there any way to determine whether the purpose of comprehensive assessment has been advanced by the MDS?

Improvements in nursing homes since OBRA 87 reflect changes in many levels. Staff qualifications, the variety of technical and rehabilitative services offered, adherence to standards of documentation, sanitation, and resident rights have all improved. How much is difficult to assess, however, because before OBRA 87 there was no documentary source. However, there are now studies that ask whether the MDS quality indicators do in fact measure quality of care. I will review several recent studies and implications for how assessment determines outcomes of care.

Any nursing home licensed to provide care under Medicare has its data available on the Nursing Home Compare website noted previously. Under various demonstration projects, nursing homes are provided with a percentile rank of their performance on each indicator compared with other nursing homes. The idea is that nursing homes scoring poorly will institute measures to improve their ranking. Let us examine several of the specific indicators in this regard.

There is little disagreement that pain is underrecognized and undertreated in the long-term care population.[7-9] CMS therefore has required routine pain assessment for all residents beginning in November 2002. However, there is little convincing evidence that this standard has had any effect on pain recognition or management in nursing homes. There are two MDS items assessing pain frequency, and intensity, but evaluators have little specific guidance on how to perform an assessment. Furthermore, the impact of dementia or other communication disorders can make it difficult for untrained staff to recognize pain.[10]

In this example, the indicators are unable to discriminate between good and poor performance and nursing home management may be unfamiliar with interpreting numeric quality data. A low reported prevalence of pain could indicate either good pain management or failure to recognize pain at all. For this reason, as shown in the example mentioned previously, facilities should adopt a systematic approach to assessment, with internal incentives for excellent documentation. Then the MDS assessment could be supplemented with specific tools, for example, especially those designed to assess cognitively impaired residents, for internal self-auditing. Assessments built into daily nursing procedures and not only recalled at MDS time would improve reliability if not validity of the data that are submitted to CMS. There are, for example, several pain scales, such as the analogue scales commonly used in hospitals, as well as pain scales developed specifically for use in cognitively impaired patients.[11,12]

Some authorities have suggested that the higher prevalence of several of the quality indicators, such as pain, probably indicates better care than that at facilities reporting lower prevalence of these "poor-quality" indicators.[6,13] There have been few rigorous studies, but a pattern is emerging that suggests an expanded role for MDS-independent assessments. For example, although the RUG mechanism allows for case-mix adjustment, the quality indicators are not adjusted. Therefore, a facility taking high-risk patients is evaluated no differently than one taking residents at intrinsically low risk. The quality indicator for pressure ulcers properly discriminates between facility-acquired and imported wounds. It attempts to adjust for case mix by counting new wounds in high-risk residents separately from those in low-risk residents. However, researchers examining the MDS data in conjunction with institutional-level data found relatively little to reliably differentiate the quality of care given in high- and low-incidence facilities.[14] The problem is compounded by the paucity of evidence-based clinical guidelines to recommend best practices in wound care.[15] Wound prevention remains the more troublesome problem because there is little evidence to support current guidelines.[16] Therefore, assessments of pressure ulcer risk, prevention, and care need further work before any specific quality indicator can be accepted at face value.

In addition to pain and pressure ulcer risk, weight is another critically important assessment, the sixth vital sign, in long-term care. The importance of rigorously standardized weighing procedures cannot be overestimated. There is an explicit trigger in MDS regarding weight changes of 5% and 10% within 30 days and 6 months. A panoply of automatic responses takes place that involves both notification of physicians, required nutritional assessments, and orders for nurses to give pharmaceutical protein–calorie supplements and other unproven nutritional additives in addition to already long lists of medications.

Often enough, the weight change is in error because of a change in procedure or calibration of scales. The baseline weight may have been transcribed from an inaccurate hospital record in which the patients were simply asked what they weighed. Furthermore, it is unfortunate that by the time weight loss has occurred, the underlying process is well advanced. Weight gain is good for residents with previous weight loss, failure to thrive, or low body mass index. Conversely, weight loss may be unavoidable for patients with end-stage diseases, including cancer and chronic renal, liver, heart and lung failure and, equally as important, end-stage dementia. As with pain and pressure ulcers, facility-level weight trends may reflect care or case mix. As a first step, weight changes need to be accurately assessed by prognosis. One scheme uses the classification intended versus unintended, desirable versus undesirable, and potentially reversible versus irreversible. Thus, assessments that categorize weight changes by underlying physiology focus nutritional interventions on cases that can show improvement and direct care plans more appropriately for those that will not.[17]

Assessments that identify nutritional risk early should take preference over weight loss as a nutritional indicator. Documentation of intake is useful, however, only if nursing assistants are trained properly. Dietitians have developed a variety of dining alternatives with positive effects on resident intake, and thus, the appropriate intervention may not be at the individual level but at the institutional level. The MDS does not address this possibility.

A standardized weight protocol must begin with a designated weight technician.[18] A certified nursing assistant (CNA) is appropriate. Weights should be taken on the same scale for all residents because transfers between floors can cause sudden weight changes. The scale should be calibrated frequently. There should be a designated wheelchair of known weight for all nonambulatory residents because individual residents' wheelchairs can migrate between rooms or be customized with addition or subtraction of positioning devices. Residents should be weighed on the same day of the week and at the same time of day each month wearing light indoor clothing and no shoes. Furthermore, renal dialysis patients should be weighed only on return from dialysis to establish their dry weight as the reference. Any variation of 5% total body weight should require a repeated weight. Physicians' documentation should include an assessment of the desirability of the change and an estimate of prognosis for improved weight. Often, however, physicians do not respond to mild weight loss, and dietary and nursing staff must determine the cause of weight loss. Is it due to the natural course of irreversible disease such as late-stage dementia or cancer? Hospice referral may be the appropriate intervention. Patients can stop eating because of treatable causes such as a urinary tract infection, gastroesophageal reflux disease, and mouth pain or as a side effect of a large number of commonly used medications. A patient requiring assistance with eating because of dementia, Parkinson's disease, or blindness requires a different intervention. The weight loss RAP makes several general suggestions, but a structured nursing assessment such as the nursing Nutrition in Long-Term Care Facility (LTCF) checklist includes sequential evaluations of effectiveness.[17]

Depression is very likely considerably underrecognized and undertreated in nursing homes for many of the same reasons that pain is underrecognized. This includes staff training in recognition of depression, particularly vegetative signs, and of inability to recognize depression in cognitively impaired residents.[19] However, once again, MDS documentation of depression does not reliably predict medical intervention. There are several short, validated depression scales that are useful for cognitively intact residents. However, there is no validated depression scale comparable to the pain scales developed for cognitively impaired residents. Further research is needed to determine reliable assessments for depression in severely cognitively impaired patients and to determine how best to implement these in nursing homes.[20]

*Every third Friday of the month, a 240-bed Medicare/Medicaid facility, Windsor Gardens Convalescent and Alzheimer Care Center, holds the monthly quality improvement/quality assurance meeting. In attendance are the administrator, the director and assistant directors of nursing, the medical director and all of the department heads (housekeeping, recreation, dementia unit, dietary, nutrition, medical records, social services, patient relations, marketing, admissions, and representatives from the laboratory and pharmacy contractors). Each department presents a summary of activities for the previous month: timeliness of activities, meal service, weight changes, feeding tubes, and nursing reports about falls, Foley catheters, and wound care. Departments that had fewer adverse events compared with the previous month are applauded; departments with more events report that they will continue to monitor and set goals to decrease the number of falls, late meals, or charts missing face sheets. None presents an analysis of why the results are better or worse or defines a specific plan to determine the reasons and follow-up with a plan.*

*Then the administrator distributes the quarterly summary of qual-
ity indicators. The facility is flagged on three indicators, those in
which the facility scores in the lowest 5% of reporting facilities:
untreated depression, bed bound residents, and low-risk pressure
ulcers. A discussion ensues. It is concluded that they are doing a
good job because there is very little depression. The medical director asks how the prevalence of depression is ascertained. The MDS
coordinator states she asks the social services coordinator who asks
the floor nurses to report if any of their residents are depressed. The
MDS Section 3.4E identifies specific signs and symptoms that the
social services coordinator was unaware of. Neither has had any
in-service training on the clinical signs of depression. It is determined that the pharmacy should print a monthly summary of the
residents on prescribed antidepressants with or without a diagnosis
of depression documented on the chart. Second, the consulting psychiatrist can provide an additional list of residents he has seen.
Third, CNAs will be given pocket cards with the MDS questions
and be asked to consult it when working with residents who may
have recently lost loved ones or who are exhibiting signs of vegetative symptoms, weeping, verbalizations of worthlessness, hopelessness, guilt, or withdrawal. A nursing supervisor will compare the
lists.*

*Similarly, for bed-bound residents, the indicator was calculated on
very small numbers. The small number of bed-bound patients
seemed out of keeping with the degree of debility of residents on the
skilled nursing  and exceptional care floors. Examining the numbers, the numerator of 4 and denominator of 37, clearly represents
an incomplete census. The MDS coordinator counted residents as
bed bound only if they were never up in a chair or Geri chair. The
definition of bed bound was reviewed. The implications for case mix
for the facility were discussed. Clearly, the staff was doing a good
job mobilizing a far greater number of totally dependent residents
than the facility was credited. The CNAs could give a precise count
of which residents required total assist.*

*Finally, the prevalence of pressure ulcers in low-risk residents was
more complex. Overall, the facility had done well in terms of a low
incidence of facility-acquired ulcers, but the indicator had picked
up a single resident readmitted from a local hospital intensive care
unit with over 30 ulcers of various stages and severity. Thus, the
numerator (ulcers) and the denominator (residents) gave a false
impression of wound care quality over a period of time. A review of
12 months retrospectively indicated no decrement in performance*

*overall. However, the medical director reported several cases, con-*
*firmed by the patient services coordinator of families complaining*
*about dressings not being changed on weekends. The nursing di-*
*rector agreed to look into weekend wound coverage. The result was*
*that the two wound care specialists had days off staggered, and a*
*third nurse was offered extra hours to fill in on days when only one*
*specialist was available.*

Two final nursing home quality indicators are related: the urinary incontinence indicator and late-loss activities of daily living (ADLs). The rationale behind the indicators was that attentive care could reverse or at least delay the onset of these debilities. Continence is one of the ADLs and one most proximately associated with decisions to institutionalize. Outpatient medicine trials suggested that a great deal of the urinary incontinence experienced by older persons could be medically treated or behaviorally managed. For incontinence associated with immobility and with progressive neurologic impairment, toileting assistance and timed voiding are the interventions of choice. One study compared patient self-report and direct observation of caregiving to medical record documentation of care. For urinary incontinence, timed toileting was documented but not often observed by trained observers or resident self-report.[21,22] Similarly, late-loss ADLs tended to be documented, but there was little correspondence between the care plan and care given.[23,24]

## SUMMARY AND CONCLUSIONS

The core of geriatric assessment in nursing homes is, by legislation, the MDS. The MDS is comprehensive, highly structured, and quantifiable. It is at the center of a process model of care focused on individual residents. The process is defined as a comprehensive assessment with the MDS that triggers focused assessment with the RAPs and Keys. This is used to develop a structured care plan that is to be reviewed at predefined intervals. There is no intrinsic reason to exclude other accepted assessment tools, but the principal limitation of the MDS is that it serves at least three different purposes: individual care planning, billing support documentation, and facility-level quality monitoring. A wise management consultant once said, "All systems perform perfectly to produce exactly what they were designed to produce." What are needed to improve care in nursing homes are not more individual resident assessments, but better, empirically derived, evidence-based interventions. Finally, evaluation processes should reward facility-level problem solving and distinguish between internal problems with care and resource limitations affecting care (e.g., staffing shortages.) A new focus on building organizational capacity would improve the quality of individual care in nursing homes.[2]

## REFERENCES

1. Institute of Medicine. *Improving the Quality of Care in Nursing Homes.* Washington, DC: National Academy Press; 1986:74.

2. Institute of Medicine. *Improving the Quality of Long Term Care.* Washington, DC: National Academy Press; 2001.

3. Ouslander JG. The Resident Assessment Instrument (RAI): Promise and pitfalls. *J Am Geriatr Soc.* 1997;45:975–976.

4. CMS News. *Enhanced Set of Quality Measures Now Available at Medicare's Easier-to-Use Nursing Home Compare.* Accessed January 22, 2004. Available from www.cms.hhs.gov/media/press/release

5. American Geriatrics Society (AGS) Position Statement. *Measuring Quality of Care in Nursing Home Residents* (Considering Unintended Consequences; approved 2002). Available from www.americangeriatrics.org/products/positionpapers/unintended_conseq.shtml

6. Mor V, Angelelli J, Jones R, et al. Inter-rater reliability of nursing home quality indicators in the US. *BMC Health Services Res.* 2003;3:20.

7. Won AB, Lapane KL, Vallow S, Schein J, Morris JN, Lipsitz LA. Persistent nonmalignant pain and analgesic prescribing patterns in elderly nursing home residents. *J Am Geriatr Soc.* 2004;52:867–874.

8. Cadogan MP, Schnelle JF, Yamamoto-Mitani N, Cabrera G, Simmon SF. A minimum data set prevalence of pain quality indicator: Is it accurate and does it reflect differences in care processes? *J Gerontol Series A Biol Sci Med Sci.* 2004;59:281–285.

9. Engle VF, Graney MJ, Chan A. Accuracy and bias of licensed practical nurse and nursing assistant ratings of nursing home residents' pain. *J Gerontol Series A Biol Sci Med Sci.* 2001;56:M405–M411.

10. Fisher SE, Burgio LD, Thorn BE, et al. Pain assessment and management in cognitively impaired nursing home residents: Association of certified nursing assistant pain report, Minimum Data Set pain report and analgesic medication. *J Am Geriatr Soc.* 2002;50:152–156.

11. Warden V, Hurley AC, Volicer L. Development and Psychometric Evaluation of the Pain Assessment in Advanced Dementia (PAINAD) Scale. *J Am Med Dir Assoc.* 2003; 4:50–51.

12. Villaneuva MR, Smith TL, Erickson JS, Lee AC, Singer CM. Pain Assessment for the Dementing Elderly (PADE): Reliability and validity of a new measure. *J AM Med Dir Assoc.* 2003;4(1):1–8.

13. Mukamel DB, Watson NM, Meng H, Spector WD. Development of a risk-adjusted urinary incontinence outcome measure of quality for nursing homes. *Med Care.* 2003;4194:467–478.

14. Bates-Jensen BM, Cadogan M, Osterweil D, et al. The Minimum Data Set pressure ulcer indicator: Does it reflect differences in care processes related to pressure ulcer prevention and treatment in nursing homes? *J Am Geriatri Soc.* 2003;51:1203–1212.

15. *Treatment of Pressure Ulcers.* Clinical Guideline No. 15. AHCPR Pub. No. 95-0652; December 2004. Available from www.ncbi.nlm.nih.gov/books

16. *Pressure Ulcers in Adults: Prediction and Prevention.* Clinical Practice Guidelines No. 3. AHCPR Pub. No. 92-0047; May 1992. Available from www.ncbi.nlm.nih.gov/books

17. Council for Nutrition. *Clinical Guide to Prevent and Manage Malnutrition in Long-Term Care.* Council for Nutrition, Clinical Strategies in LTC. *Programs in Medicine,* 2000. Available from www.ltcnutrition.org/PDF/clinicalMalnutritionGuide.pdf

18. Simmons SF, Garcia ET, Cadogan MP, et al. The Minimum Data Set weight-loss quality indicator: Does it reflect differences in the care processes related to weight loss? *J Am Geriatr Soc.* 2003;51:1410–1418.

19. Jones RN, Marcantonio ER, Rabinowitz T. Prevalence and correlates of recognized depression in US nursing homes. *J Am Geriatr Soc.* 2003;51:1404–1409.

20. Simmons SF, Cadogan MP, Cabrera GR, et al. The Minimum Data Set depression quality indicator: Does it reflect differences in care processes? *Gerontologist.* 2004;44: 554–564.

21. Stevenson KB, Moore JW, Sleeper B. Validity of the Minimum Data Set in identifying urinary tract infections in residents of long-term care facilities. *J Am Geriatr Soc.* 2004;52:707–711.

22. McConnell ES, Pieper CF, Sloane RJ, Branch LG. Effects of cognitive performance on change in physical function in long-stay nursing home residents. *J Gerontol Series A Biol Sci Med Sci.* 2002;57:M778–M784.

23. Schnelle JF, Cadogan MP, Yoshii J, et al. The Minimum Data Set urinary incontinence quality indicators: Do they reflect differences in care processes related to incontinence? *Med Care.* 2003;41:909–922.

24. Schnelle JF, Bates-Jensen BM, Levy-Storms L, et al. The Minimum Data Set prevalence of restraint quality indicator: Does it reflect differences in care? *Gerontologist.* 2004;44:245–255.

# 17

## Assessment at the Time of Hospitalization

Marilyn Lopez

## AGING SOCIETY

### Overview

In 2000, older adults (people over the age of 65 years) represented 12.4% of the population. By 2030, this percentage is expected to increase to 20% as baby boomers start turning 65 in 2011.[1] The aging of American older cohorts and its effects on health care centers require strategies and programs to ensure best practices for the hospitalized older population. This chapter describes geriatric assessment and management at the time of hospitalization by using evidence-based practice (EBP) in designing an interdisciplinary geriatric model of care as well as an expansion of the advanced practice nurse's role.

In 2000, hospitalized older patients represented approximately 40% of discharges and used almost one half of the hospital days of care and expenditures.[2,3] Eighty percent of Americans 65 years old and older have a chronic illness or functional disability as compared with those 75 years old and older with three or four chronic health conditions.[2] Forty-four percent of hospitalized older people will experience at least one unexpected clinical event while hospitalized.[2] Furthermore, older persons often present with multiple co-morbid challenges and are often dependent in activities of daily living (ADLs) requiring the critical expertise of clinicians in maximizing functional recovery and disease management throughout hospitalization and along the continuum of care.

## Evidence-Based Practice (EBP)

Since 1979, the rate of hospitalization among older persons has increased by 23%; concurrently, the rate of hospitalization among all other groups has decreased.[4] According to the National Center for Health Statistics (2003), hospitals rarely have programs that target older patients.[5] With limited nursing resources and nursing care that needs to be delivered efficiently and effectively, it is important to think about creative ways to assure better processes and care outcomes. Comprehensive care provided to older persons is aimed at enhancing practice and dovetailing education with procedural changes by using EBP at the bedside.

EBP refers to practice that integrates the best available external and internal clinical evidence from systematic research with individual clinical expertise and the preferences of the patient.[6] Many of the concepts of EBP have long been used in nursing to develop protocols and pathways or to conduct research utilization as well as research-based practice projects.[6] Sometimes the work is done on a case-by-case basis, but more often, it is an elaborate process undertaken to develop guidelines or recommendations that can be applied broadly within a hospital department or across clinical specialties.[6]

The Internet is a major resource for clinicians to learn about EBP as well as how to find the best evidence for practice. Websites are used for finding practice recommendations and/or guidelines that have been developed by others using an evidence-based approach.[6] Identifying web-based resources allows nurses to exchange information in caring for older adults. In addition, this gives nurses the ability to evaluate research strengths and weaknesses as well as the most current best evidence in making decisions about the care of older adults.[7] The challenge for nurses and other clinicians is to be able to present evidence-based information to patients in a format that informs them of all the possible outcomes, including risks and benefits.[7] On the other hand, outcome measures such as discharge readiness are becoming increasingly important in relationship to health care quality and patient safety. Clearly, EBP is a logical approach in providing the best possible outcomes with the most cost-effective use of resources.

The hospital is a precarious environment for older adults who are particularly susceptible to adverse drug reactions, falls, infection, and the consequences of immobility. Goals focus on raising the standards of nursing care through geriatric education, focused nursing assessment, evidence-based protocols, and outcomes that take into consideration optimal function and comfort, as well as dignity.[8] Therefore, nurses as well as advanced practice nurses need to expand their roles in attaining expert skills to embed geriatric evidence-based nursing practice in a care delivery system geared toward the growing magnitude of older persons in need of health care services.

## Acute Care Geriatric Model Design

Given the profile of this patient population, how do we design a program suited to an acute care setting based on evidence-based medicine and evidence-based nursing practices? Geriatric expertise is vital no matter where older persons reside—whether in the emergency room, surgery, medicine, oncology, or other specialty services. Clinical issues identified by clinicians include a variety of syndromes such as cognitive impairment, sensory needs, nutrition, skin integrity, incontinence, and functional decline. In order to implement and sustain a geriatric program, a design needs to achieve best practice that is sensitive to the unique needs of this population. Acute care organizations throughout the country have adopted and tailored geriatric models of care by incorporating education, training that uses the expertise of advanced practice nurses in implementing and integrating the clinical, psychosocial, and financial aspects that influence care needed by older patients and their families.

A recent study demonstrated that an advanced practice nurse-centered discharge planning and home care interventions for at-risk hospitalized older persons reduced readmissions, lengthened the time between discharge and readmission, and decreased the costs of providing health care.[9] Other academic medical centers participating in a nationwide initiative Nurses Improving Care to Hospitalized Elders (NICHE) project funded by the Hartford Foundation, including Yale-New Haven Hospital, New England Medical Center, University of Virginia Medical Center, and NYU Medical Center (NYUMC), have identified a need to customize and refine geriatric assessments and protocols. NICHE was conceptualized in collaboration with the Educational Development Center, Inc. of Newton, MA, and has been implemented in over 100 sites nationally.[10] Goals aim to identify and develop best practices in nursing care of older adults and infuse these practices at the bedside in providing care to older patients throughout the continuum of care. An exemplar of best practice was demonstrated through a Geriatric Resource Nurse (GRN) model at NYUMC that included immediate access to unit-based expert geriatric nurses, the development of their own clinical expertise, and later the opportunity for professional advancement along the clinical leadership ladder.[11]

At NYUMC, the GRN role development begins with interested staff nurses and a unit-based educational and training program. In the GRN model, unit-based registered nurses volunteered to take a lead role in identifying older persons at risk for functional decline and incorporating geriatric concepts into practice.[12] The inception of practice changes and role development begin with unit-base educational sessions and case studies. Case studies are presented on interdisciplinary grand rounds and conferences along with the expertise of a geriatric nurse practitioner. The object of the case studies, conferences, and discussions is to provide knowledge and skills for staff nurses to become first-line experts in the field of nursing care for the older adult.

The needs of geriatric patients are captured through a systematic assessment, collection of clinical information, geriatric grand rounds presentations, and the use of evidence-based approaches for geriatric clinical problems. An example of systematic review to capture potential and existing geriatric problems in hospitalized older persons was first introduced by Dr. Fulmer called "SPICES" (sleep problems, problems with eating and feeding, incontinence, confusion, evidence of falls, skin breakdown).[12] Continual refinement of tool development and self-learning modules has also been designed and tailored to benefit the needs of individual organizations such as the University of Virginia and North Memorial Health Care in Robbinsdale, Minneapolis.[13,14]

Central to a comprehensive assessment is discharge planning, which is aimed at attaining continuity of care.[15] The process should ensure a prompt and well-organized medical and nursing discharge plan in the acute environment and after hospitalization. Therefore, crucial to discharge planning is efficient transitions from hospital to home in meeting continual medical, functional recovery and preventing adverse relapse encountered in readmissions.[15]

Most recently, NYUMC has designed a comprehensive geriatric program to incorporate an admission assessment tool, which identifies older adults who have an increased risk for further health complications in the hospital and at home after discharge. The NYUMC tool is called "SHARING." The "SHARING" tool identifies older persons exhibiting the following: *s*kin breakdown, *h*earing/visual impairments, *a*lteration in mental status, *r*estraint alternatives, *i*ncontinence, *n*utritional needs, and *g*uarding gait needs.[11] After the patient is discharged, a SHARING follow-up phone call program facilitates the transition from hospital to home and aims to prevent readmissions.

NYUMC as well as numerous NICHE hospital sites have also incorporated evidence-based tools into admission assessments to identify high-risk older adults and prompt early interventions. Screening instruments are used to assess cognition, delirium, ADLs, independent activities of daily living, as well as assessing function, that is, Mini-Mental State Examination, Cognitive Assessment Method, and Instrumental Activities of Daily Living (IADL). ADL tools are part of nursing admission assessments and documentation systems.[16–19]

Depending on the needs of the organization, evidence-based tools are implemented and tailored to meet the needs of patients, families, and the constant changing health care demands to achieve successful clinical outcomes. Without strong assessment skills, the nurse is unable to plan the required care of the older person and further evaluate physiologic and psychologic changes. It is important to have supportive leadership and clinical experts in providing skills required to facilitate assessment, integrate the information collected, and communicate this information to other staff involved in the care of the older population.[20]

In many NICHE sites where the GRN model is practiced, educational sessions include didactic information on advanced nursing care of hospitalized older persons. The format for these sessions is formal all-day conferences presented by advanced practice nurses. Other expertise is available through university faculty as well as guest experts in the field of gerontologic care. Formal lecture presentations may be 30 to 40 minutes long with additional time for discussion. Case studies are presented as a collaborative effort among interdisciplinary team members to identify older persons who are at high risk for functional decline.

Incentives for the geriatric expert unit staff nurse need to be incorporated into a clinical ladder advancement. Financial reward compensation for board certification as well as other incentives to publish program outcomes has been overwhelmingly motivational in many NICHE sites. Accomplishments are well documented in participating NICHE sites through conferences, composing abstracts for research studies, exhibiting program outcome poster presentations, as well as contributing to research journals. The GRN model has provided several benefits in acute care institutions: The nursing staff has become more sensitive to the needs of geriatric patients. Geriatric nursing practice has improved, and critical groups of nurses now work together to formulate a program of nursing research in older person care.[21,22] Therefore, the approach formed the core strategy of the new model geriatric care.

## CARE ISSUES

### Common Geriatric Problems in the Acute Care Setting

Functional decline occurs in 25% to 60% of older persons after entering acute care because of the interaction of patients' existing comorbidities with the hospital environment.[23] The initial assessment of physical function should include documentation of a patient's ability to perform ADLs and IADLs.[18] The Katz ADL scale assesses a patient's ability to perform related functions: bathing, dressing, toileting, transferring, continence, and eating. The IADL tool evaluates the ability in tasks such as telephone use, shopping, transportation, budget management, adhering to medication regimens, cooking, housekeeping, and laundry.[19]

The "Up and Go" test is a performance-based measure that can be easily administered in any setting. The patient is asked to rise from a sitting position, walk 10 feet, turn, and return to the chair and sit.[24] Patients performing the task in less than 20 seconds are generally independent. Patients who take longer than 30 seconds to complete this test tend to be more dependent and are at a high risk for falls.[24] Moreover, care planning needs to incorporate physiotherapy early in an admission episode to improve strength, endurance, and mobility. Older patients admitted to an acute care setting have specialized needs vital to a plan of care that needs to be recognized promptly at admission by clinicians in order to maintain and optimize ADL function.

Malnutrition occurs in as many as 40% of patients in acute care settings.[25] The most accurate evidence of malnutrition in a patient is hypocholesterolemia and hypoalbuminemia.[26] Assessment of malnutrition involves a dietary history, daily caloric intake, the availability of food, the use of nutritional and herbal supplements, and the adequacy of the patient's diet. In addition, malnutrition increases the risk of pressure ulcer development and delays wound healing and possibly results in diminished tensile strength in healing wounds as well as increased wound dehiscence.[27]

Skin breakdown is often an iatrogenic complication of hospitalization and increased length of stay, as well as a contributor to mortality and morbidity.[28] The prevalence of pressure ulcers is as high as 23% for hospitalized patients.[25] It is generally agreed that pressure ulcers are preventable. The Braden Scale for predicting pressure sore risk is the most widely used tool by acute care institutions to identify at-risk patients on admission for skin breakdown. The Braden tool in the acute care environment assesses risk within 48 hours or when there is a condition change in the following six areas: sensory perception, skin moisture, activity, mobility, nutrition, and friction/shear.[29] Braden score items range from 6 to 23. Scores of 16 or less indicate a high risk, whereas scores of more than 16 indicate moderate to no risk for the general population.[30,31]

Older patients over the age of 65 years may have extensive nutritional needs, require assistance with ADLs, and have problems with continence. Urinary incontinence affects up to 31% of hospitalized patients 65 years old and older.[32] Incontinence is associated with a decreased ability to perform ADLs and is strongly linked with pressure ulcer development.[32] Interventions aim to maintain skin integrity with the proper use of skin care products and incontinence products to wick urine from skin.[20] The nursing plan of care necessitates evaluation of current medications that can cause incontinence. Additionally, establishing a regular toileting schedule along with a daily bladder diary and bowel-tracking diary optimizes care delivery.

The decision to use an indwelling urinary catheter should be made with the knowledge that it may involve the risk of producing side effects and possibly contribute to disease when used inappropriately.[33] The incidence of bacteriuria in patients with an indwelling urinary catheter may be directly linked to the duration of catheterization. Of patients with bacteriuria, 10% to 25% will develop symptoms of local urinary tract infections, and approximately 3% will develop bacteremia, a serious and possibly life-threatening complication.[33] Moreover, the use of indwelling urinary catheters is associated with lower survival and a longer length of stay.[34]

In the United States, more than $400 million is spent yearly on over-the-counter laxatives.[35] Bowel management is an essential component of the patient's overall health status and should be addressed using the same degree of concern in evaluation and treatment of other body systems and functions.[36] Constipation is a concern for older individuals with poor dentition, inadequate diet, immobility, dehydration, polypharmacy, depression, dementia, metabolic imbalances, and co-morbid illnesses.[35] Constipation is estimated to affect 25% of the older adults and is responsible for more than 2.5 million physician visits every year.[37] Nearly 50% of all patients older than 65 years reported using laxatives.[38] Bowel management should take into consideration the specific needs of the older patient. Additionally, constipation may be a consequence of the administration of pharmacologic agents, which are introduced for the alleviation or prevention of other pathophysiologic conditions.[39] Clinicians can aid in the prevention of bowel complications and can establish a regimen review periodically.

Visual impairment is usually disregarded and misjudged in the older hospitalized adult. An essential item that requires attention at admission is the potential loss of vision or the need of assistive devices for effective communication that increases the need for maintaining independent functioning. Visual impairment is an important cause of activity limitation and disability and places the older adult at greater risk for falls, hip fractures, and other injuries.[40]

Pain is not part of the normal aging process. Pain was defined by the North American Nursing Diagnosis Association in 1992 as "a state in which an individual experiences and reports the presence of severe discomfort of an uncomfortable sensation."[40] Pain can be divided into the following categories: (1) acute pain after an injury or surgery, (2) chronic malignant pain resulting from a progressive, possibly fatal, disorder such as cancer, and (3) chronic nonmalignant pain representing a progressive disorder that does not directly result in death, such as osteoarthritis.[40] Examples of more commonly used pain assessment tools include Visual Analogue Scales (VASs), Numerical Rating Scales (NRSs), and Verbal Descriptor Scales (VDSs).[40] VASs have 10-cm horizontal or vertical lines with a marker on each end indicating the absence of pain on one end and worst pain possible at the other end. NRS patients are asked to rate their pain intensity on a 0 to 5, 0 to 10, or 0 to 100 scale. Zero represents the absence of pain, and the highest number of the scale represents the worst possible pain. A VDS has a list of words that indicates pain for increasing levels of intensity. In using the VDS scale, patients are asked to choose the adjective that best describes their past or present pain.

Nonverbal or cognitively impaired older adults pose assessment challenges.[40] Cognitively impaired older persons may fail to interpret sensations as painful, are often less able to recall their pain, and may not be able to communicate verbally with staff; therefore, older adults are frequently undertreated for pain.[41] Clinicians may need to rely more on nonverbal cues, such as facial grimaces or bracing restlessness, for individuals who are unable to communicate verbally.

A recent use of an observational tool used in acute care settings is the Nonverbal Pain Indicator (NPI). The NPI tool captures the presence of a pain indicator, which is scored as a 1, and the total number of indicators are summed for those occurring at rest, with movement, and overall. There are no cutoff scores with the NPI. The presence of any of the behavioral indicators of pain warrants further investigation, treatment, and monitoring by clinicians.[41] Therefore, development of new tools for cognitively impaired and nonverbal older patients continues to require astute observation and research.

## Acute Medical and Functional Recovery

Health in older persons is best measured in terms of function. Forty percent of all older patients experience a functional decline as a result of hospitalizations.[2] Older persons are mostly prone to adverse drug reactions, falls, infection, and the effects of immobility. These complications are recognized as iatrogenic events. The term "iatrogenesis" refers to any adverse physical or mental condition caused by the effects of treatment.[2] Up to 75% of older people experience a decrease in their functional ability from hospital admission to discharge, which often results in the need for home health care services, dependent community living, or long-term care facility placement.[42]

The incidence of fractures also increases exponentially with age. Hip fractures are the most severe in terms of morbidity.[43] Hip fractures are a serious consequence of falls in the older population. More than 90% of hip fractures in persons over 70 years of age are caused by falls.[44] Falls are common among the older population and are the leading cause of injury-related deaths and hospitalization. Morbidity coupled with falls comprises physical injury, psychologic trauma, and a loss of independence with early institutionalizations.[43]

Delirium, dementia, depression, and protein–energy malnutrition are also very common and frequently undetected in a hospitalized older adult. Comprehensive geriatric assessment and planning to optimize functional and medical recovery involve looking at high-risk factors that include cognitive status, depression, malnutrition, ADL/IADL function, and financial disability. Cognitive impairment in older persons prolongs hospital recovery of ADL and IADL function. Delirium may affect 60% of frail older people in the hospital.[45] Forty-five percent of hospitalized, cognitively impaired older adults have been found to develop delirium accounting for longer lengths of stay, a higher rate of complications, and increased cost of care.[45] The Confusion Assessment Method tool distinguishes delirium, also known as reversible confusion, from other types of cognitive impairment.[17] Interventions to reduce adverse events such as delirium may include orienting patients frequently, reducing sleep deprivation by limiting vital signs during the night, walking patients when possible, ensuring that patients' sensory aids are functioning, and avoiding dehydration.

Depression is not a natural part of aging. However, depression can be common in late life. Collectively, major depression and minor depression are reported in 13% of community-dwelling older adults, 24% of older medical outpatients, and 43% of both acute care and nursing home-dwelling adults.[46] The Geriatric Depression Scale has been used extensively with older adults. Essentially, patients are asked 30 questions, answering with yes and no regarding how they feel that day. Scores of 0–9 are normal, 10–19 indicate mild depression, and 20–30 severe depression.[47] This tool is useful in assessing baseline depression in older adults and comparing later scores in a hospital episode.

In physical assessment, the presence of muscle wasting should be correlated with laboratory tests such as serum and total cholesterol levels, and lymphocyte count should be added.[26] In addition, prealbumin is the earliest laboratory indicator of nutritional status and has become known as the ideal marker for malnutrition.[48] Generally, albumin is considered a late indicator of malnutrition.[49] Albumin has a half-life of 20 days as compared with prealbumin, which has a half-life of 2 days, making prealbumin a more timely and sensitive indicator. Patients should also be assessed for oral pathology, ill-fitting dentures, problems with speech or swallowing, medication use that might cause anorexia or dysgeusia, and financial and social problems that may be contributing factors to malnutrition.[26]

To improve outcomes, prevention is a key element in the care of older patients. Older adults are particularly more prone than younger adults to experience a "cascade iatrogenesis," which is a sequence of adverse events that begins with a single problem such as a medication error, aspiration, skin breakdown, or a fall.[2] The goal of intervening to alter the incidence of "cascade iatrogenesis" in hospitalized older patients demands early assessment of potential problems and interventions to preserve functional mobility.[2]

Medication assessment is necessary for use of sedatives, hypnotics, narcotics, anticholinergics, glycemic agents, diuretics, and other pharmacologic agents, placing the older patient at risk. Other clinical indicators such as serum values, oxygenation, and other therapeutic drug regimens should be monitored closely. In addition, assess for alternatives and need for restraints, tubes, catheters, and intravenous lines whenever possible. Geriatric patients in the hospital are more vulnerable to the risks associated with physical and chemical restraints.[50] Additionally, it is important to ensure that undernourished patients eat frequent meals and incorporate oral supplements as needed in a plan of care.

An estimated 25% to 40% of all US medication prescriptions are written for older people.[51] Older patients are more likely than younger persons to have four or more prescribed medications.[52] A component of a thorough geriatric assessment is a medication review and recognition of medication adverse drug effects. This assessment requires coordination and knowledge of drug reactions and costs. Iatrogenic drug reactions average 20% to 25% for hospitalized older persons.[42] Differences in how drugs are absorbed, metabolized, and excreted in older persons alter their response to medications and increase the need for close monitoring of drug therapy. Older adults' susceptibility to drug-induced health problems is also a reflection of the estimated hospital admission rates for drug-related problems and toxicity ranging between 10% and 33%.[51] In addition, the lack of financial resources for medications, groceries, and household utilities can impact both a decline in function and morbidity and mortality after discharge.

Family is an important health care resource for older patients in planning for medical and functional recovery. Family members have an important role in easing an older person's hospital stay by being physically present, providing familiar voices and items, and maintaining usual family routines and life patterns in the hospital.[53] Interventions need to be coordinated to accomplish increased communication between family caregivers and health care providers as well as identification of specific caregiving activities for families in order to improve outcomes for hospitalized older persons.

## Multidisciplinary Care of the Older Adult

The health care environment has been extremely influenced by higher patient acuity, cost-containment measures, an increase in lawsuits, and increased expectations by an educated generation of health care consumers.[54] In the acute care setting, individual experts from different disciplines come together to care for patients. Each team member contributes his or her special skills and experience in addressing the task at hand. Mobilization of resources, with interdisciplinary team members, focuses on the clinical, functional, psychosocial, and financial elements influencing care. Multidisciplinary geriatric consultation teams provide comprehensive assessment and make recommendations regarding prevention and management of common geriatric syndromes.

Team goals are to preserve function and medical recovery by preventing nosocomial complications such as falls, delirium, and functional decline. A geriatric team may have at least one physician, an advanced practice nurse certified in gerontology, a social worker, a nutritionist, a pharmacist, and other specialty team members contributing individual expertise of patient needs. Team members are empowered in their designated roles to contribute to an optimized patient experience and enhance productivity of these interactions leading to better outcomes, both functional and clinical.[55]

Cohesive health care teams have five key characteristics: clear goals with measurable outcomes, clinical and administrative systems, division of labor, training of all team members, and effective communication.[56] A unified and effective multidisciplinary team is critical and associated with positive clinical outcomes and increased patient and family satisfaction. The demand for quality care requires a group of diverse clinicians who communicate with each other regularly about the care of a defined group of patients and who participate in that care. Interdisciplinary team rounds are a coordination strategy to generate and integrate an interdisciplinary plan of care for patients and their families.[57] These activities outline shared pertinent information, approaches for dealing with difficult and long-standing patient problems, identification of barriers to care and potential solutions, and the identification of individual and team learning needs.[58] In addition, team activities must consider not only the patient clinical outcomes, but also customer service ratings and financial outcomes.[54]

## NURSING PRACTICES

### Role of the Expert Staff Nurse

In a clinical ladder, organization at each level commensurates with the nurse's education, demonstrated expertise, and experience. Tailoring a geriatric model of care focuses on the third and fourth clinical levels that are comparable to Benner's stages of "competent" and "proficient nurse." Emphasis is on the nurses' use of analysis to connect situations to an appropriate action that focuses on the problem at hand.[59] Efforts at the bedside need to address all levels of staff nursing and advanced practice nursing. There is also a growing demand to incorporate best practices and geriatric certifications among staff nurses as well as advanced practice nurses in all specialty practices in the care of the older patient. Nurse-to-nurse expert consultation is essential in providing seamless care across services and institutional settings.

At NYUMC, nurses achieve a senior staff nurse, a nurse clinician, or senior nurse clinician title through a clinical ladder program which formally supports and recognizes the development of clinical expertise, such as geriatric nursing. The continual pursuit of educational advancement skills into practice is important. The expert staff nurse is identified as a GRN by other staff and team members. A GRN is identified as a unit role model as well as first-line educator in assessing, intervening, and evaluating geriatric syndrome management. A success of a GRN model is the recruitment of staff nurses who care for older adults and use the expertise of an advanced practice nurse to integrate select geriatric core competencies into his or her nursing care.

Key initiatives from NICHE site programs include creating, using, and refining EBP tools as well as protocols in assessment of the older adult at risk for acute confusion, urinary incontinence, falls, restraints, as well as other prevalent syndromes unique to an organization. At numerous NICHE sites, alternative treatment options have shown to decrease medical orders for restraints and the amount of time patients require restraints. The development of alternatives to restraints includes the assessment and prevention of falls, reorientation, using nonpharmacologic alternatives to restraints, the use of sensory and assistive devices (hearing aid, glasses, walkers, canes, etc.), and involving family/hospital volunteers at the bedside in a plan of care.

Incorporating the skills of nursing attendants is an integral part of a geriatric assessment and management. A comprehensive plan of care involves nursing attendants participating in rounds, conferences, and case studies in coordinating toileting, restraint alternatives, and mealtime routines that may potentially decrease functional incontinence, immobility, and the risk of malnutrition. A GRN's participation in interdisciplinary rounds addresses the need to have accountability and responsibility for care coordination. GRNs are encouraged to present patients to the interdisciplinary team, coordinate various referrals, and identify interventions that support the comprehensive patient and family plan of care. The GRN model has demonstrated in several NICHE sites an increase in interdisciplinary staff knowledge, sensitivity, and creativity in caring for our older adults and their families across the continuum.

## Focused Geriatric Case Management

According to the January 2002 Case Management Advisor, companies are using their data to predict patterns of high use in the future and get case managers involved earlier.[60,61] The larger insurers are looking for innovative ways to work with their data and to identify which patients can benefit from more intensive services early on. Nevertheless, a complication from chronic illness consumes a significant proportion of the nation's health care dollars.[60,61] Payers, providers, and employers are looking at ways to avoid hospitalization and improve health maintenance.[8] Managed care has placed increasing pressure on hospitals to provide cost-effective and high-quality care and to reduce house staff. This development has encouraged teaching hospitals to employ nurse practitioners.[62] In addition, increasing acuity and age among the inpatient population combined with the need to reduce length of stay suggest a need to re-examine the delivery of care in the acute care setting.

Hospital-based nursing case management has been acknowledged as a viable advanced practice role for nurses.[8] The role of the advanced practice nurse to integrate case management skills is part of the solution to manage complex multiple chronic issues as our population ages.[8] Advanced practice nurses have a pivotal role in identifying an at-risk population such as geriatrics with focus on disease management. A common and challenging example is high-risk older groups who have dementia and multiple co-morbid illnesses; who are dependent in ADLs, living alone, requiring complex patient and family teaching; and who are financially challenged and in need of postdischarge follow-up care.

To manage patient care, a health care system requires reliable systems to evaluate medical needs. In addition, this also necessitates the assessment of the level of care and services provided tracking patient care as patients move across the continuum of care.[8] With a limited number of geriatricians and nurses in the field of geriatrics, advanced practice nurses in a variety of specialty areas are seeking certification in geriatrics.[63] Advanced practice nurses function as part of a team and bring advanced skills to a greater collaboration with payers and providers and an increased flow of information among all parts of the health care system.[8]

Advanced practice nurses are critical members of the health care team that involves getting people through the system more efficiently and eliminating delays in clinical testing, resource utilization, and achieving clinical daily outcomes. This is crucial in optimizing acute functional recovery and minimizing iatrogenesis in the high-risk older population. At NYUMC, a follow-up phone call program facilitates the transition from hospital to home, prevents readmissions, and promotes wellness through education and the use of community resources. Further analysis of this process should include specialty service standardized assessment instruments, electronic communication, increased community outreach education, training, continuity, and expanded service options for patients who do not meet the homebound requirements.[64]

## Advanced Practice Role

Approximately 4,200 nurses had been certified in geriatric care since 1991.[63] In 2003, few people were enrolled full-time in programs to become certified gerontologic nurse specialists.[63] Given the minimal number of trained professionals in the field of geriatrics and the growing population of older adults, it is likely that advanced practice nurses, especially those specializing in adult and family practice, are caring for many older adults. Considering the large number of older adults served by all specialty nurses, the geriatric competence of all nurses will need to be enhanced.[63] This includes the knowledge, skills, and attitudes of nearly 400,000 registered nurses who belong to more than 450 national specialty nursing associations.[65] Nevertheless, the expertise of geriatric nurse practitioners has been preferred and used by a number of acute care institutions to provide expert consultation as well as designing and implementing programs that meet the needs of hospitalized older persons.

Advanced practice nurses are in a pivotal role in meeting the challenges of acute care for the hospitalized older population in the new millennium. Institutions are recognizing the need to foster and sustain institutional geriatric educational and training programs such as NICHE. Opportunities aim at conducting bedside research as well as identifying areas for future study. Future areas for research can include further analysis of securing medication compliance, health promotion and prevention, reducing unnecessary hospital resources, that is, avoiding readmission, cost containment, and decreasing length of stay without compromising quality care. Most importantly, resources need to be explored that serve the financially challenged older population with no or limited prescriptive plans, dental care, and afford-able medications.

Health promotion and prevention programs are becoming more the necessity of any acute care organization that directly impacts mortality, morbidity, patient/family satisfaction as well as hospital costs. Assess-ment by expert team members aids in identifying families for outpa-tient follow-up and support programs and provides assistance in coping with hospitalization. Community outreach programs on various older population topics, as well as individual counseling, aid in readiness to learn programs on self-management of disease such as diabetes, chronic obstructive pulmonary disease, and heart failure. Future advanced prac-tice nurses with geriatric expertise are critical to support families caring for this growing population.

As the older population increases, a new generation of baby boomers who are more involved with their care will demand more computer-related health care information. Patients and families want to know what their options are, and payer organizations will be re-quired to provide coverage.[61,62] Payers are recognizing the fact that automation is going to be the only way to remain lucrative. Advanced practice nurses' skills are essential to health care institutions through automated electronic systems that are capable of promoting standards for ordering and processing electronic prescriptions, equipment, re-sources, and follow-up teaching in chronic disease management.[66] Therefore, automation allows advanced practice nurses to focus on appropriate care, adhere to guidelines, and explain options to pa-tients.

Given the complex needs of older patients, advanced practice nurs-ing is challenged to conduct skilled, continuous geriatric assessment throughout hospitalization and after discharge to determine needs, medication reviews, and medication affordability, and in turn provide cost-effective care without compromising quality care. As we continue to meet the challenges of acute care, geriatric assessment warrants in-novative models of care and programs to ensure access to geriatric ex-perts as well as a multidisciplinary care management approach with the growing numbers of older people in the years to come. Continu-ing support to nursing staff from clinical and managerial nursing leaders and from university faculty provides knowledge, sensitivity, and awareness to identify syndromes and effectively measure out-comes and implement and evaluate care protocols. Finally, providing advanced practice nurses with specialized geriatric skills in addressing disease management, health promotion, and prevention in meeting the financially challenged high-risk older adult is critical in the viability of all institutions regardless of setting.

*Acknowledgment:* *My sincerest gratitude to NYU Medical Center and the Hartford Institute for Geriatric Nursing for their continued support towards my clinical advancement of geriatric nursing practice. I gratefully acknowledge the assistance of Kristin Lemko, RN, BSN, in the preparation of this manuscript.*

## REFERENCES

1. Federal International Forum on Aging. *Older Americans 2004: Key Indicators of Well-Being.* Washington, DC: U.S. Government Printing Office; November 2004.

2. Habel M. The hospitalized older adult. *Nurse Week.* March 2004;5(3):22–24.

3. Landsfeld S, Rooke A. Hospital care geriatrics. *Ann Long Term Care.* 2004;12:19–24.

4. Naylor, M. Nursing counts: Delirium, depression often overlooked: Hospitalized elders require special care. *Am J Nurs.* 2003;103:116.

5. American Hospital Association. *Health Statistics,* 2001 ed. Chicago Health Forum; 2001.

6. DeGeorges K. Untangling the web of evidence-based health care. *AWHONN Lifelines.* 1999;3:47–48.

7. Closs SJ, Cheater FM. Evidence for nursing practice: A clarification of the issues. *J Adv Nurs.* 1999;30:10–17.

8. McKendry M, Van Horn J. Today's hospital-based case manager: How one hospital integrated/adopted evidence-based medicine using InterQual Criteria. *Nursing Case Management.* 2004;9:61–71.

9. Naylor MD, Brooten D, Campbell R, et al. Comprehensive discharge planning and home follow-up of hospitalized elders: A randomized clinical trial. *JAMA.* 1999;28:613–620.

10. Fulmer T, Mezey M, Botrell M et al. Nurses Improving Care for Healthsystem Elders (NICHE): Using outcomes and benchmarks for evidence-based practice. *Geriatr Nurs.* 2002;23:127.

11. Lopez M, Delmore B, Ake J, et al. Implementing a geriatric resource nurse model. *J Nurs Admin.* 2002;32:577–585.

12. Fulmer T. SPICES: An overall assessment tool of older adults. *MEDSURG Nurs.* 2002;11:44–45.

13. Lee KV, Fletcher K. Sustaining the geriatric resource nurse model at the University of Virginia. *Geriatric Nurs.* 2002;23:128–132.

14. Guthrie PF, Edinger G, Schumacher S. TWICE: A NICHE Program at North Memorial Health Care. *Geriatr Nurs.* 2002;23:133–138.

15. Smith S. Discharge planning: The need for effective communication. *Nurs Stand.* 1996;10:39–41.

16. Folstein MF, Folstein SE, McHugh PR. "Mini-Mental State": A practical method for grading the cognitive state of patients for the clinician. *J Psychiatr Res.* 1995;12:189–198.

17. Inouye SK, Van Dyck CH, Balkin S, et al. Clarifying confusion: The cognitive assessment method: A new method for detection of delirium. *Ann Intern Med.* 1990;113:941–948.

18. Katz SF, Moskowitz RW, Jackson BA, et al. Studies of illness in the aged: The Index of ADL: A standardized measure of biological and psychological function. *JAMA*. 1963;185:914–919.

19. Lawton MP, Brody EM. Assessment of older people: Self-Maintaining and instrumental activities of daily living. *Gerontologist*. 1969;9:179–186.

20. Olenek K, Skowronski T, Schmaltz D. Geriatric nursing assessment: A holistic approach to patient care incorporating the "giants of geriatric nursing" and patient psychosocial issues can improve nursing assessment. *Gerontol Nurs*. 2003;29:5–9.

21. Fulmer TT. The geriatric nurse specialist role: A new model. *Nursing Manage*. 1991; 22:91–93.

22. Fulmer TT. Grow your own experts in hospital elder care. *Geriatr Nurs*. 1991; 12:64–66.

23. Palmer RM. Acute hospital care of the elderly: Minimizing the risk of functional decline. *Clev Clin J Med*. 1995;62:117–128.

24. Posiadlo D, Richardson S. The timed "Up and Go": A test of basic functional mobility for frail elderly persons. *J Am Geriatr*. 1991;39:142–148.

25. Himes D. Protein–calorie malnutrition and involuntary weight loss: The role of aggressive nutritional intervention in wound healing. *Ostomy Wound Manage*. 1999;45: 46–55.

26. Robertson RG, Montagnini M. Geriatric failure to thrive. *Am Fam Physician*. 2004; 15;70:343–350.

27. Zulkowski K. A conceptual model of pressure ulcer prevalence: MDS + items and nutrition. *Ostomy Wound Manage*. 1999;45:36–44.

28. Nelson EA, Bradley MD. Dressings and topical agents for arterial leg ulcers (Cochrane Review). *The Cochrane Library*. Issue 4. Chichester, UK: John Wiley and Sons; 2003.

29. Ayello E, Braden B. How and why to do pressure ulcer risk assessment. *Adv Skin Wound Care*. 2002;15:125–132.

30. Braden B, Bergstrom N. Predictive validity of the Braden Scale for Pressure Score Risk in a nursing home population. *Res Nurs Health*. 1994;17:459–470.

31. Bergstrom N, Braden B, Boynton P, Bruch S. Using a research-based assessment scale in clinical practice. *Nurs Clin North Am*. 1995;30:539–551.

32. Iqbal P, Casteleden CM. Management of urinary incontinence in the elderly. *Gerontology*. 1997;43:151–157.

33. Saint S. Clinical and economic consequences of nosocomial catheter-related bacteriuria. *Am J Infect Control*. 2000;28:68–75.

34. Landefeld S, Rooke GA. Hospital Care Geriatrics. *Annal Long-Term Care*. 2004;12: 19–24.

35. Pekmezaris R, Aversa L, Wolf-Klein G, et al. The cost of chronic constipation. *Am Coll Med Direct*. 2002;3:224–228.

36. Salcido R. Bowel problems in older adults. *Topics Geriatr Rehab*. 2000;16:92–96.

37. Harris MS. The evaluation and treatment of constipation. *Pract Gastroenterol*. 1998;22:12–17.

38. Wilson JAP. Constipation in the elderly. *Clin Geriatr Med*. 1999;15:499–509.

39. Richmond JP, Wright ME. Review of the literature on constipation to enable development of a constipation risk assessment scale. *Clin Effect Nurs*. 2004;8:11–25.

40. Forrest J. Assessment of acute and chronic pain in older adults. *J Gerontol Nurs.* 1995;21:15–20.

41. Horgas AL. Assessing pain in persons with dementia. Try this: Best practices in nursing care for hospitalized older adults. *John Hartford Geriatr Nurs Alzheimer's Assoc.* 2003;1.

42. Zulkowuski K. Examination of care-planning needs for elderly newly admitted to an acute care setting. *Ostomy Wound Management.* 2000;46(1):32–38.

43. Broadhurst KCM, Wilson MT, Kinirons AW, et al. Clinical pharmacology of old age syndromes. *Clin Pharmacol.* 2003;56:261–272.

44. McElhinney J, Koval K, Zuckerman JD. Falls and the elderly. *Arch Am Acad Orthopaed Surg.* 1998;2:60–65.

45. Britton A, Russell R. Multidisciplinary team interventions for delirium in patients with chronic cognitive impairment. *The Cochrane Library.* 2004(2).

46. Kurlowicz L. The Geriatric Depression Scale: Try this: Best practices in nursing care to older adults. *Hartford Institute Geriatr Nurs.* 1999;4.

47. Yesavage JA, Brink TL, Rose TL, et al. Development and validation of a geriatric depression screening scale: A preliminary report. *J Psychiatr Res.* 1982;17:37–49.

48. Beck F, Rosenthal TC. Prealbumin: A marker for nutritional evaluation. *Am Fam Physician.* 2002;65:1575–1578.

49. Collins N. The difference between albumin and prealbumin. *Adv Wound Skin Care.* 2001;14:235–236.

50. Fletcher K. Use of restraints in the elderly. *Clin Adv Pract Acute Crit Care.* 1996;7: 611–620.

51. DeMaagd G. High-risk drugs in the elderly population. *Geriatr Nurs.* 1995;16: 198–207.

52. Hall M, Owings MF. Division of Health Care Statistics. *2000 National Hospital Discharge Survey.* Advance Data 329. Department of Health and Human Services. Hyattsville, Maryland.

53. Li H, Melnyk B, McCann R, et al. Improving outcomes of hospitalized elders and family caregivers. *Nat Inst Health/National Inst Nurs Res.* 2003;26:284–299.

54. Sierchio GP. A multidisciplinary approach for improving outcomes. *J Infus Nurs.* 2003;26:34–43.

55. Schaefer J, Davis C. Case management and the chronic care model: A multidisciplinary role. *Case Manage.* 2004;9:96–103.

56. Grumback K, Bodenheimer T. Can health care teams improve primary care practice? *JAMA.* 2004;291:1246–1251.

57. Smith S. Discharge planning: The need for effective communication. *Nurs Stand.* 1996;10:39–41.

58. Margo H, Gagner S, Goering M, et al. Interdisciplinary rounds: Impact on patients, families, and staff. *Clin Nurse Spec.* 2003;17:133–142.

59. Benner P. From Novice to Expert: Excellence and Power in Clinical Nursing Practice. Menlo Park, California. Addison Wesley Publishing; 1994.

60. New year heralds increased need for care managers in health care. Case Management Advisor. American Health Consultants. 2002;13(1):1–12.

61. Changing health care environment can make discharge planning a juggling act. Case Management Advisor. American Health Consultants. *Hospital Case Management.* April 2003;11:49–64.

62. Kovner CP, Harrington C. Nursing counts: Acute care nurse practitioners. *Am J Nurs.* 2001;101:61–62.

63. Stotts N, Deitrich CE. The challenge to come: The care of older adults. *Am J Nurs.* 2004;104:40–47.

64. Bowles K, Foust J, Naylor M. Hospital discharge referral decision making: A multidisciplinary perspective. *Appl Nurs Res.* 2003;16:134–143.

65. Mezey M, Fulmer T. The future history of gerontological nursing. *J Gerontol A Biol Sci Med Sci.* 2002;57:M438–M441.

66. Wakefield B. Enhancing care for older individuals through telehealth. *J Gerontol Nurs.* 2003;29:4.

# Section IV
## Specialty Topics for Clinicians

# 18

# *Adherence to Medical Treatment*

Hillary R. Bogner and Monica Crane

Adherence is "the extent to which a person's behavior (in terms of taking medications, following diets, or executing lifestyle changes) coincides with medical or health advice."[1] "The term compliance is troublesome to many people because it conjures up images of patient or client sin or serfdom."[1] Here the focus is on several patient-level factors, but physician and treatment factors are associated with adherence as well (Table 18–1). Indeed, there are system and health policy issues, such as the availability of health insurance coverage, that relate to adherence that are not shown in Table 18–1.

Adherence is a multifaceted concept. Patients may be adherent to some components of their therapeutic regimen but not to others (takes medicine but does not follow diet or exercise recommendations), may follow instructions to take medicine for one condition but not for others (takes medicine for congestive heart failure but not for depression), or may follow instructions at some times but not at others (takes antihypertensive only when feeling "tense"). Haynes et al.[2] and others[3,4] reviewed the factors associated with adherence to medical regimens. Generally, the efforts to predict nonadherence from patient demographic variables alone have not been fruitful; however, features of the medical regimen (e.g., side effects, costs, number of medications), aspects of the clinical setting (e.g., the time to the refer-

**Table 18–1** Patient, Physician, and Treatment Factors Potentially Associated with Adherence to Medical Regimens, not Necessarily Listed in Order of Importance. Characteristics May Not Be Independently Associated with Adherence.

### *Patient*

Demographic variables (age, gender, ethnicity, and level of educational attainment)
Functional status
- Activities of daily living
- Instrumental activities of daily living

Past experiences
- Personal experience with health care
- Past experience of family or friends with health care

Cognitive functioning
- Memory
- Attention
- Executive functioning/planning

Cultural beliefs and norms about illness and its treatment
Efficacy beliefs
- Outcome–efficacy beliefs (treatment can change the outcome)
- Self-efficacy beliefs (personal efforts can achieve adherence)

Health beliefs about
- Perceived threat of illness
- Risks and benefits of action
- Medications

Personality variables
- Neuroticism (vulnerability and adherence factor)
- Extroversion, agreeableness, conscientiousness, openness to experience (adherence factors)

Social support
- Provides emotional support that improves adherence
- Provides instrumental support, such as transportation, that improves adherence
- Negative feedback may increase stigma and diminish adherence

Physical illness
- direct effect of physical illness on adherence to and outcomes of treatment
- Beliefs and cognitions about physical illness
- Use of multiple medications increases complexity of regimen

Severity of illness
- Number of symptoms
- Interference with functioning

Co-morbid psychiatric conditions
- Anxiety and depression
- Substance abuse (especially alcohol misuse and abuse)

---

**Physician**

---

Patient–physician communication skills
Beliefs about illness and its treatment
- Effectiveness of treatment
- Treatment of illness in older patients is worthwhile and effective

Beliefs about patient interaction
- Telling patients about side effects of medications
- Providing cues that permit the patient to reveal nonadherence to the regimen

Cultural competence in managing illness
- Knowledge of prevalence and incidence of illness across ethnic groups
- Understanding how response to medicines might vary with ethnicity
- Values eliciting the culturally held beliefs and attitudes about illness and its treatment

Concordance between the cultural beliefs and norms of the patient and of the physician
Comfort in dealing with older patients

---

**Treatment**

---

Complexity of the regimen (including the total number of medications taken)
Side effects of medicines that are unpleasant or that interfere with functioning
Age-related changes in drug metabolism and drug–drug interactions
Costs of therapy
- Medication costs
- Costs of medical supplies and visits with specialists (including transportation costs)

Geographic proximity of the primary care office to the specialist office
Time between the primary care visit and the appointment with the specialist
Ethnic differences in pharmacokinetics and pharmacodynamics that affect side effect
  profiles and efficacy

---

ral appointment), and beliefs of the patient about the illness and its treatment do appear to play a role. Other factors, such as personality, have received less attention. Patient knowledge of a condition is not enough to change adherence behavior.[5–7]

Complicating the matter, nonadherence to medicine can be intentional as well as nonintentional.[2] It is commonly assumed that failure to adhere to a medical regimen occurs unintentionally on the patient's part because of lack of understanding or forgetting or for other reasons. Underlying this assumption is that the patient wants to fulfill the requirements of the regimen and that culpability for failure to do so rests entirely with the patient. However, nonadherence to medications and other therapeutic regimens may be intentional. In other words, intentional nonadherence ("intelligent noncompliance")[8] reflects a conscious decision on the part of the patient to stop or modify the treatment.[9] The determinants of these two forms of nonadherence—nonintentional and intentional—are probably different, and thus the interventions to address each may differ as well. The physician and clinical setting probably also play a role in the ability and willingness of the patient to adhere to the recommended regimen. Evidence shows that intentional nonadherence to medical therapy is common in older persons. For example, assessing 372 prescriptions from 111 older adults in at-home interviews, two thirds of the cases of nonadherence were intentional, and only 15% were thought to be due to "forgetting."[10] In a study of hospitalized older persons, 11% of the 315 drug-related admissions were due to noncompliance with medication, and in about one third of the cases, the nonadherence was intentional (e.g., the patient stopped treatment because side effects were not tolerated).[11]

## COGNITIVE FUNCTION

Normal cognitive changes associated with aging are related to a general slowing of overall cognition, which can be modified by physical health, medications, and activity. With a slowed intellectual response time, a nondemented older patient will likely require more time in problem-solving and timed tasks.[12] Also, low health literacy is more prevalent among older adults, which can impact ability to adhere to medications and written instructions.[13] However, the prevalence of dementia increases with age, and thus, it is important to identify patients with cognitive impairment. This is important particularly at earlier stages in a neurodegenerative disease when a patient may not have environmental support systems (spouse, family member, or caregiver) in place.

Cognitive impairment has been associated with a decreased ability to adhere to medication regimens.[14,15] An assessment of executive function, attention and calculation, learning and memory, language, as well as visuospatial function, will help the clinician understand which cognitive activity is impeding a patient's ability to adhere to medications. For example, cognitive tasks related to medication adherence include (1) comprehending the instructions, (2) using working memory to integrate instructions across medications to formulate an adherence plan, (3) remembering the plan or writing it down, and (4) remembering the prospective act of actually taking the medicine as prescribed.[16–18] These tasks require intact cognitive (memory, attention) and executive (planning behaviors) processes.

Particularly important to medication regimens is executive functioning, which involves orchestration of elemental functions into complex goal-directed behavior, and maintaining goal-behavior in the face of internal and external distractions. Executive control is thought to be a function of circuits between frontal lobes and limbic structures. Anterior subcortical lesions involving the frontocaudate projections and the caudate nucleus appear to be associated with depression and impaired initiation of spontaneous behavior.[19] Dysexecutive functioning may be particularly important when the cue for the desired behavior is poorly specified,[20] such as taking medication.

## SOCIAL SUPPORT

Emotional support and regimen-specific support have been shown to increase the adherence to the medical regimen across a variety of medical conditions.[21-24] High social support also reflects personal characteristics, including relationship orientation and skills needed to form a positive treatment relationship with the physicians and others involved in care.[25,26]

## BELIEFS ABOUT ILLNESS AND ITS TREATMENT

The beliefs and ideas of patients regarding illness and its treatment have been cast into a number of frameworks, including the health beliefs model,[27-28] the theory of reasoned action,[29] the theory of planned behavior,[30] the transtheoretical stage model,[31] and the self-regulatory model of illness.[32,33] The self-regulatory model posits cognitive and emotional processing, occurring in parallel, and consisting of evaluation of health threat, coping strategies, and appraisal of the outcomes of decisions.[33] Each model has its strengths and weaknesses, but no single model accounts for a large amount in the variance of health outcomes. Nevertheless, lay concepts of disease appear to affect adherence to therapy in conditions such as hypertension, although physicians do not generally assess and try to correct the symptom models of patients.[34] Patients may adhere to some components of a medical regimen, but not others, depending on their illness representation.[35] There is increasing awareness that patient notions of illness are critical to providing culturally competent and effective health care.[36,37] Failure to elicit ideas about illness can result in poor communication, a lack of adherence to prescribed therapy, or refusal to undergo tests or thera-peutic procedures.

## INTERVENTIONS

Despite the advances in the number of pharmacotherapeutics, few studies have looked at interventions to increase adherence,[38] and even fewer studies have looked at the effect of improved adherence.[39] Given that a decline in speed and processing is the most characteristic change seen with aging, increased patient education may be the first step to improve adherence to regimens. In one study, an education program improved adherence to an antidepressant regimen as well as a response to treatment.[40] Best medication adherence requires nearly all aspects of cognitive function; therefore, multifaceted education programs, or multiple interactions between the provider and patient may allow the patient to overcome a specific area of cognitive diffi-culty. Other literature[41] suggested that multifaceted interventions and interventions tailored to the patient's problem area with adherence resulted more often in improved compliance.

Patients with mild memory loss may benefit from mnemonic aids such as making lists, and using reminders as cognitive tools (self-cueing) (Table 18–2).[42] Some literature suggests that persons over the age of 70 years demonstrated improved adherence when provided with aids to planning and organization.[16,18] Other strategies to help patients adhere to medications include the use of pillboxes and blister packs (premade in the pharmacy). These tools are helpful in aiding

---

**Table 18–2** Helpful Hints

| *Helpful Hints* |
| --- |

Pillboxes
Mail-order pharmacy
 • Some will prepare pillboxes, blister packs, and/or prefilled syringes
Pharmacy call to remind patient to refill medication
Refrigerator medication charts
Having patients equate taking medication along with an activity  e.g., brushing their teeth or making breakfast
Engaging the help of family members

memory as well as allowing for more facile access to pills (as compared with childproof bottles). In addition, polypharmacy increases the risk of adverse drug events, drug interactions, and poor adherence. Providers can request patients to bring in medications for a periodic review to identify unnecessary medications.

## CONCLUSION

Older adults are at risk for adverse health consequences of nonadherence. With the "graying" of our society, there is a need for further research to examine programs that improve adherence in older adults, as well as improve other outcome measures such as decreased morbidity and mortality, and quality of life.

### REFERENCES

1. Haynes RB. Introduction. In: Haynes RB, Taylor DW, Sackett DL, eds. *Compliance in Health Care.* Baltimore: Johns Hopkins University Press; 1979.

2. Haynes RB, Taylor DW, Sackett DL. *Compliance in Health Care.* Baltimore: Johns Hopkins University Press; 1979.

3. Kaplan RM, Simon HJ. Compliance in medical care: Reconsideration of self-predictions. *Ann of Behav Med.* 1990;12:66–71.

4. Coons SJ, Sheahan SL, Martin SS, Hendricks J, Robbins CA, Johnson JA. Predictors of medication noncompliance in a sample of older adults. *Clin Ther.* 1994;16: 110–117.

5. Becker MH. Patient adherence to prescribed therapies. *Med Care.* 1985;23: 539–555.

6. Mazzuca SA. Does patient education in chronic disease have therapeutic value? *J Chron Dis.* 1982;35:521–529.

7. German PS, Klein LE, McPhee SJ, Smith CR. Knowledge of and compliance with drug regimens in the elderly. *J Am Geriatr Soc.* 1982;30:568–571.

8. Weintraub M. Intelligent noncompliance and capricious compliance. In: Lasagna L, ed. *Patient Compliance.* New York: Futura Publishing Company; 1976:39–47.

9. Gordis L. Conceptual and methodologic problems in measuring patient compliance. *Compliance in Health Care.* Baltimore: Johns Hopkins University Press; 1979:23–48.

10. Cooper JK, Love DW, Raffoul PR. Intentional prescription nonadherence (noncompliance) by the elderly. *J Am Geriatr Soc.* 1982;30:329–333.

11. Col N, Fanale JE, Kronholm P. The role of medication noncompliance and adverse drug reactions in hospitalizations of the elderly. *Arch Intern Med.* 1990;150:841–845.

12. Hultsch DF, Hertzog C, Dixon RA, Small BJ. *Memory Change in the Aged.* Cambridge: Cambridge University Press; 1998.

13. Chew LD, Bradley KA, Flum DR, Cornia PB, Koepsell TD. The impact of low health literacy on surgical practice. *Am J Surg.* 2004;188:250–253.

14. Maddigan SL, Farris KB, Keating N, Wiens CA, Johnson JA. Predictors of older adults' capacity for medication management in a self-medication program: A retrospective chart review. *J Aging Health.* 2003;15:332–352.

15. Rosen MI, Beauvais JE, Rigsby MO, Salahi JT, Ryan CE, Cramer JA. Neuropsychological correlates of suboptimal adherence to metformin. *J Behav Med.* 2003;26: 349–360.

16. Park DC. Applied cognitive research. In: Craik FIM, Salthouse TA, eds. *The Handbook of Aging and Cognition.* Hillsdale, NJ: Lawrence Erlbaum Associates; 1992: 449–493.

17. Park DC, Morrell RW, Frieske D, Blackburn AB, Birchmore D. Cognitive factors and the use of over-the-counter medication organizers by arthritis patients. *Hum Factors.* 1991;33:57–67.

18. Park DC, Kidder DP. Prospective memory and medication adherence. In: Brandimonte M, Einstein GO, McDaniel MA, eds. *Prospective Memory: Theory and Applications.* Mahwah, New Jersey: Lawrence Erlbaum Associates; 1996:369–390.

19. Coffey CE, Figiel GS, Djang WT, Weiner RD. Subcortical hyperintensity on magnetic resonance imaging: A comparison of normal and depressed elderly subjects. *Am J Psychiatry.* 1990;147:187–189.

20. Glisky EL. Prospective memory and the frontal lobes. In: Brandimonte M, Einstein GO, McDaniel MA, eds. *Prospective Memory: Theory and Applications.* Mahwah, NJ: Lawrence Erlbaum Associates; 1996:249–266.

21. Young P, Dewse M, Fergusson W, Kolbe J. Respiratory rehabilitation in chronic obstructive pulmonary disease: Predictors of nonadherence. *Eur Respir J.* 1999;13: 855–859.

22. Peyrot M, McMurry JF, Kruger DF. A biopsychosocial model of glycemic control in diabetes: Stress, coping, and regimen adherence. *J Health Soc Behav.* 1999;40: 141–158.

23. Schlenk EA, Hart LK. Relationship between health locus of control, health value, and social support and compliance of persons with diabetes mellitus. *Diabetes Care.* 1984;7:566–574.

24. Garay-Sevilla ME, Nava LE, Malacara JM, et al. Adherence to treatment and social support in patients with non-insulin dependent diabetes mellitus. *J Diabetes Complications.* 1995;9:81–86.

25. Sarason IG, Sarason BR, Shearin EN. Social support as an individual difference variable: Its stability, origins, and relational aspects. *J Pers Soc Psychol.* 1986;50: 845–855.

26. Muran JC, Segal ZV, Samstag LW, Crawford CE. Patient pretreatment interpersonal problems and therapeutic alliance in short-term cognitive therapy. *J Consult Clin Psychol.* 1994;62:185–190.

27. Rosenstock I. The health belief model and preventive behaviour. *Health Educ Monographs.* 1974;2:354–386.

28. Strecher VJ, Rosenstock IM. The health belief model. In: Glanz K, Lewis FM, Rimer BK, eds. *Health Behavior and Health Education: Theory, Research, and Practice.* 2nd ed. San Francisco: Jossey-Bass Publishers; 1997:41–59.

29. Ajzen I, Fishbein M. *Understanding Attitudes and Predicting Social Behaviour.* Englewood Cliffs, NJ: Prentice Hall; 1980.

30. Ajzen I. From intentions to actions: A theory of planned behaviour. In: Kuhl J, Beckmann J, eds. *Action Control: From Cognition to Behaviour*. Heidelberg: Springer-Verlag; 1985.

31. Prochaska JO, Redding CA, Evers KE. The transtheoretical model and stages of change. In: Glanz K, Lewis FM, Rimer BK, eds. *Health Behavior and Health Education: Theory, Research, and Practice*. 2nd ed. San Francisco: Jossey-Bass Publishers; 1997:60–84.

32. Skelton JA, Croyle RT, eds. *Mental Representation in Health and Illness*. New York: Springer-Verlag; 1991.

33. Leventhal H, Meyer D, Nerenz D. The common sense representation of illness danger. In: Rachman S, ed. *Contributions to Medical Psychology*. Oxford: Pergamon Press; 1980.

34. Meyer D, Leventhal H, Gutmann M. Common-sense models of illness: The example of hypertension. *Health Psychology*. 1985;4:115–135.

35. Leventhal H, Cameron L. Behavioral theories and the problem with compliance. *Patient Educ Couns*. 1987;10:117–138.

36. Stewart M, Brown JB, Weston WW, McWhinney IR, McWilliam CL, Freeman TR. *Patient-Centered Medicine: Transforming the Clinical Method*. Thousand Oaks, California: Sage Publishers; 1995.

37. Mouton CP, Esparza Y. Ethnicity and geriatric assessment. In: Gallo J, Fulmer T, Paveza GJ, Reichel W, eds. *Handbook of Geriatric Assessment*. Gaithersburg, Maryland: Aspen Publishers; 1999:13–27.

38. Haynes RB, McKibbon KA, Kanani R. Systematic review of randomised trials of interventions to assist patients to follow prescriptions for medications. *Lancet*. 1996;348:383–386.

39. Vik SA, Maxwell CJ, Hogan DB. Measurement correlates, and health outcomes of medication adherence among seniors. *Ann Pharmacother*. 2004;38:302–312.

40. Akerblad AC, Bengtsson F, Ekselius L, von Knorring L. Effects of an educational compliance enhancement programme and therapeutic drug monitoring on treatment adherence in depressed patients managed by general practitioners. *Intern Clin Psychopharmacol*. 2003;18:347–354.

41. van Eijken M, Tsang S, Wensing M, de Smet PA, Grol RP. Interventions to improve medication compliance in older patients living in the community: a systematic review of the literature. *Drugs Aging*. 2003;20:229–240.

42. Park DC, Morrell RW, Frieske D. Medication adherence behaviors in older adults: Effects of external cognitive supports. *Psychological Aging*. 1992;7:252–256.

# 19

# Developing and Managing a High-Functioning Interdisciplinary Team

Eugenia L. Siegler

B ecause comprehensive geriatric assessment encompasses so many domains, providers with varied areas of expertise and different assessment tools often struggle to shape their observations into a complete picture of the individual patient. The format that seems to best meld disparate points of view is the interdisciplinary team.

## CASE VIGNETTE

*In its weekly meeting, the geriatric team discussed the case of Mrs. AM, an 87-year-old widow who had undergone a comprehensive new patient assessment earlier that month. Formerly independent, she had been referred by her internist because of deterioration in her health that did not appear to be due to her underlying medical conditions. The geriatric fellow presented the case. The nurse practitioner, social worker, geriatric psychiatrist, and dietitian each briefly presented individual evaluations based on a combination of interviews and specific assessment tools. The social worker, who was leading the meeting, then guided an interactive discussion that determined the patient's most important problems and a care plan to address them. The fellow documented the meeting's findings in*

431

*the patient's chart and agreed to present a follow-up of the recom-*
*mendations 4 weeks later.*

Although we have granted the interdisciplinary team an almost mythic status, its very size and diversity often precludes it from functioning as efficiently or effectively as the one the vignette depicts. Nonetheless, teams offer the best opportunity to combine the expertise of multiple health professionals, and when they do work, they provide not just a forum for case discussion, but also emotional support for those who are caring for very needy patients.

Teams, which are described in both the medical and business literature, have been defined as "a small number of people with complementary skills who are committed to a common purpose, set of performance goals, and approach for which they hold themselves mutually accountable."[1] Teams can be composed of members from one profession (unidisciplinary) or several (multidisciplinary). We tend to reserve the term "interdisciplinary" for those multidisciplinary teams that show healthy—and even contentious—interactions when problem solving and foster shared decision making.[2]

Interdisciplinary teams have been likened to marriages because they represent a union of different individuals and require attention and energy to maintain that union. Unlike married couples (ideally), members of teams come and go; although this turnover can add life and new ideas, it is inherently destabilizing and one of the greatest challenges to a team's growth and function.

## EVIDENCE FOR EFFECTIVENESS OF TEAMS

Health care teams are most useful when they are responsible for patients with complex medical and social problems. Unfortunately, studies demonstrating that teams improve patient outcomes are notoriously difficult to conduct; proving that the team is responsible for a positive effect may be nearly impossible when so many variables are involved in the care of complex patients. In addition, the literature on interdisciplinary teams lacks consistent terminology and methods.[3] A few studies have attempted to examine the collaborative process itself. A Cochrane review of nurse–physician collaboration[4] cited two studies, both in inpatient hospital wards[5,6] and concluded that interventions that increase collaboration improve process measures such as length of stay and satisfaction,[5] but not outcomes such as mortality. Another Cochrane review of collaboration, this time of multidisciplinary approaches to inpatient rehabilitation of older persons with hip fractures, was unable to document statistically significant improvement in outcomes for collaborative team care, largely because of the heterogeneity of the studies.[7]

Of the areas especially germane to functional assessment teams, ACE (Acute Care for Elders) Units include interdisciplinary team rounds among their distinguishing features (other features include prepared environment, patient-centered care, discharge planning, medical director review, and oversight of patient care).[8] Although some studies have been equivocal,[9,10] ACE units appear to improve at least short-term functional outcomes of the inpatients they serve.[11,12] In the primary care setting, effective teamwork can improve clinical outcomes and patient satisfaction.[13]

## PRACTICAL MATTERS: CREATING AND MAINTAINING TEAMS

Health care teams are not a recent phenomenon. Those interested in the history of teams can consult a number of sources; Tsukuda[14] in particular offered an insightful view of teams' progress over the last century. She describes certain themes that, although not necessarily evidence based, recur throughout the literature (p. 33):

- Team care improves the quality of care.
- Successful teams must be developed; they do not just happen.
- Team work is difficult, requiring active learning and practice of specific knowledge and skills.
- Team development takes time.
- Teams need administrative and financial support to succeed.
- Team education must take place at all levels.

Practically speaking, therefore, although every team is unique and has its own life and history, team growth and development are to some degree predictable. Because teams are dynamic, understanding group process increases the likelihood that members can form and maintain a healthy team. Drinka and Clark[15] described five phases of team formation (p. 18–27). These phases are neither unidirectional nor monolithic; teams can move back and forth between different phases, and individual team members may be in a different phase from the rest of the team.

- Forming: A team begins, and all participants are on good behavior.

- Norming: The team develops goals and a sense of purpose.
- Confronting: Conflicts that have been suppressed begin to surface; individuals begin to exert more power and to debate in a constructive manner.
- Performing: The team is at its most effective, efficient, and creative.
- Leaving: This may refer to individual members who depart or to a team that disbands.

Teams work if their members prepare for and address inherent weaknesses. In their analysis of 1,220 surveys of team members in 26 PACEs (Programs of All-Inclusive Care of the Elderly), Temkin-Greener et al.[16] documented that leadership, communication, coordination, and conflict management predicted team cohesion and effectiveness. Team process requires constant attention, and focusing on these factors increases the chances that a team will survive and thrive.

After clinicians have determined that a team will be a helpful addition to patient care, creating the team and its forum for interaction requires a number of steps:

*Determine the purpose(s) of the team.* Too often, we form teams because that is what geriatric specialists are supposed to do. Before starting a team, ask whether it is truly necessary. Keep in mind that teams are expensive. If an eight-member team meets weekly for an hour, can it honestly say it has accomplished the equivalent of a day's worth of work?

*Teams form for a variety of reasons.* These include but are not limited to (1) development or modification of care plans, (2) teaching, (3) development of creative solutions for difficult problems, and (4) meeting Center for Medicare and Medicaid Services (CMS) requirements. Teams may have more than one purpose; many interdisciplinary teams serve both educational and care management functions. Participants must clearly understand the team's purpose(s) if they are to understand their own roles and to monitor the team's effectiveness.

*Determine the team membership in advance.* The purpose of the team should determine its membership. There is no advantage to including representatives over every discipline if they will not be active participants. Most outpatient assessment teams will have physicians, nurses, and social workers as core members; rehabilitation teams, which tend to develop comprehensive, short-term care plans, may also include representatives of each of the therapies, as well as other disciplines such as pharmacy and nutrition. Occasionally, a core team may be established, with "special guests" invited to discuss specific patients they serve. Table 19–1 outlines the skills and training of professionals who often serve on interdisciplinary teams.

*Decide on the frequency, timing, etiquette, and location of meetings.* Do not ignore the obvious. Convenience and a comfortable setting promote team effectiveness. Lunch does not.

*Designate one individual to be responsible for the meetings.* The organizer must determine which cases will be presented, who will present them, and what materials (charts, consultants' notes) must be available. This can be a responsibility designated to one individual or can rotate among individual team members.

*Use a formal meeting format.* This may seem unnecessary and overly rigid, but structure enhances a meeting's effectiveness immeasurably. One such format is the "Seven Step Meeting Process" (Executive Learning, Inc, http://www.elinc.com).

1. Clarify objectives. Ensure that all team members understand the purpose of the meeting; most will be devoted to case discussion, but some meetings may have other objectives: scheduling, housekeeping tasks, evaluations, etc.
2. Review roles. These roles can and should rotate among team members. Determine who will assume these roles for this meeting. Clarify when the timekeeper should provide warnings.
   a. Timekeeper
   b. Recorder
   c. Leader
   d. Facilitator
3. Review agenda and determine how much time will be devoted to each item.
4. Discuss cases and other items on the agenda. Adhere scrupulously to the agreed-on timeline.
5. Review the meeting record. Have the recorder recap the items. Review the care plans that the team has generated.
6. Plan next steps and next meeting agenda.
7. Evaluate the meeting. Do not skip this; it is an essential step in team process. Do not fail to set aside time to review the team's effectiveness. In the early phases of team formation, try going around the table to ensure that everyone comments. That step may not be needed in a well-functioning team, but each meeting should have a clear opportunity for reflection and change.

*Devote some meetings to the team itself.* Like our relationships, gardens, or automobiles, teams require ongoing maintenance. Teams are

**Table 19–1** Members of Interdisciplinary Teams

| Discipline | Practice Roles/Skills | Education/Training |
|---|---|---|
| **Nurse** | | |
| Registered nurse | Planning for optimal functioning, coordination of care, teaching, direct and indirect patient care. | Registered nurse with associate degree: 2 years of training. BS, registered nurse: 4 years in college. MS, registered nurse: 4 years in college and 2 years of postgraduate specialty study. |
| Nurse practitioner | Health assessment, health promotion skills, histories and physicals, ordering conducting and interpreting some lab and diagnostic tests; teaching and counseling. | Master's degree with defined specialty area such as gerontology or palliative care. |
| **Physician** | | |
| General requirements | Treatment of diseases and injuries, provision of preventive care; diagnosis, prescription, treatments, surgery. | 4 years of medical or osteopathic school after college, plus 3–7 years of graduate medical education (internship, residency, fellowship). |
| Geriatrician | Special training in diagnosis, treatment, and prevention of disorders in older people; psychosocial and biomedical aspects of aging. | 1–2 years of postgraduate fellowship training; most have passed an exam to hold a Certificate of Added Qualifications in geriatrics. |
| Psychiatrist | Assessment and treatment of mental, emotional, and behavioral symptoms and illnesses. | Residency training in psychiatry; may also include fellowship training (e.g., in geriatric psychiatry). |
| Physician assistant | Provide medical care under the supervision of licensed physicians; provide a broad range of diagnostic and therapeutic services. | 2-year physician assistant program after Bachelor's degree; most have health care experience before entering physician assistant program. |
| Social worker | Assessment of individual and family psychosocial functioning and provision of care to help enhance or restore capacities; this can include locating services or providing counseling. | 4-year college degree leads to a Bachelor's of Social Work; 2 years of graduate work to a Master of Social Work. |

| Discipline | Practice Roles/Skills | Education/Training |
|---|---|---|
| Psychologist | Assessment, treatment, and management of mental disorders; psychotherapy with individuals, groups, and families. | Graduate training usually lasts 5 years beyond undergraduate training. |
| Pharmacist | Assists with determination and revision of a patient's medications to achieve an optimal regimen that suits individual's medical and therapeutic needs; information resource of patient and medical team. | Baccalaureate program is 5 years. Pharmacists may also hold a doctoral degree (Pharm.D.). |
| Occupational therapist | Uses therapies to help individuals achieve independence; occupational therapists focus on improving activities of daily living; they also perform environmental assessments and recommend and teach use of adaptive equipment. | BS or MS in occupational therapy with minimum of 6 months' field work. |
| Speech/language pathologist | Assess speech and language development and treat language and speech disorders. They also evaluate and treat people with swallowing disorders. | Master's or doctoral degree. |
| Physical therapist | Have expertise in the examination and treatment of musculoskeletal and neuromuscular problems that affect movement and function. | 4 year college degree or master's degree. |
| Chaplain | Provide visits and ministry to patients and family. | Master's degree in theology, plus a minimum of 1 year of clinical supervision. |
| Dietitian | Evaluate the nutritional status of patients; work with family members, patient, and team to determine appropriate nutritional goals for patient. | BS in food and nutrition; MS also available. Registered Dietitian must pass the national exam of the American Dietetic Association. |

Modified from *GITT Curriculum Guide*, 2003, p. 86

composed of people who, if they devote real effort, can create something that is useful, exciting, and fun. People can also be lazy, angry, tired, bored, uninterested, or even pathologic; such counterproductive behaviors can destroy any team. Only if time is devoted to self-examination can the team learn to identify its problems, solve them before they become intractable, and function again.

## TEAM TRAINING

Setting aside time for team process, although necessary, is not sufficient if team members do not know how to work together. Team skills are not intuitive; health care professionals must learn them, and most educators value these skills, at least in theory.[17,18] A number of well-established programs are designed to train health care teams and geriatric teams in particular.[14] The Department of Veterans Affairs sponsors Interdisciplinary Team Training Programs (http://www. va.gov/oaa/AHE_ITTP.asp) and the Health Resources and Services Administration has underwritten team training through its Geriatric Education Centers (http://bhpr.hrsa.gov/interdisciplinary/gec.html) and Area Health Education Centers (http://bhpr.hrsa.gov/ahec/). The John A. Hartford Foundation funded the Geriatric Interdisciplinary Team Training program, which has developed a broad literature based on experiences of its original sites,[19] and training materials are available on its website (http://www.gitt.org/).

Needless to say, formal team training is expensive and logistically cumbersome. Even when there is institutional support and time for training, gaining buy-in from all parties may be difficult. The experiences of the Geriatric Interdisciplinary Team Training program reflect this; Reuben et al.[20] have documented that the "disciplinary split" (the "tradition, culture, and regulatory requirements" unique to each profession) remains a serious barrier to team training, with physicians, in particular, demonstrating the least enthusiasm for the process. Finding ways to educate trainees in a cost-effective and efficient manner remains one of the greatest challenges for those who teach and work in teams.

## CONCLUSIONS

Assessment tools are most useful when they guide subsequent decision making. The complex patient who requires assessment in multiple domains presents special challenges; the identified needs may come into conflict or may be too overwhelming for a single provider to manage. By working together, providers may be able to devise solutions that none alone could have foreseen or implemented. That is the idea and the ideal behind the interdisciplinary team. Even experienced and motivated clinicians must expend significant energy creating and maintaining these teams, but those of us who love this kind of collaboration feel that we have been amply rewarded.

## REFERENCES

1. Katzenbach JR, Smith DK. The discipline of teams. *Harvard Business Review.* 1993;March–April:111–120.

2. Siegler EL, Whitney FW. What is collaboration? In: Siegler EL, Whitney FW, eds. *Nurse-Physician Collaboration: Care of Adults and the Elderly.* New York: Springer; 1994:3–10.

3. Schofield RF, Amodeo M. Interdisciplinary teams in health care and human services settings: Are they effective? *Health Social Work.* 1999;24:210–219.

4. Zwarenstein M, Bryant W. Interventions to promote collaboration between nurses and doctors. *Cochrane Database Syst Rev.* 2000; The Cochrane Library(3,2004):CD000072.

5. Curley C, McEachern JE, Speroff T. A firm trial of interdisciplinary rounds on the inpatient medical wards: An intervention designed using continuous quality improvement. *Med Care.* 1998;36(8 Suppl):AS4–AS12.

6. Jitapunkul S, Nuchprayoon C, Aksaranugraha S, et al. A controlled clinical trial of multidisciplinary team approach in the general medical wards of Chulalongkorn Hospital. *J Med Assoc Thai.* 1995;78:618–623.

7. Cameron ID, Handoll HH, Finnegan TP, Madhok R, Langhorne P. Co-ordinated multidisciplinary approaches for inpatient rehabilitation of older patients with proximal femoral fractures. *Cochrane Database Syst Rev.* 2001(3):CD000106.

8. Palmer RM, Counsell S, Landefeld CS. Clinical intervention trials: The ACE unit. *Clin Geriatr Med.* 1998;14:831–849.

9. Harris RD, Henschke PJ, Popplewell PY, et al. A randomised study of outcomes in a defined group of acutely ill elderly patients managed in a geriatric assessment unit or a general medical unit. *Australian N Z J Med.* 1991;21:230–234.

10. Counsell SR, Holder CM, Liebenauer LL, et al. Effects of a multicomponent intervention on functional outcomes and process of care in hospitalized older patients: A randomized controlled trial of Acute Care for Elders (ACE) in a community hospital. *J Am Geriatr Soc.* 2000;48:1572–1581.

11. Landefeld CS, Palmer RM, Kresevic DM, Fortinsky RH, Kowal J. A randomized trial of care in a hospital medical unit especially designed to improve the functional outcomes of acutely ill older patients. *N Engl J Med.* 1995;332:1338–1344.

12. White SJ, Powers JS, Knight JR, et al. Effectiveness of an inpatient geriatric service in a university hospital. *J Tennessee Med Assoc.* 1994;87:425–428.

13. Grumbach K, Bodenheimer T. Can health care teams improve primary care practice? *JAMA.* 2004;291:1246–1251.

14. Tsukuda RA. A perspective on health care teams and team training. In: Siegler EL, Hyer K, Fulmer T, Mezey M, eds. *Geriatric Interdisciplinary Team Training*. New York: Springer; 2000:21–37.

15. Drinka TJK, Clark PG. *Health Care Teamwork: Interdisciplinary Practice and Teaching*. Westport, CT: Auburn House; 2000.

16. Temkin-Greener H, Gross D, Kunitz SJ, Mukamel D. Measuring interdisciplinary team performance in a long-term care setting. *Med Care*. 2004;42:472–481.

17. Counsell ST, Kennedy RD, Szwabo R, Wadsworth NS, Wohlgemuth C. Curriculum recommendations for resident training in geriatric interdisciplinary team care. *J Am Geriatr Soc*. 1999;47:1145–1148.

18. Boaden N, Leaviss J. Putting teamwork in context. *Med Educ*. 2000;34:921–927.

19. Siegler EL, Hyer K, Fulmer T, Mezey M. *Geriatric Interdisciplinary Team Training*. New York: Springer; 1998.

20. Reuben DB, Levy-Storms L, Yee MN, et al. Disciplinary split: A threat to geriatrics interdisciplinary team training. *J Am Geriatr Soc*. 2004;52:1000–1006.

## ADDITIONAL REFERENCES

Heinemann GD, Zeiss AM, eds. *Team Performance in Health Care: Assessment and Development*. New York: Kluwer Academic/Plenum Publishers; 2002.

Hyer K, Flaherty E, Fairchild S, et al. *Geriatric Interdisciplinary Team Training: The GITT Kit*, 2nd ed. New York: John A. Hartford Foundation; 2003.

# Assessing Disaster Preparedness and Response

Ian Portelli and Terry Fulmer

The constant looming threat of a next disaster is a matter of worldwide concern. Whether it is an international/national terrorist event (e.g., biological, chemical, nuclear, or radiologic) or natural (e.g., tsunami), disruption and chaos is ensured.[1-4] The appalling mass casualty terrorist acts of September 11, 2001, on the World Trade Center and the Pentagon left everyone feeling vulnerable—especially older adults. Terrorism and disaster are a constant worry that looms over everyone and can be a cause of distress for the nation's physical, psychologic, and socioeconomical stability.[5,6]

This chapter focuses on health assessment for older adults as related to disaster. Preparation and response of older persons are reviewed, with an emphasis on the role of clinicians as they provide health care to older adults.

## DEFINITION AND TYPOLOGY OF A TERROR DISASTER

A terror disaster is a hazard[a] to the community/population. September 11, 2001, is a graphic example of how communities can be

---

[a] *Hazard* is a phenomenon that has the potential to affect human life and activity adversely, for example, earthquake, volcanic eruption, economic collapse, political crisis, epidemic, landslide, and deforestation.[13]

defined at risk[b] or vulnerable,[c] in spite of the high level of security and capacity[d] in place. Different organizations define the term disaster in a variety of ways, often closely associating it to organizational mandates. However, disaster caused by terrorism is commonly defined as a traumatic event defined by its capacity to evoke terror, fear, helplessness, or horror in the face of a threat to life or serious injury.[7] It is human caused, intentional, interpersonal violence.[7] These disasters can be caused by bombings, contamination, and weapons of mass destruction (biological, chemical, nuclear, or radiologic).[7]

Terrorist events can resemble disasters (and are dealt with as such) because of the impact on people and the environment. Terrorism is a tool of a criminal that is used to affect entire populations through random events, thereby conveying a message of terror and fear that stops normal life patterns.[8] Although terrorist attacks appear suddenly, they are often rooted in a strong political, social, and economic context. In case of terrorism, high-risk targets can be identified among military and civilian government facilities, international airports, large cities, and high-profile landmarks. Terrorists might also focus their target onto large public gatherings, water and food supplies, utilities, and corporate centers.[7]

Looking into terrorism and borrowing from disaster research, a descriptive outline of a representative typology can be generated:[8]

1. Incubation—a long-term warning stage of a terrorist act that could be before or after a terrorist act[8]
2. Impact—on occurrence of a terrorist act[8]
3. Immediate postimpact—priority action taken right after immediate first defense/alert of impact[8]
4. Recovery—disaster relief (transitional shift toward reorientation)[8]
5. Reorientation—resetting the clock and setting new guidelines, standards, and benchmarks[8]

---

[b] *Risk* is the expected severity of a disaster. The level of risk will depend on the potential impact of the hazard, the vulnerability level of people, and their capacity to cope with the situation.[13]

[c] *Vulnerability* is related to the degree to which people are susceptible to loss, damage, suffering, and death. Vulnerability includes various factors, including, among others, physical, economic, social, political, and religious factors.[13]

[d] *Capacity* refers to the internal and external resources people, households, and communities have to cope within situations that threaten their lives and well-being.[13]

## THE IMPACT OF DISASTER IN OLDER ADULTS

Terrorist acts are serious traumatic events that can create new physical and psychologic barriers for older adults.[4] How older adults and their communities are affected by disasters is closely related to their capacities and vulnerabilities. Vulnerability is the degree to which people are susceptible to loss, damage, suffering, and death. Being vulnerable generally comprises physical, economic, social, and or political weaknesses.[4]

The older adult population is often classified as a "special" or "at-risk population" that is vulnerable to major and minor effects of disaster.[4,9] Signs and symptoms exhibited by an older adult may be similar to other people in the community but may be heightened by pre-existing physical and psychologic conditions of the older individual. After a disaster, common recurring symptoms documented in literature include re-experiencing an increase in physiologic arousal, emotional disturbance, psychologic numbing, and behavioral avoidance.[9-11] Clinicians need to be alert to symptoms that cannot be explained by health conditions and consider the disaster effects. Clinicians, disaster workers, and family members need to be familiar with community-based agencies that can assist with care, training, information, and support of the older adults (e.g., the national aging network collaborative).[4,11]

Reports show that during the September 11, 2001, attacks on the city of New York, emergency workers believed that all buildings in lower Manhattan had been evacuated, when in reality some older adults and people with disabilities were not. This part of the community had no electricity (and, therefore, no television, lights, elevators, refrigerators, etc.), no running water, and no information about what was happening or what they should do.[12] Within 24 hours after the 9/11 terrorist attacks, animal advocates were on the scene rescuing pets, but some frail older adults waited for up to 7 days for medical teams to rescue them.[12] Clinicians need to document carefully the living situation of their older clients and to help determine whether they can evacuate in disaster events.

## PREDISASTER PREPAREDNESS FOR OLDER ADULTS

Federal Emergency Management Agency (FEMA)[13] defined mitigation as "the cornerstone of emergency management." It describes any step taken to reduce the likelihood of a disaster occurring or, in the

event of a disaster, on lessening its impact. Mitigation has become a
cornerstone in state and federal disaster programs over the past few
years, primarily because of the overwhelming success of mitigation
activities nationwide.[13] Mitigation describes an ongoing effort at the
federal, state, local, and individual levels to lessen the impact of disasters on families, homes, communities, and state/national economy.
Furthermore, it is the ongoing effort to lessen the impact that disasters have on people's lives and property through damage-prevention
plans, processes, and insurance.[13] One example is the airline security changes since September 11, 2001.

Emergency management planning specific to the older adult is vital. A strong specific preparedness plan is required before an emergency. Older persons can increase their level of safety by learning how
to protect one's self and cope with disaster. Even if physical limitations are present in the older adult, a protection plan can be generated
and tailored to each older person's capacity. A basic disaster checklist
is shown in Table 20–1.[14]

Clinicians can have a major impact on their older patients by helping them consider in advance what they will need. The older person
should have medical and general supplies assembled to last 7 days,
storing and labeling them accordingly, using an easy to carry container (e.g., backpack or duffle bag) that can be used for evacuation.
Clinicians can help older adults prepare by helping them set up a
medical supply kit (Table 20–2).[14]

In case of a disaster, older adults may need to evacuate their current location. Coordinating with a home care provider, an apart-

---

**Table 20–1** Basic Disaster Checklist for Older Adults[14]

- Assemble a disaster supply kit with batteries, water, etc.
- Arrange for someone to check on you in the event of a disaster.
- Plan and practice the best escape routes from your home.
- Plan for transportation if you need to evacuate to a shelter (e.g., Red Cross).
- Find the safe places in your home for each type of emergency.
- Have a plan to signal the need for help.
- Post emergency telephone numbers near the telephone.
- If you have home health care service, plan ahead with your agency for emergency procedures.
- Teach those who may need to assist you in an emergency how to operate necessary equipment. Be sure that they will be able to reach you.

**Table 20–2** Medical and General Kit[14]

**Medical Kit**
- First-aid kit
- Prescription medicines (7-day supply), list of medications including dosage, list of any allergies
- Extra eyeglasses and hearing-aid batteries
- Extra wheelchair batteries, oxygen
- List of the style and serial numbers of medical devices such as pacemakers
- Medical insurance and Medicare cards
- List of doctors and relatives or friends who should be notified if you are injured
- Any other items you may need

**General Kit**
- Battery-powered radio and flashlight with extra batteries for each
- Change of clothing, rain gear, and sturdy shoes
- Blanket or sleeping bag
- Extra set of keys
- Cash, credit cards, change for the pay phone
- Personal hygiene supplies
- Phone numbers of local and nonlocal relatives or friends
- Insurance agent's name and number
- Other items one wants to include

ment building supervisor, or an organization for evacuation procedures is extremely important. Clinicians need to be knowledgeable regarding how to obtain assistance for special transportation. Physicians and nurses can prepare instruction documents regarding appropriate clothing, sturdy shoes, the disaster supplies kit, and locking the house. Using travel routes specified or special assistance provided by local officials without taking short cuts (as they may be unsafe) would be the next step. A communication plan should be in place.

In the days, weeks and sometimes months after a disaster, older adults whose lives have been disrupted must make many important decisions. Older adults may be overwhelmed by the volume of information given to them in a short period of time.[14] Older adults are at high risk for emotional stress after a disaster. Reactions caused by or aggravated by disasters can include depression, irritability, anger, trouble sleeping or eating, family discord, restlessness, and substance abuse. Identifying these problem areas and getting help may prevent serious problems in the future.

## THE EFFECTS OF TERRORISM ON THE OLDER ADULT

Older adults will respond to disasters in a variety of ways, given the unique nature of individuals. However, slower physical reaction times and sensory impairment will impact the response capacity. Older adults with cognitive impairment will be especially vulnerable, and advanced care planning must take place.

Older adults are likely to have chronic health conditions that may worsen in a disaster. Heart conditions, depression, arthritis, and dementia may be exacerbated, and clinicians should instruct older patients on what to expect. Table 20–3 describes reactions that may occur in a disaster.[15]

## POSTDISASTER ISSUES FOR OLDER ADULTS

Post traumatic stress disorder (PTSD) is the most prevalent postdisaster ailment and is characterized by episodes of helplessness, shortness of breath, disorientation, agitation, and fear.[16,17] Sensations and symptoms can mimic health attacks.[17] Clinicians should be aware

**Table 20–3** High-Level Categorization of Reactions to a Disaster[15]

| | |
|---|---|
| Emotional (feeling) reactions | Feelings of shock, disbelief, anxiety, fear, grief, anger, resentment, guilt, shame, helplessness, hopelessness, betrayal, depression, emotional numbness (difficulty having feelings, including those of love and intimacy, or taking interest and pleasure in day-to-day activities) |
| Cognitive (thinking) reactions | Confusion, disorientation, indecisiveness, worry, shortened attention span, difficulty concentrating, memory loss, unwanted memories, repeated imagery, self-blame |
| Physical (bodily) reactions | Tension, fatigue, edginess, difficulty sleeping, nightmares, being startled easily, racing heartbeat, nausea, aches and pains, worsening health conditions, change in appetite, change in sex drive |
| Interpersonal reactions | Neediness, dependency, distrust, irritability, conflict, withdrawal, isolation, feeling rejected or abandoned, being distant, judgmental, or overcontrolling in friendships, marriages, family, or other relationships |
| Spiritual (meaning) reactions | Wondering why, why me, where was God; feeling as if life is not worth living, loss of hope |

that PTSD can not only be seen in subjects directly exposed to the disaster but also in older adults that are made aware of the disaster because it triggers past trauma[18] and experiences that can lead, as Lantz and Buchalter[16] stated, to "disabling anxiety." The clinician should inform and prepare the older adult for a long-lasting psychologic recovery.[19,20]

Depression may be another serious sequelae after a disaster. Feelings of depression may be even stronger if the older adult feels that no one understands him or her. The clinician should be aware of symptoms of depression, which may include (1) suicidal ideation, (2) isolation, (3) sudden changes in weight, (4) insomnia, and (5) alcohol or drug abuse (including prescription drugs).[21,22] As a consequence of the aging process, older adults may experience multiple losses, including a loss of physical/sexual attractiveness, hearing, sensory and motor skills, memory, spouse, relationships, control over the environment, work roles, and independence.[4,9,10] Clinicians should be sensitive to signs of depression among older victims because losses sustained from the disaster may add to ones already present and may lead to depression. This may also be reflected in an inappropriate attachment to specific items or property. This may lead to transfer trauma, that is, when an older adult is dislocated without use of proper procedures, resulting in ailments and even death. The psychologic tasks associated with adjusting to new surroundings and routines can lead to aggravation, depression, increased irritability, serious illness, and even death in a frail older person.[9,10]

In case of a disaster, environmental factors (e.g., chronic disease) may affect the ability of an older person to remember information or to act appropriately. An older person may not be able to remember disaster instructions/plans. The role of the clinician includes assessing the older adult for age-related impairment of temporal and spatial memory.[4,10] Older adults may also respond in a slower manner to calls for disaster relief, due to age-related changes in cognitive and motor activity. Some older adults will experience no immediate reaction. They may be energized by a stressful situation and not react until weeks or months later. The reaction time may also slow down and lead to difficulties in comprehension of alerts and broadcasts. Therefore, clinicians may need to provide outreach and instruction to older patients in regard to what to do. Delayed responses could be related to medication or age-impairing nervous or psychomotor ability.[9,10]

Older persons may fear that they will lose their independence if they ask for assistance. The fear of being placed in a nursing home may be a barrier to accessing services. Assurance by the clinician and building a strong information base are essential.[10] When institutionalized, the older adults' sense of control changes as they are not used to being guided by rules and medical staff.[9,10] Therefore, older adults may fear that if placed in a nursing home they will never return to their previous home. Clinicians should express sensitivity when dealing with older adults and provide reassurance that they are there to provide services.[10] Clinicians can assist older persons after disaster by aiding older persons in locating essential services, whereas crisis counselors can assist older persons in grieving over disaster-associated losses. Education and information are the best ways to deal with this situation.[9,10] A large portion of older adults who have a lower educational level (compared with the general population) could present with literacy issues, which could result in difficulties in completion of applications, self-assessment questionnaires, or understanding directions.[4,9,10]

Older adults are more susceptible to the effects of heat or cold. Clinicians should be aware that this becomes more critical in disasters when heat and air conditioning may be unavailable or unserviceable.[4,9,10] The capacity of the central nervous system and body regulator apparatus to maintain the constant state of body temperature changes with aging; thus, older persons are at risk of hypothermia and hyperthermia.[23]

Con artists, scammers, or dishonest contractors target older persons, particularly after a disaster. They are often ready to take advantage of the misfortunes of others, using home repair to victimize and abuse the condition in which the older person is living.[14] These issues need to be addressed in shelters and in housing arrangements or before clinical discharge. Education at disaster centers about these crimes may help to prevent further victimization.

Older adults are not a homogenous group. Sociocultural and religious factors play a role. What might be acceptable to an 85-year-old person may not be to a person of 65.[10] The diversity of an older population must be kept in mind, and individualized plans will be essential for an optimum health care delivery.[9,10] The older population presents with challenges for disaster clinicians and relief workforce. Older adults are commonly stereotyped as the frail (especially in the case of a disaster)[24] However, older adults reflect "successful aging" and are described by Rowe and Kahn[25] as "multidimensional, encompassing three distinct domains: avoidance of disease and disability, maintenance of high physical and cognitive functions, and sustained engagement in social and productive activities" (p. 443). It is erroneous to draw conclusions or categorize all older adults as frail when studies document resiliency and robustness for many in their later years.[24] These older adults may do well after disaster.

## ASSESSMENT AFTER DISASTER

The DeWolfe[26] Population Exposure Model (Figure 20–1) has been used across all age groups and is useful for assessing older adults after a disaster event.[26]

The experience of a disaster is overwhelming for any age group, even if no evidence of physical harm (symptoms or wounds affecting ability to function) was incurred. Stress can exacerbate a current medical condition that in older adults could trigger a life-threatening event.[14,28] The American Red Cross and Centers for Disease Control and Prevention[14,28] have documented that after a disaster an older adult may experience symptoms and disorders that clinicians need to review. The following main categories are suggested: (1) psychologic and emotional, (2) physical, (3) cognitive, and (4) behavioral issues (Table 20–4).[14,28] Thorough assessment by the clinician will ensure that older adults are diagnosed and triaged appropriately.

Table 20–4 documents that the normal response to a disaster varies depending on the physical, mental, and behavioral changes that occur as a response to the hazard, that is, the sympathetic nervous system (noradrenergic—flight or fight) or the parasympathetic (conservation–withdrawal) response. Lipkin et al.[29] suggested a tripartite response to a disaster, which proves to be an essential structure for an assessment. Thereby, assessing the psychologic, instrumental (rational and irrational attempts to eradicate the threat), the social, and altruistic effect on the older adult would result in a holistic assessment in case of a disaster.[29]

The International Society for Traumatic Stress Studies[15] documents how some older adults are more vulnerable than others, especially when the older person has prior experience or had other underlying traumatic events in life, for example, accidents, abuse, assault, combat, emargination, and chronic medical illnesses. With such clients, the clinician needs to encourage discussion and provide constant orienting information and assurances regarding the situation. The clinician needs to engage with the older adult and assist in building a support structure around the patient while assessing the reliability of the family or client support group.[30]

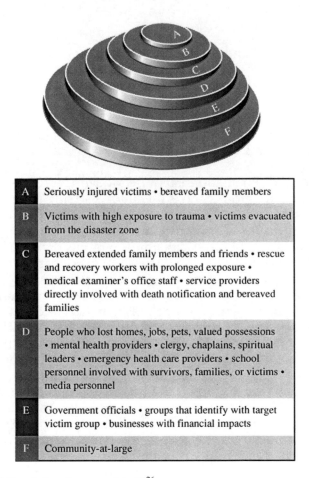

| A | Seriously injured victims • bereaved family members |
| B | Victims with high exposure to trauma • victims evacuated from the disaster zone |
| C | Bereaved extended family members and friends • rescue and recovery workers with prolonged exposure • medical examiner's office staff • service providers directly involved with death notification and bereaved families |
| D | People who lost homes, jobs, pets, valued possessions • mental health providers • clergy, chaplains, spiritual leaders • emergency health care providers • school personnel involved with survivors, families, or victims • media personnel |
| E | Government officials • groups that identify with target victim group • businesses with financial impacts |
| F | Community-at-large |

**Figure 20–1** Population Exposure Model[26]

"Victims are forever changed by the experience of terrorism."[31] After an older adult has experienced disaster, his or her life changes forever. Feelings of loss may remain present for a long time.[24,32,33] Therefore, during assessment, it is important to offer practical suggestions. A comprehensive assessment, including observation by mental health specialists, can help reduce stress symptoms and promote postdisaster adjustment.[15] Addressing the basic needs of shelter, food and water, sanitation, privacy, and opportunities to sleep (at least briefly) is crucial.[15,34,35] Avoiding alcohol and other drugs as a coping mechanism is

**Table 20–4** Older Adult's Assessment Needs[14,27]

### 1. Psychologic and Emotional
A. Anxiety
B. Fear
C. Grief
D. Denial
E. Loss of emotional control
F. Sense of failure
G. Blaming others or self
H. Feeling overwhelmed
I. Irritability, restlessness, overexcitability
J. Depression, moodiness, crying
K. Anger, blaming
L. Feelings of apathy, diminished interest in usual activities
M. Feelings of isolation, detachment, estrangement
N. Feelings of guilt about surviving
O. Denial or constriction of feelings
P. Flashbacks or unwelcome memories of the disaster
Q. An exaggerated reaction to being startled
R. Recurrent nightmares about the disaster or about other traumatic events
S. Inability to fall or stay asleep
T. Sleeping excessively

### 2. Physical
A. Difficulty breathing
B. Shock symptoms
C. Dizziness
D. Profuse sweating
E. Thirst
F. Visual difficulties
G. Clenching of jaw
H. Rapid heart rate
I. Headaches
J. Weakness
K. Nausea, upset stomach, other gastrointestinal problems
L. Muscle soreness
M. Hot or cold spells; sweating or chills
N. Numbness or tingling in body parts
O. Heavy feeling in arms and/or legs
P. Feeling a "lump" in the throat
Q. Chest pains
R. Trouble catching your breath; rapid breathing
S. Tremors
T. Fatigue
U. Increase in allergies, colds, or flu
V. Heart palpitations
W. Nonspecific aches and pains

### 3. Cognitive
A. Poor concentration
B. Mental confusion
C. Slowness of thought
D. Inability to express oneself verbally or in writing
E. Forgetfulness
F. Inability to make judgments and decisions
G. Loss of ability to think of alternatives or prioritize tasks
H. Disorientation
I. Heightened or lowered alertness
J. Poor problem solving
K. Memory problems
L. Nightmares
M. Difficulty identifying familiar objects or people

### 4. Behavioral
A. Hyperactivity
B. Outbursts of anger or frequent arguments
C. Loss of objectivity
D. Withdrawal, social isolation, distancing oneself from others
E. Increased use of alcohol, tobacco, or other drugs
F. Avoidance of activities or places that remind one of the disaster
G. Family problems
H. Temporary loss or increase of appetite
I. Change in sexual functioning

important in the older adult. Assisting the older adult in re-establishing old routines is a practical way to ease his or her tension.[30,36]

Common psychosocial symptoms detected in diagnosis and treatment in case of a terrorist attack are acute stress disorders, acute PTSDs, and chronic PTSDs (Table 20–5).[28,29,37] Key symptoms to look for in an assessment, as described by the DSM-IV,[38] include the exposure to the traumatic event, persistent re-experiencing of the event, avoidance of stimuli associated with the trauma and reduced responsiveness to the environment, increased arousal not present before trauma. Symptoms must be present for at least 1 month and can cause significant impairment in social, occupational,[39] and areas of function. PTSDs may be complicated by other underlying neurologic and physical disorders, and thus, a differential diagnosis might show evidence of depression, adjustment disorders, obsessive compulsive disorders, schizophrenia, anxiety, or alcohol/substance abuse.[22,40] A psychiatric consultation is needed.[29] The clinician's main role is to differentiate between the normal and abnormal response to the disaster,[41] provide the support and comfort needed, and effectively diagnose the underlying stressors leading to the illness[42] while identifying high-risk individuals and follow-up with proper treatment, care, and referral.[16,29]

The National Center for PTSD (NCPTSD)[43] focuses on the assessment and evaluation for PTSD, stating that it can vary widely depending on the type of evaluation. An experienced clinician may take as little as 15 minutes to get a feel for the experience that an older adult has incurred and to determine whether treatment for PTSD is needed. Meanwhile, a PTSD-specific assessment may take eight or more 1-hour sessions, especially if information is necessary for disability or legal claims.[43] Questions are structured to explore traumatic experiences and symptoms that the older person experiences. Evaluations that are more thorough are likely to involve detailed, structured interviews, self-report questionnaires, and psychologic tests to record thoughts and feelings.[43] The Clinician Administered PTSD Scale (CAPS) was developed by National Center for PTSD staff and is among the most widely used types of interviews.[43]

The Clinician Administered PTSD Scale format includes looking into frequency and intensity of the core PTSD symptoms and of some common associated symptoms, which may have important implications for treatment and recovery.[43] The Structured Clinical Interview for DSM is another tool that is widely used and it assesses a range of psychiatric disorders including PTSD. Some other instruments essential for postdisaster assessments include Anxiety Disorders Interview Schedule-Revised, the

**Table 20–5** PTSD: Six Criteria for Diagnosis[40]

**1. TRAUMATIC EVENT**

The patient has been exposed to a traumatic event in which both of the following were present:

- Patient experienced, witnessed, or was confronted with event(s) that involved actual or threatened death or serious injury to self or others.
- Patient's response involved intense fear, helplessness, or horror.

**2. RE-EXPERIENCE OF THE EVENT**

The event is persistently experienced in one or more of these ways:

- Recurrent and intrusive distressing recollections, including images, thoughts, or perceptions
- Recurrent distressing dreams
- Acting or feeling as if the event were recurring (i.e., a sense of reliving the experience, illusions, hallucinations, and flashbacks, including those that occur on awakening or when intoxicated)
- Intense psychologic distress at exposure to cues that symbolize or resemble an aspect of the traumatic event
- Physiologic reactivity on exposure to cues that symbolize or resemble an aspect of the traumatic event

**3. AVOIDANCE**

Persistent avoidance of stimuli associated with the trauma and numbing of general responsiveness (not present before the trauma), as indicated by three or more of these:

- Efforts to avoid thoughts, feelings, conversations associated with the trauma
- Efforts to avoid activities, places, people that arouse recollection of the trauma
- Inability to recall an important aspect of the trauma
- Markedly diminished interest or participation in significant activities
- Feeling of detachment or estrangement from others
- Restricted range of affect (e.g., unable to experience loving feelings)
- Sense of a foreshortened future (e.g., not expecting to have a career, marriage, or normal life span)

**4. AROUSAL**

Persistent symptoms of increased arousal (not present before the trauma), as indicated by two or more of these:

- Difficulty falling or staying asleep
- Irritability or outbursts of anger
- Difficulty concentrating
- Hypervigilance
- Exaggerated startle response

**5. DURATION**

Symptoms must be present for more than 1 month.

**6. FUNCTIONAL IMPAIRMENT**

The disturbance causes clinically significant distress or impairment in social, occupational, or other important areas of functioning.

PTSD-Interview, the Structured Interview for PTSD, and the PTSD Symptom Scale Interview.[43] Self-reporting assessments can be more time and cost-effective but may not be as efficient as a clinician's thorough analysis of the situation, usually including a single score representing the amount of distress an individual is experiencing.[43] The PTSD Checklist is a good example of a relevant self-reporting checklist being used both in the military and civilian populations. Other self-reporting measures include the Event Scale-Revised, the Keane PTSD Scale of the MMPI-2, the Mississippi Scale for Combat Related PTSD and the Mississippi Scale for Civilians, the Posttraumatic Diagnostic Scale, the Penn Inventory for Posttraumatic Stress, and the Los Angeles Symptom Checklist.[43]

Two assessment instruments of psychosocial response to bioterrorism assessment tools are shown in Figures 20–2 and 20–3.[29]

| Communication Skills | Done |
|---|---|
| Prepare | |
| Open | |
| Gather Information | |
| Start open ended | |
| Do not interrupt | |
| Use nonleading questions | |
| Ask questions individually | |
| Avoid medical jargon | |
| Actively listen (appropriate use of silence) | |
| Encourage patient to reveal all concerns through **verbal** and nonverbal encouragement ("tell me **more,** anything else," lean forward) | |
| Summarize | |
| Elicit and Understand Patient's Perspective | |
| Use of Relationship Building Skills | |
| Use appropriate nonverbal behavior (made eye contact, **attentive,** and open posture, reassured patient with a **touch** when appropriate) | |
| Recognize and name emotions | |
| Use PEARLS* statements to respond to emotions | |
| Patient Education | |
| *Ask* what patient already knows | |
| *Tell* information clearly; do not alarm ("you have PTSD") or give false reassurances | |
| **Ask patient** if he/she understands and encourage questions | |
| Negotiate and Agree on Plan | |
| Manage Flow | |
| Close | |

*PEARLS: Partnership, Empathy, Apology, Respect, Legitimize/Normalize, Support

³**Low risk**— no current thoughts, no plans
**Intermediate risk**— current thoughts, no plans
**High risk**— current thoughts with plans

†Subjective Units of Distress (1–100 self reported)

| Content | Done |
|---|---|
| PTSD Screening (SNAP) | |
| "Do you find yourself jumpier or more easily startled?" (**S** = Startle) | |
| "Are you less emotional than you would expect?" (**N** = Numbness) | |
| "Are you having trouble sleeping or concentrating?" (**A** = Arousal) | |
| "Are you having frequent unwelcomed thoughts about the event?" "Are you having nightmares?" ( **P** = Persistence) | |
| Depression Screening | |
| In the past 2 weeks, have you had a depressed mood most of the day? | |
| In the past 2 weeks, have you a loss of interest or pleasure in most activities? | |
| Alcohol and Substance Abuse Screening ( +CAGE) | |
| Have you ever had a problem with drugs? | |
| Do you drink alcohol? How much this week? | |
| Have you ever felt you ought to Cut down on your drinking? | |
| Have people Annoyed you by criticizing your drinking? | |
| Have you ever felt bad or Guilty about your drinking? | |
| Have you ever had a drink first thing in the morning to steady your nerves or get rid of a hangover (Eye-opener)? | |
| Suicide Risk Assessment³ | |
| Have you had any thoughts that life is not worth living or that you would be better off dead? | |
| This past week have you had thoughts about hurting or even killing yourself? If yes, what have you thought about? Have you actually done anything to hurt yourself? | |
| Education/Intervention | |
| Deliver Diagnosis— "I think you are suffering from..." | |
| Demystify— "Let me tell you what this means" | |
| Education about meaning of symptoms, normal responses to trauma, expectations for symptom resolution | |
| Discuss nonpharmacologic symptom specific treatments—(i.e., calm breathing, sleep hygiene) | |
| Discuss pharmacologic treatments | |
| Discuss referrals (i.e., CBT, exposure therapy) | |
| Plan for symptom monitoring (SUDS†) and follow-up | |

**Figure 20–2** Psychosocial Aspects of Bioterrorism: Interview Skills Checklist[44]

| Areas of Focus | Acute Stress | Disorder Acute PTSD | Chronic PTSD |
|---|---|---|---|
| Onset Following Trauma | Within 26-days<br>or<br>Anytime | Immediately<br>or<br>Anytime | Immediately<br>or<br>Anytime |
| Duration | 2—30 days | Up to 3 months | 3 months-<br>years |

$\longleftarrow$ —————————————————————————————— $\longrightarrow$

| | |
|---|---|
| Screening Questions—SNAP | • *Startle*—Do you find yourself jumpier or more easily startled?<br>• *Numbness*—Are you less emotional than you would expect?<br>• *Arousal*—Are you having trouble sleeping or concentrating?<br>• *Persistence*—Are you having frequent or unwelcome thoughts about the event? Are you having nightmares? |

$\longleftarrow$ ————————————— $\longrightarrow$

| | |
|---|---|
| Diagnostic Criteria (PTSD) | • Experienced horrific event—direct or indirect<br>• Persistent symptoms (prolonged over 3 months)<br>• Re-experienced event<br>• Avoidant behaviors<br>• Aroused responses to negatively conditioned elements of the experience<br>• Co-morbidity: Two-Question Depression Screen, Alcoholism and Substance Abuse—CAGE Questions |
| Rating Scales | • Clinically Administered PTSD Scale Part 2 (CAPS-2)<br>• Davidson Trauma Scale (DTS)<br>• Impact of Event Scale (IES)<br>• Critical Global Impressions (CGI-S) and (CGI-I) |

$\longleftarrow$ —————————————————————————————— $\longrightarrow$

| | |
|---|---|
| Stress Disorder Treatments | **Exposure Therapy**—*Education to normalize symptoms*<br>• **Calm Breathing**—to teach how to calm self when tense or stressed<br>• **Putting the experience in perspective**—recounting tauma memories<br>• **Approaching safe situations**—those that have been avoided because they are reminiscent of trauma<br>**Cognitive restructuring**<br>• To help survivors identify and evaluate their perceptions about the trauma, about how dangerous the world is, and about their ability to cope with stress<br>**Cognitive Behavior Therapy**—*Reinforcing the half-full glass*<br>• Show the patient how thoughts affect his/her feelings<br>• Awareness of negative thoughts that distress or are self-defeating<br>• Challenge negative thoughts and substitute positive ones |

$\longleftarrow$ —————————————————————————————— $\longrightarrow$

| | |
|---|---|
| Medications | Few high-quality studies, none in **disaster** per se<br>If symptoms warrant: *SSRI, TCA, MAOI, Benzodiazepine* |

**Figure 20–3** Management of Psychosocial Responses to Bioterrorism[29]

Assessment should include stress factors that could outlast the vulnerability state in the older adult. During massive disasters, casualties or survivors may be directly exposed to or witness events that may make them more vulnerable to serious stress reactions.[15] Being aware of these risk factors is important and could ease the assessment process.[15] Some examples could be loss of family, neighborhood, or community; life-threatening danger or physical harm; exposure to horrible death, bodily injury, or bodies; extreme environmental or human violence or destruction; a loss of home or valued possessions; a loss of communication with or support from important people in one's life; intense emotional demands; extreme fatigue, weather exposure, hunger, or sleep deprivation; extended exposure to danger, loss, emotional/physical strain; and exposure to toxic contamination (such as gas, fumes, chemicals, radioactivity, or biological agents).[15]

Emphasis on postassessment maintenance or re-establishment of communication with family, peers, and counselors in order to talk about the experiences is crucial for the older person's well-being. It is also a prerequisite to identify key resources such as the Federal Emergency Management Agency, the Red Cross, the Salvation Army, local and state health departments for health, housing, and basic emergency assistance.[45] Identifying local cultural or community supports helps maintain or re-establish normal activities such as attending religious services.

## CONCLUSION AND RECOMMENDATIONS

Disaster preparedness and care planning for older adults are integral features of geriatric assessment. Referral to experts as needed is important for those of us who do not feel prepared in this new area of health assessment. For all clinicians, the focus of a health assessment must be on the needs of the older adult, and sometimes simply asking the question "Do you feel ready if there were to be a disaster?" may set the stage for the next steps in the care-planning process.

### REFERENCES

1. Kron S, Mendlovic S. Mental health consequences of bioterrorism. *Israel Med Assoc J*. 2002;4:524–527.

2. Ursano RJ, Norwood AE, Fullerton CS. *Bioterrorism: Psychological and Public Health Interventions*. New York: Cambridge; 2004.

3. Ursano RJ. Uniformed Services University of the Health Sciences. Center for the Study of Traumatic Stress. *Planning for Bioterrorism: Behavioral & Mental Health Responses to Weapons of Mass Destruction & Mass Disruption*, 1st ed. Bethesda, MD: Center for the

Study of Traumatic Stress, Department of Psychiatry, Uniformed Services University of the Health Sciences; 2000.

4. Oriol W. *Psychosocial Issues for Older Adults in Disasters: A Guide for Health and Mental Health Professionals.* Washington, DC: Substance Abuse and Mental Health Services Administration, Center for Mental Health Services, Emergency Services and Disaster Relief Branch; 1999.

5. Karwa M, Bronzert P, Kvetan V. Bioterrorism and critical care. *Crit Care Clin.* 2003;19:279–313.

6. Karwa M, Currie B, Kvetan V. Bioterrorism: Preparing for the impossible or the improbable. *Crit Care Med.* 2005;33(1 Suppl):S75–S95.

7. US Department of Homeland Security. *Are You Ready? An In-Depth Guide to Citizen Preparedness.* U.S. Department of Homeland Security; Washington, DC; 2004.

8. Wilkins WL, Vultee F. *Disasters that Communicate: A Proposal for Definition and Research Agenda.* University of Missouri School of Journalism; 2005. Available from http://www.colorado.edu/hazards/o/jan05/jan05c.html (Accessed February 20, 2005).

9. Department of Health and Human Services Centers for Disease Control and Prevention. Terrorism Preparedness and Emergency Response; CDC 2004. Available from http://www.bt.cdc.gov/ (Accessed February 20, 2005).

10. US Administration on Aging and Kansas Department on Aging. The Disaster Preparedness Manual: Impact of Disaster on Older Adults; 2003. Available from http://www.dmhas.state.ct.us/trauma/olderadults.pdf (Accessed February 20, 2005).

11. Valdez A, Brewster L, Wilder G, Wagner R, Mendez R, Schmidt M. *Emergency Preparedness Manual for the Aging Network.* Kansas Department of Aging; Washington DC; 1995.

12. O'Brien N. Emergency preparedness for older people. Issue Brief, January–February 2003, International Longevity Center-USA; 2003. Available from www.ilcusa.org/_lib/pdf/epopib.pdf (Accessed February 20, 2005).

13. Federal Emergency Management Agency (FEMA) Mitigation. US Department of Homeland Security; 2005. Available from http://www.fema.gov/hazards/terrorism (Accessed February 20, 2005).

14. American Red Cross. Special Needs & Concerns. Disaster Preparedness for Seniors. American Red Cross; 2005. Available from http://redcross.org/services/disaster/beprepared/seniors.html (Accessed February 20, 2005).

15. The International Society of Traumatic Stress Studies (ISTSS). Mass Disasters, Trauma, and Loss; 2005. Available from http://www.istss.org/terrorism/disaster_trauma_and_loss.htm (Accessed February 20, 2005).

16. Lantz MS, Buchalter EN. Posttraumatic stress disorder: When older adults are victims of severe trauma. *Clin Geriatr.* 2003;11(04).

17. Connecticut Community Care, Inc. *First 9/11: Now Post Traumatic Stress Disorder.* Connecticut Community Care, Inc. Bristol, CT; 2002:1–4.

18. Cook JM. Traumatic exposure and PTSD in older adults: Introduction to the special issue. *J Clin Geropsychol.* 2002;8:149–152.

19. APA Working Group on the Older Adult. What practitioners should know about working with older adults. *Prof Psychol Res Pract.* 1998;29:413–427.

20. Butler LD, Koopman C, Azarow J, Desjardins JC, Hastings TA, Spiegel D. Distress and resiliency in coping with the tragedy of 9/11/01. Paper presented at the annual meeting of the International Society of Traumatic Stress Studies (ISTSS), Baltimore; 2002 November.

21. Cook JM, Arean PA, Schnurr PP, Sheikh J. Symptom differences of older depressed primary care patients with and without history of trauma. *Int J Psychiatry Med*. 2001;31: 415–428.

22. Office for Victims of Crime (OVCRC). OVC Handbook for Coping after Terrorism. Office for Victims of Crime, Victims and Family Assistance; 2002. Available from http://www.ojp.usdoj.gov/ovc/publications/infores/cat_hndbk/cat_hndbk_2.htm (Accessed February 20, 2005).

23. Harvey BS. Hyperthermia. *N Engl J Med*. 1993;329:483–487.

24. Myrna L. The frail and the hardy seniors of 9/11: The needs and contributions of older Americans. The Public as an Asset, Not a Problem, A summit on leadership during bioterrorism, Johns Hopkins University Center for Civilian Biodefense Strategies; 2003. Available from www.hopkins-biodefense.org/pages/events/peoplesrole/lewis/lewis_trans. html (Accessed February 20, 2005).

25. Rowe JW, Kahn RL. Successful aging. *The Gerontologist*. 1997;37:433–440.

26. DeWolfe DJ. Unpublished manuscript. Population Exposure Model and text excerpted from Mental Health Interventions Following Major Disasters: A Guide for Administrators, Policy Makers, Planners and Providers. Rockville, MD: Substance Abuse and Mental Health Services Administration. Partial text is available of page 12 of the following online manual; 2004. Available from http://www.mentalhealth.org/publications/allpubs/KEN95-0011/default.asp (Accessed January 20, 2005).

27. US Department of Health and Human Services, Substance Abuse and Mental Health Services Administration (SAMHSA) Mental Health All-Hazards Disaster Planning Guidance; 2003. Available from http://www.mentalhealth.org/publications/allpubs/SMA03-3829/part_two.asp (Accessed February 20, 2005).

28. Centers for Disease Control and Prevention (CDC). Emergency Preparedness and Response; CDC; 2004. Available at http://www.bt.cdc.gov/ (Accessed February 20, 2005).

29. Lipkin M, Zabar S, Kalet A. Psychosocial Response to Bioterrorism: Diagnosis and Treatment. Fact sheet prepared by NYU School of Medicine, Decision of Primary Care; 2002. Available from http://chip.med.nyu.edu/datafiles/chipsite/psychosoc/cd/ToolsHandouts/ReactiontoTraumaPocketCard.doc (Accessed February 20, 2005).

30. Nathanson M. Reactions of the elderly to trauma. *Disaster Preparedness and Mental Health Among Elderly*. New York University: New York; 2004.

31. US Department of Justice OVC Handbook for Coping after Terrorism. A guide to healing and recovery. Office for Victims of Crime, Victims and Family Assistance; 2002. Available from http://www.ojp.usdoj.gov/ovc/publications/infores/cat_hndbk/NCJ190249.pdf (Accessed February 20, 2005).

32. Cook JM, Riggs DS, Thompson R, Coyne JC, Sheikh JI. Posttraumatic stress disorder and current relationship functioning among World War II ex-prisoners of war. *J Fam Psychol*. 2004;18:36–45.

33. Butler AS, Panzer AM, Goldfrank LR, Institute of Medicine. Committee on Responding to the Psychological Consequences of Terrorism Board on Neuroscience and Behavioral Health. *Preparing for the Psychological Consequences of Terrorism: A Public Health Strategy*. Washington, DC: National Academies Press; 2003.

34. Centers for Disease Control and Prevention (CDC). Helping People Cope with a Traumatic Event; CDC; 2004. Available from http://www.cdc.gov/masstrauma/factsheets/professionals/coping_with_trauma.htm (Accessed February 20, 2005).

35. Horowitz MJ. *Stress Response Syndrome,* 4th ed. Northvale, NJ: Aronson; 2002.

36. Schlenger WE, Caddell JM, Ebert L, Jordan BK, Rourke KM. Psychological reactions to terrorist attacks: Findings from the National Study of Americans' Reactions to September 11. *JAMA.* 2002;288:581–588.

37. Galea S, Ahern J, Resnick H, et al. Psychological sequelae of the September 11 terrorist attacks in New York City. *N Engl J Med.* 2002;346:982–987.

38. Widiger TA, American Psychiatric Association, Task Force on DSM-IV. *DSM-IV Sourcebook,* 1st ed. Washington, DC: American Psychiatric Association; 1994.

39. Reissman DB, Klomp RW, Kent AT, Pfefferbaum B. Exploring psychological resilience in the face of terrorism. *Psychiatr Ann.* 2004;33:627–632.

40. Cuervo-Rubio R. VA Trainee Pocket Card Department of Veterans Affairs; 2005. Available from http://www.va.gov/oaa/pocketcard/geriadv.asp (Accessed February 20, 2005).

41. Bonder B, Wagner MB. *Functional Performance in Older Adults,* 2nd ed. Philadelphia: FA Davis; 2001.

42. Andresen E, Rothenberg B, Zimmer JG. *Assessing the Health Status of Older Adults.* New York: Springer Pub.; 1997.

43. National Center for PTSD (NCPTSD) Measuring PTSD; 2005. Available from http://www.ncptsd.org/facts/treatment/fs_lay_assess.html (Accessed February 20, 2005).

44. NYU School of Medicine, Decision of Primary Care. Psychosocial Aspects of Bioterrorism: Interview Skills Checklist; 2002. Available from http://chip.med.nyu.edu/datafiles/chipsite/psychsoc/cd/ToolsHandouts/InterviewSkillsChecklist.doc (Accessed February 20, 2005).

45. Zunin LM, Myers D. *Training Manual for Human Service Workers in Major Disasters,* 2nd ed. Washington, DC: Department of Health and Human Services, Substance Abuse and Mental Health Services Administration, Center for Mental Health Services; 2000.

# *Index*

461

CPSIA information can be obtained at www.ICGtesting.com
Printed in the USA
LVOW091622260812

295927LV00004B/5/P